Key D...
Psychi...
Health...

For Elsevier:

Commissioning Editor: Steven Black
Development Editor: Catherine Jackson
Project Manager: Emma Riley
Senior Designer: Sarah Russell
Illustration: Gillian Murray

Key Debates in Psychiatric/Mental Health Nursing

John R. Cutcliffe PhD BSc(Hons) Nrsg RMN RGN RPN RN
David G. Braithwaite Professor of Nursing, University of Texas (Tyler), USA;
Adjunct Professor of Psychiatric Nursing, Stenberg College International School of Nursing,
Canada; Director, Cutcliffe Consulting

Martin F. Ward RMN RNT CertEd Dip Nurs NEBSS Dip MPhil
Independent Mental Health Nursing Consultant; Coordinator of Mental Health Nursing Courses,
University of Malta; Chair of the Expert Panel, HORATIO – Psychiatric Nurses in Europe

With Forewords by
Sandra P. Thomas PhD RN FAAN
Professor and Director, PhD Program in Nursing, University of Tennessee, Knoxville, USA; Editor-in-Chief, 'Issues in
Mental Health Nursing'
Antony Sheehan DSci(Hons) MPhil BEd(Hons) RN DipHsm CertEd (FE)
Director of Care Services, Department of Health Professor of Health and Social Care Strategy, University
of Central Lancashire, UK

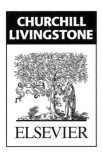

CHURCHILL
LIVINGSTONE

ELSEVIER

EDINBURGH   LONDON   NEW YORK   OXFORD   PHILADELPHIA   ST LOUIS   SYDNEY   TORONTO   2006

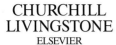

CHURCHILL
LIVINGSTONE
ELSEVIER

ISBN-13: 978-0-443-07391-5
ISBN-10: 0-443-07391-0

British Library Cataloguing in Publication Data
A catalogue record for this book is available from the British Library.

Library of Congress Cataloging in Publication Data
A catalog record for this book is available from the Library of Congress.

Note
Knowledge and best practice in this field are constantly changing. As new research and experience broaden our knowledge, changes in practice, treatment and drug therapy may become necessary or appropriate. Readers are advised to check the most current information provided (i) on procedures featured or (ii) by the manufacturer of each product to be administered, to verify the recommended dose or formula, the method and duration of administration, and contraindications. It is the responsibility of the practitioner, relying on their own experience and knowledge of the patient, to make diagnoses, to determine dosages and the best treatment for each individual patient, and to take all appropriate safety precautions. To the fullest extent of the law, neither the Publisher nor the Authors assume any liability for any injury and/or damage to persons or property arising out or related to any use of the material contained in this book.

Working together to grow
libraries in developing countries

www.elsevier.com | www.bookaid.org | www.sabre.org

ELSEVIER   BOOK AID International   Sabre Foundation

ELSEVIER   your source for books, journals and multimedia in the health sciences

www.elsevierhealth.com

The publisher's policy is to use **paper manufactured from sustainable forests**

Printed in China

The Publisher's Policy is to use Paper manufactured from sustainable forests.

Contents

Foreword   *Sandra P. Thomas*   viii
Foreword   *Antony Sheehan*   x
Preface   xiii
List of Contributors   xvii
Acknowledgements   xxi

Chapter 1:   Introduction – debate within psychiatric/mental health nursing:
              its nature, its place and its necessity   *John R. Cutcliffe & Martin F. Ward*   1

DEBATE 1:   What's in a name? Are we 'psychiatric' or 'mental health' nurses?

              Editorial   22
Chapter 2:   The case for 'psychiatric' nurses   *Phyllis du Mont*   24
Chapter 3:   The case for 'mental health' nurses   *Mary Chambers*   33
Commentary: *John Collins*   46

**DEBATE 2:   Reconciliatory or recalcitrant: should psychiatric/mental health
              nursing strive for independence from or be closely allied to
              psychiatric medicine?**

              Editorial   54
Chapter 4:   Psychiatry and psychiatric nursing in the New World Order   *Peter Morrall*   56
Chapter 5:   Declaring conceptual independence from obsolete professional
              affiliations   *Liam Clarke*   70
Commentary: *Jon Allen*   84

**DEBATE 3:   Heterogeneous or homogeneous: should psychiatric/mental health
              nursing have a specialist or generic preparation?**

              Editorial   90
Chapter 6:   Generic nurses: the nemesis of psychiatric/mental health nursing?
              John R. Cutcliffe & Hugh P. McKenna   92
Chapter 7:   Debating the integration of psychiatric/mental health nursing content in
              undergraduate nursing programmes   *Olive Younge & Geertje Boschma*   107
Commentary: *Stephen Tilley*   119

DEBATE 4:   Practice or theory centred: should psychiatric/mental health nursing be located within higher education and have a theory emphasis, or should it be practice oriented?

Editorial   130

Chapter 8:   The case for maintaining P/MH nurse preparation within higher education   *Ben Hannigan & Michael Coffey*   132

Chapter 9:   Theory versus practice – gap or chasm? The preparation of practitioners: academic and practice issues   *Linda Marie Lowe*   144

Commentary: *Maritta Välimäki*   158

DEBATE 5:   Dealing with violence and aggression in psychiatric/mental health nursing: the cases for 'control and restraint' and 'de-escalation'

Editorial   166

Chapter 10:   Managing violence – a contemporary challenge for psychiatric/mental health nurses: the case for 'control and restraint' *James Noak, Sean Conway & John Carthy*   168

Chapter 11:   Issues and concerns about 'control and restraint' training: moving the debate forward   *Andrew McDonnell & Ian Gallon*   181

Commentary: *Malcolm Rae*   195

DEBATE 6:   Expansion or diminution of our character, essence and core: the matter of nurse prescribing in psychiatric/mental health nursing

Editorial   204

Chapter 12:   Gently applying the brakes to the beguiling allure of P/MH nurse prescribing   *Tom Keen*   206

Chapter 13:   Psychiatric/mental health nurses as non-medical prescribers: validating their role in the prescribing process   *Katharine P. Bailey & Steve Hemingway*   220

Commentary: *Dawn Freshwater*   235

DEBATE 7:   Caring for the suicidal person – the modus operandi: engagement or observation?

Editorial   240

Chapter 14:   Considering the care of the suicidal client and the case for 'engagement and inspiring hope' or 'observations'   *John R. Cutcliffe & Phil Barker*   242

Chapter 15:   Close observations: the scapegoat of mental health care? *Martin F. Ward & Julia Jones*   257

Commentary: *Peter Campbell*   272

DEBATE 8:   The standardisation of psychiatric/mental health nursing: eliminating confusion or settling for mediocrity?

	Editorial	278
Chapter 16:	In support of standardisation *Susan McCabe*	280
Chapter 17:	Against standardisation *Gary Rolfe*	292
Commentary:	*Wendy Austin*	306

DEBATE 9:   An appropriate, useful and meaningful research paradigm for psychiatric/mental health nursing: the qualitative–quantitative debate

	Editorial	312
Chapter 18:	Qualifying psychiatric/mental health nursing research *Chris Stevenson*	314
Chapter 19:	'Pro' quantitative methods (on being a good craftsperson) *Nigel Wellman*	323
Commentary:	*Philip Burnard*	336

DEBATE 10:   The proper focus: should psychiatric/mental health nursing have a humanistic or biological emphasis?

	Editorial	342
Chapter 20:	Psychiatric/mental health nursing: biological perspectives *Kevin Gournay*	344
Chapter 21:	Biological psychiatry versus humanism: why taking meaning seriously in mental health practice is not inferior *Michael Clinton*	356
Commentary:	*Bryn Davis*	369

| | Subject Index | 376 |

Foreword

Sandra P. Thomas

Her name was Toby. She was lying, naked, on a bare mattress in the floor of a dingy seclusion room reminiscent of a prison cell. The attendants told me that she had been placed there three days ago, after violent acting out on the ward. I, a 19-year-old student, was outside the door peering in at her through a small grimy window, from which the staff made its periodic observations. Her hair was a dull brown, greasy and matted. There was no flicker of curiosity in her eyes as I slowly unlocked the door. I had no clue what I was to do with Toby, my first psychiatric patient. Didactic instruction had been appallingly brief and entirely disease-focused. Therefore, I knew what paranoid schizophrenia was, but what should I actually *do* with Toby? Mercifully, common sense and basic nursing knowledge led to my first 'interventions': I took Toby to the shower, assisted with a shampoo, and helped her select appropriate warm garments from her meagre state-issued wardrobe. We were going outside into fresh air. I don't recall asking anyone's permission to take Toby out of the locked ward. We students only saw a supervisor once or twice a day anyway. After a week of orientation, we had been assigned to wards, bereft of instructors or registered nurse role models. Terrified of the patients, most of the students huddled in the nurses' station except for the specified times of dispensing medication (usually Thorazine concentrate, mixed in juice, which patients swallowed with exaggerated gulps because they knew the students had been warned to watch them closely).

As we walked through a long, dimly lit tunnel in the basement, making our way to the building's exit, Toby spoke for the first time: 'Aren't you afraid? There is nobody down here.' There was a strange glint in her eyes. For the first time, I realized that I was indeed quite alone, with a patient viewed as dangerous. Relying solely on intuition, and perhaps the hubris of youth, I felt no fear. Indeed, throughout the 3 months that I worked with Toby, I never feared her. Our outings took us all over the campus of the massive 2,000-bed psychiatric hospital. We walked past the building where electroshock therapy was administered in barbaric, assembly-line, fashion, in a huge room where patients watched others have their grand mal seizures while waiting their own turn. We walked past the tuberculosis unit, the chaotic admissions hall, and the geriatric complex, from which the stench of urine was unmistakable. Sometimes we even dared go near an off-limits building housing the patients with black skin, which did not admit students of the white race for clinical experience in the 1950s.

Gradually, I began to hear about Toby's dreams, the violent images and rivers of blood. I learned about her rape at the age of 4, the genesis of those rivers of blood. I began to understand her paranoia, her propensity for violence. From her psychiatrist I received a grim prognosis; recovery was not in the lexicon of psychiatry at the time. I mined her data for my 'case study', the magnum opus of the psychiatric rotation, for which I received an A. But I also connected with her as one human being to another. While working with Toby, I experienced the gamut of emotions. I was horrified by her history, intrigued by the psychodynamics, and completely helpless to make her better. Although Hildegard Peplau had already published her seminal book, 'Interpersonal Relations in Nursing', in 1952, I did not know of it. I knew nothing about the principles of establishing 'therapeutic relationships'. I was stumbling along on instinct and good intentions. Such was my introduction to psychiatric nursing nearly 50 years ago.

Fast forward 25 years. Now I am a master's prepared clinical specialist in P/MH nursing. I work on an adult inpatient unit that provides topnotch acute care. Every patient has a registered nurse as admission interviewer and developer of the care plan. Goals are formulated, and all charting by the multidisciplinary team during a patient's hospital stay pertains to his or her progress toward attaining those goals. Patients have the same primary nurse throughout the hospitalization. All staff members are RNs or psychiatric techs (who tend to be bright young men and women majoring in psychology in college). All patients have 1:1 interaction time with their primary nurse each day, various group therapies and psychoeducational sessions led by nurses, and evening groups with their families, also led by nurses. Length of stay tends to be about 3 weeks, with the final week devoted to intensive planning for aftercare and return to the community. Frequent staff meetings facilitate a united approach when there are patients adept at splitting and manipulating us. The psychiatrists who admit to the unit are extremely respectful of the nurses, never interrupting our 'sacred' 1:1 interaction time with patients or asking us to perform wifely duties such as carrying their charts, calling their offices, or fetching them coffee. It is truly a therapeutic milieu. Toby would have gasped in amazement.

Fast forward 25 years once again. Now I am an academician and researcher, a 'senior scholar', if you will, invited to contribute a foreword for this book. Dutifully, I begin to read. 'Duty' soon gives way to absorption, then admiration and pride in the progress of my specialty. The erudite and cogent arguments of the chapter authors display a sophistication within psychiatric nursing that I could never have imagined when I plunged ahead with Toby as a novice nurse, without guidance of theory (or empirical evidence about 'best practices'). The progress of psychiatric nursing – in my lifetime – is simply stunning.

The engaging and stimulating debates in this book, emanating from both sides of the big pond, will create ripples in that pond for quite some time. The 10 debates address what we specialists in P/MH nursing call ourselves, how we are prepared for practice and research, who we might align ourselves with (and why), which paradigms and standards ought guide our practice, and which epistemology should undergird our science. The reader will consider the merits of arguments articulated by a bevy of brilliant writers, who sweep one along with vivid verbiage and compelling facts – with a sprinkling of audacious heresy here and there. Readers will decide for themselves whether we are a specialty group in disarray, 'on the path to professional suicide' (as McCabe fears), or poised to achieve clinical and scientific excellence in the 21st century. The chapters will undoubtedly provoke disagreement as well as nods of consensual validation. If you are provoked to take pen in hand and enter the debates, all the better. I am confident that nothing would please the editors more! In fact, as editor of a P/MH journal that explicitly encourages submission of controversial pieces, I am often dismayed at the *lack* of rebuttal and debate that takes place among my colleagues.

Ultimately, the product of our lively debates must be improved services to consumers. The well-documented worldwide toll of mental morbidity is dreadful. Despite continuing debates – which are a sign of the maturity and vigor of P/MH nursing – surely there is also universal *agreement* that patients need improved care delivery systems, access to evidence-based treatments, and expert care from their psychiatric nurses. Toby deserved so much more than what I could offer her 50 years ago. How might her experience differ in the 21st century?

Reference

Peplau H E 1991 Interpersonal relations in nursing: A conceptual frame of reference for psychodynamic nursing, New York, Springer (originally published 1952).

Foreword

Antony Sheehan

It is a great pleasure to write this foreword. When I read the draft of this book I felt a tremendous sense of excitement. From a distinguished list of contributors has come one of the finest publications in this area which I have read. Some of the writers and commentators are people whom I have respected and looked up to throughout my professional career. Reading what all the contributors have written produces a warm glow. How wonderful to be so stimulated!

Readers will be challenged and provoked, yet ultimately delighted by this book's contents. At a time of continuing change – in both service intervention arrangements and also priorities – this book's contribution to practitioners' professional development will be hugely significant.

As to the relevance and immediacy of the topic, I would make my point by commenting in a very personal way. As I have progressed in the Service I have come to respect more and more my base training as a Mental Health Nurse. Indeed, I not only value this – on a par with almost all else – but I consider it to have been one of the most significant achievements in my life. The reasons for this are many and various. They are also very personal. Of relevance, however, is the deep sense of pride which my training and work as a Nurse has imparted, for when I reflect on the many brilliant practitioners with whom I have worked over the years, I recognise a common quality which they all possessed. This was the fervent belief that we must strive endlessly for improvement – for ourselves, in our practice and for our clients who entrust themselves to our care.

This now provides the link with what I wish to say about this book. The quality I have so admired in those who have inspired me is that theirs was an intention to constantly question what we were doing and if possible to discover better ways of doing it. Some of this was born of frustration and restlessness associated with poor practice. Some of it was instinctive – their knowing that betterment was always possible. On the other hand, a constant limitation was the paucity of opportunity to mount sensible challenge and debate. However, notwithstanding these constraints, their ultimate motivation was always the needs of others, never themselves. The unspoken proposition was that every person relying on our care deserved our wholehearted effort – applied with a motivation which acknowledged that there was always something new or different that could be done to assist a person in their difficulty, hopefully bringing improvement leading to stabilisation and/or recovery.

This book adopts a debating approach. Here we should reflect that, classically, a defining feature of a profession is that it is built upon a body of knowledge and learning. This should never stop evolving. How better to ensure this than that people contribute their ideas in such dialectic, because, by the Oxford Dictionary's definition, dialectic will 'test the truth of opinions . . . by discussion and logical disputation'.

My statement here gives an obvious hint. Readers will find this book challenging in that writers adopt positions and raise debate by making statements with which readers, variously, may agree. At the same time they make assertions with which some may disagree or want to take issue. However, as Cutcliffe and Ward rehearse in their opening chapter, freedom of speech – and by implication, the raising of controversy by testing opinions and questioning conventional views – is very much the hallmark of free societies. Within these, it is not only in the interest of professionals that they partake in examination and debate, but for the interests of the wider community, it is their duty. It is perhaps a strange paradox to have to defend critical debate when, in mental health work in particular, one of the most crucial and important features in nursing practice is good, effective communication.

The topics and themes selected encompass all the fundamental questions and issues. These range from defining and re-defining role(s), training, function and remit and in the final chapter, a wise and provocative treatment of philosophical positioning. Here, Gourney and Clinton – assisted by Davis' commentary – revisit the vitally important challenge of biological versus humanistic determinants of mental ill health and problems.

Thus the reader is taken on a journey of mind-stretching questions where, in part if not in whole, the challenge is that of deciding on the answers!

A significant thought which I would also like to share is the appropriateness of this book so close on the heels of the Chief Nursing Officer's recent review report (2006) concerning Mental Health Nursing, *From Values to Action*.

In this the CNO reminds us that mental health nurses are the largest profession working in mental health today. She goes on to record (on page 3) how service users and carers want MHNs to 'have positive human qualities as well as a range of technical knowledge and skills'. Encouraged by Professor Louis Appleby's remark that 'Mental Health Nursing is at the heart of modern mental health care', with the Healthcare Commission also affording the CNO's report the status of being 'an important contribution to modernising and improving the quality and care for service users' (on page 3 of the Report), the opportunity may be grasped to link the thinking and debate stimulated by this book with the vision for mental health nursing as advanced in the CNO's report.

Significantly, the CNO adopts an approach which both recognises and is driven by 'values'. The confrontation of topics raised in this book's debates must likewise be values-driven.

So to my concluding remarks. I recommend with enthusiasm this book to would-be readers. It is a solid and significant contribution to the ongoing development of mental health nursing. I warmly applaud the writers whose ideas provide such a vital contribution and stimulus to the various debates which accompany the broader question of mental health nursing development.

Finally I pay tribute to these contributors' ongoing work and interest in this area. In the very finest traditions of professional practice I consider that they and their ideas are a tremendous credit to nursing.

Reference

Department of Health 2006 From values to action: The Chief Nursing Officer's review of mental health nursing. Department of Health, London.

Preface

It is difficult to imagine free societies without the presence and influence of debate. Such is the value of debate and freedom of speech that are a prerequisite for genuine debate, that these practices are written into the constitutions, customs and practices of many countries. Further, national and local government systems and procedures have been developed and refined over the years in order to enable, even facilitate, debate. Indeed, one might argue that effective, contemporary, democratic government is founded upon and predicated by the need for debate.

Rather than being restricted to the higher echelons of national (Federal) government, or isolated to the few wisest and most erudite amongst us, debate resides within the purview of 'everyman'. It is both, one might suggest, our 'right' and simultaneously our 'duty'. In these days where freedom, democracy and the liberty to debate are perhaps 'taken for granted', it is worth remembering the cost that many have paid throughout history to uphold and maintain our rights to free speech and debate. Lest we all become too blasé, it is worth considering what society can look like when the right to debate is removed.

Autocracy, dictatorships, empires, oppressive regimes – each of these is synonymous with the absence of freedom of speech, where the only debate that occurs is arguably tokenistic, synthetic and lacking in meaning. Before those lucky individuals, who live in a world where debate is possible, become too complacent and self-congratulatory, we ought to recognise and acknowledge that they have their own barriers to debate. Some of these might be described as residing in the individual – one's levels of confidence and anxiety; the belief that one has nothing worthwhile or interesting to say; the expectation that someone else, perhaps wiser and more bold, will debate in one's stead; and the fear of 'losing face' and feeling a sense of shame amongst our peers. These are perhaps 'intra-personal' reasons why one may be reluctant to engage in meaningful debate. Other barriers might be described as residing in our society: individuals, groups, authorities and corporations who are reluctant to relinquish their power; governments who wish to retain a sense of control; and systems that might collapse like a 'house of cards' if their philosophical basis were debated and shown to be fundamentally flawed. Each of these might be described as 'extra-personal' reasons why one is prevented or prohibited from engaging in meaningful debate.

Nevertheless, even within the two principal formal areas that are perhaps most relevant to this book, health care and academia, there are factors and processes that can hinder and those that can encourage debate. Yet, in reading this book, the Editors believe that the nature, value and absolute necessity of debate for all involved in both formal areas will become clearer. Accordingly, we believe there are at least eight reasons why there is a need for this book on the 'Key Debates in Psychiatric/Mental Health Nursing', and summarise these as follows:

1 P/MH nurses have to deal with uncertainty on a daily basis. They have to make difficult decisions, often when conflicting evidence and/or philosophies/ideologies exist. Thus, there is a clear need to provide these people with the most complete, balanced and thought-provoking information possible in order better to inform their subsequent practice-related decisions.

2 P/MH nurses have a professional (and moral) duty to act in the role of client advocate; implicit in such a role is the requirement to construct and present arguments/debates.

3 Given that P/MH nursing has often been described as a 'broad church', one in which aspirant nurses need to locate themselves, rather than adopting a philosophical, theoretical and practice 'stance' based on one-sided 'position' statements, here P/MH nurses will be able to review contrasting and sometimes opposing 'sides' of the debate, juxtaposed with one another, and should therefore be able to draw their own conclusions.

4 Debate is an immensely useful educational tool. Thus, engaging in debate can become one of the mediums through which P/MH nurses engage in 'lifelong' learning.

5 Debate can indicate new questions and areas for research and practice development.

6 Engaging in debate can lead to more cogent, evidence-based decision-making.

7 P/MH nurses have a professional and moral obligation to debate the developmental direction(s) that their discipline should take.

8 Debate, especially when it embraces a wide range of views, evidence and opinions, reminds each of us of the uncertain nature of the world, of health care and, especially, of mental health care. Therefore, engaging in debate helps to prevent us from becoming rigid, dogmatic and unthinking practitioners, educationalists, researchers or managers. It can help to thwart each of us from being beguiled by the allure of certainty.

In putting together a book that focuses on 'key debates', and recognising and operating within word and space limits, the Editors would like to point out that difficult choices had to be made around which debates to include and which to leave out. The Editors wish to emphasise that in no way is this list of debates meant to be exhaustive or representative of the only issues that warrant debate. Understandably, the choice of which debates to include reflects, at least in part, the views, values and, to some extent, the interests of the Editors. The idiosyncrasies of the Editors notwithstanding, we believe the debates will have currency and meaning for the majority of P/MH nurses. They have been selected in part as a result of our communication with the international community of P/MH nurses; as a result of searching the extant literature for ongoing debates; as a result of the introduction of some mental health care policy; and, in part, in an attempt to capture practice, policy, education and research related debates. Accordingly, the debates might be regarded as a collection of some of the key debates in P/MH nursing. Additional debates that we considered featuring in the book include: the thorny issue of nurses' holding power; the introduction of Community Treatment Orders; the increasing use of mechanical surveillance in P/MH nursing; the use of seclusion rooms; practice-level doctorates in P/MH nursing; defining and identifying P/MH nurse leaders; labelling and diagnostics; practitioner-assisted suicide; whether P/MH nursing is a profession, discipline or vocation, and whether or not it should even strive to become a profession. It is the hope of the Editors that these debates may form the cadre of a second volume.

In order to provide some additional preliminary justification for certain choices we have made in constructing this book (and at the same time, perhaps off-setting potential criticism), the Editors would like to offer the following explanations:

• The term psychiatric/mental health nurse is used throughout the book, except, of course, in the chapters that deal with the 'proper' term. Given that this issue was one of our featured debates, it was prudent not to prejudice either view by the Editors adopting one or other of these terms throughout the book.

- The Editors have chosen to use the word 'discipline' rather than 'profession' when referring to the occupational group (and status) of P/MH nurses. The Editors do not believe (a) that P/MH nursing can accurately be described as a 'profession' (applying several theories/positions of how to determine professions, e.g. trait theory, Registrar General's classification of social class, or the more postmodernist theories of professional groups as essentially and primarily self-serving groups), or (b) that P/MH nurses should even aspire to achieving professional status (again given the illuminating arguments in these postmodernist positions).
- The Editors have not stipulated a 'proper' term to be used by contributors when referring to the recipient of formal mental health care. This has been left to the individual discretion of the contributors (and the multiple terms used in this context, we believe, indicates something of the uncertainty that exists in P/MH nursing).
- The questions posed at the beginning of the debates are purposefully 'polarised' and posited as binary opposites when, in some cases, this may be a simplistic position. In some ways, it is for the reader (and the commentators) to decide whether these are indeed opposite positions.
- On assigning gender to nurses and recipients of formal mental health care, we have again left this choice to each of the contributing authors.
- The Editors deliberately restricted the contributing authors to a maximum of 25 references per chapter, and to a word limit of 5000 words. No doubt, additional, relevant, extant literature and references do exist and these could have been used to bolster the positions taken by authors. The choices of what literature to access, and what not to, remained within the purview of the authors.
- Furthermore, it is perhaps tautological to point out that the inclusion of a particular position as part of our selected debates, in no way suggests that the editors either uphold or support that position.

Finally, it would be remiss of the Editors if they did not point out that these debates and associated chapters do not constitute the 'definitive position' on any of the issues featured. We acknowledge that debating ongoing issues can (should?) be an iterative process; positions and opinions change as new evidence emerges, as the dominant discourse changes and/or as society's values evolve. To posit these chapters as the 'endpoint' to these deliberations would be de facto to prevent and inhibit debate – a counterproductive outcome for a book that wishes to avoid certainty and promote debate.

John R. Cutcliffe
Martin F. Ward   July 2005

List of Contributors

John Allen EN RMN BA(Hons) MSc

Director of Nursing, Oxfordshire Mental Healthcare NHS Trust and Buckinghamshire Mental Health NHS Trust; Chair of the Mental Health and Learning Disabilities Nurse Directors and Leads National Forum, UK

Wendy Austin BScN, MEd, PhD

Canadian Research Chair, Relational Ethics in Health Care; Professor, Faculty of Nursing, University of Alberta, Canada

Katharine P. Bailey BSN MSN APRN

Director of Adult Clinical Affairs, Northwest Centre for Family and Mental Health, Lakeville, Connecticut, USA

Phil Barker PhD RN FRCN

Visiting Professor, Trinity College, Dublin, Ireland; Director, Clan Unity Mental Health Recovery Consultancy, Dundee, UK

Geertje Boschma RN PhD

Assistant Professor, Faculty of Nursing, University of Calgary, Canada

Philip Burnard PhD RN

Vice Dean, School of Nursing and Midwifery Studies, University of Cardiff, UK

Peter Campbell BA

Honorary Lecturer, Institute of Applied Social Studies, University of Birmingham, UK

John Carthy RMN Fe.tec.

Clinical Ward Manager, Ravenswood House Regional Secure Unit, Fareham, Hampshire, UK

Mary Chambers RGN RMN DipN(Lond) RNT BEd(Hons) DPhil Cert Behavioural Psychotherapy FRSM

Professor of Mental Health Nursing and Chief Nurse, Kingston University/St George's Medical School and Southwest London Mental Health NHS Trust, London, UK

Liam Clarke RN Dip Ed DipN(Lond) Dip Rel Stud (Cantab) DPMSA(Med Phil) BA MSc PhD

Principal Lecturer for Mental Health, Faculty of Health, University of Brighton, UK

Michael Clinton PhD RN

Professor and Dean, Faculty of Nursing, and Professor, Faculty of Medicine, University of Calgary, Canada

Michael Coffey RMN RGN BSc MSc

Lecturer in Community Mental Health Nursing, School of Health Science, Swansea University, UK

John Collins MA DipEduc BA(Hons) DPSN RN RPN

Dean of Nursing, The International School of Nursing and Health Studies, Vancouver, Canada

Sean Conway RMN RGN BSc DMS CertMHP

Senior Nurse – Operations, The State Hospital, Carstairs, UK

John R. Cutcliffe PhD BSc(Hons) Nrsg RMN RGN RPN

David G. Braithwaite Professor of Nursing, University of Texas (Tyler), USA; Adjunct Professor, Stenberg College International School of Nursing, Canada; Director, Cutcliffe Consulting; Associate Editor: Journal of Psychiatric and Mental Health Nursing; Assistant Editor: International Journal of Nursing Studies

Bryn Davis RGN RMN RNT BSc PhD

Professor Emeritus Nursing Education, University of Wales, UK: Academic and Professional Nursing Consultant

Phyllis M. du Mont PhD RN

Assistant Professor of Nursing, University of Tennessee, Knoxville, USA

Dawn Freshwater PhD FRCN RN RNT DipPsych

Professor of Mental Health and Primary Care, Institute of Health and Community Studies, Bournemouth University, UK

Ian Gallon RMN SRN

Project Manager, Centre for Clinical and Academic Innovation, University of Lincoln, UK; Chair, Royal College of Nursing Mental Health Nursing Forum

Kevin Gournay CBE FRCPsych(Hon) FMedSci FRCN MPhil PhD CPsychol AFBPsS Cert Behavioral Psychotherapy

Professor of Psychiatric Nursing, Health Services Research Department, Institute of Psychiatry, London, UK

Ben Hannigan BA(Hons) MA RN

Senior Lecturer in Mental Health Nursing, School of Nursing and Midwifery Studies, Cardiff University, UK

Steve Hemingway MA BA(Hons) PGDE RMN

Lecturer in Mental Health Nursing, Department of Mental Health and Learning Disability Nursing, School of Nursing and Midwifery, University of Sheffield, UK

Julia Jones BA(Hons) PhD

Senior Research Fellow, Department of Mental Health and Learning Disability, St Bartholomew School of Nursing and Midwifery, City University, London, UK

Tom Keen RMN MSc

Senior Lecturer in Mental Health Studies, University of Plymouth, UK (Retired)

Linda Marie Lowe RGN RMW BSc(n) MHCE MPH PhD(c)

Assistant Professor of Nursing, University of Northern British Columbia, Prince George, British Columbia, Canada

Susan McCabe EdD APRN BC

Associate Professor and Director for Undergraduate Programmes, Fay W. Whitney School of Nursing, University of Wyoming, USA

Andrew McDonnell BSc MSc PhD

Clinical Psychologist, Director of Studio3 Training Systems, Bath, UK

Hugh P. McKenna RMN RGN RNT DipN(Lond) AdDipEd PhD FFN FRCSI FEANS FRCN

Dean of the Faculty of Life and Health Sciences, University of Ulster, Jordanstown UK

Peter Morrall PhD MSc BA(Hons) PGCE RN

Head of Group for Mental Health, Learning Disabilities and Behavioural Sciences, School of Healthcare, University of Leeds, UK

James Noak RN RMN MSc Cert HSM Cert Health Econ MHSM

Forensic Nurse Consultant, West London Mental Health NHS Trust, UK; Robert Baxter Research Fellow, Institute of Psychiatry, London, UK

Gary Rolfe PhD MA BSc RMN PGCEA

Professor, School of Health Science, University of Wales, Swansea, UK

Chris Stevenson RMN BA(Hons) MSc PhD

Chair in Mental Health Nursing, School of Nursing, Faculty of Science and Health, Dublin City University, Ireland

Stephen Tilley RMN BA PhD Cert Behavioural Psychotherapy

Senior Lecturer, Nursing Studies, School of Health and Social Sciences, University of Edinburgh, UK

Maritta Välimäki RN LicNSc PhD
Professor, Department of Nursing Science, University of Turku, Finland

Martin F. Ward RMN RNT CertEd Dip Nurs NEBSS Dip MPhil
Independent Mental Health Nursing Consultant; Coordinator of Mental Health Nursing Courses, University of Malta; Chair of the Expert Panel, HORATIO – Psychiatric Nurses in Europe

Nigel Wellman MSc BA(Hons) RMN
Professor of Mental Health Nursing, Thames Valley University, London, Slough and Reading, UK; Honorary Consultant Nurse, Berkshire Healthcare NHS Trust, UK

Olive Younge RN PhD CPsych
Professor, Faculty of Nursing, University of Alberta, Edmonton, Alberta, Canada

Acknowledgements

The Editors offer their most profound and sincere thanks to all of the contributors to this book. Whether you wrote a debate position, commentary or foreword, your contribution remains greatly appreciated.

This book is dedicated to Professor Phil Barker, not only because of the depth and extent of his undeniable contributions to psychiatric/nursing practice, but also because of the personal support and immensely positive influence that he provided to both of the Editors. Thank you Phil.

John R Cutcliffe & Martin F Ward

Introduction – debate within psychiatric/mental health nursing: its nature, its place and its necessity

'Just because I disagree with you doesn't mean I'm disagreeable.'

Samuel Goldwyn

The historical origins of debate: the role model of the Ancient Greeks

It is not without a distinct sense of irony that the authors note that the nature of debate is, in and of itself, a matter of debate! Even a cursory examination of resources dedicated to 'debate', for example the journal *Contemporary Argumentation and Debate,* internet debate sites such as the Debate Union (http://debate.uvm.edu/), the Debate Encyclopedia (http://en.wikipedia.org/wiki/Debate) and the Debating Union (http://www.klubdebat.uw.edu.pl/klubdebat/Eng/1_1.htm), will show that multiple definitions exist. This may not be entirely surprising given the evidence that debate has existed in democratic societies for millennia.

Perhaps the first recorded evidence of formalised debate dates back to the Ancient Greek civilisation. History records that when democracy first flourished in ancient Greece, over two thousand years ago, Athenian citizens would often meet in public assembles. Far from being an esoteric or largely pointless activity, the debate engaged in at these meetings directed the very nature of the civilisation. They decided whether or not they should go to war, how and when they should fight; they debated and subsequently created laws that directed the course of daily life for citizens. Leaders, orators and members of the general public engaged in debates that ranged from philosophical issues, such as what was morally and legally right, to more pragmatic issues, such as what would be the best way to achieve a desired outcome, what was possible, and what was prudent. Subsequent to these debates, citizens would cast their votes and thus determine the policy and actions of the state. It is important to reiterate here that these votes were always preceded by debate. This arena for public debate gave rise to now famous public orators or debaters such as Demosthenes and Aeschines. (Arguably, Demosthenes' greatest oration was delivered in 330 BC, entitled 'On the Crown'. In a review and justification of his public life, he proceeded to condemn his bitter rival, Aeschines, who was then forced into exile.) Accordingly, some of the underlying philosophy and practice of contemporary democratic societies (and organisations/disciplines within these societies) can be traced back to these formative debating practices of the Ancient Greeks. This has resulted in debate being regarded as an essential activity in democratic societies.

Today debate is still not only essential to society but also tantamount to being one of the *raison d'êtres* of academic activity (Huber 1964). Although the democratic process has changed (indeed, it would be inaccurate and misleading to suggest that there is only one democratic process) – and with that forms, processes and procedures for debate – nevertheless, debates continue. Accordingly, in a book that features a range of linked debates, it may be prudent to begin by offering some statements pertaining to our understanding of what debate is: what is its nature, purpose and value? Further, we wish to explore whom should be engaged in or concerned with debate and, given the focus of the book, whether or not psychiatric/mental health (P/MH) nurses should be, or are, involved in debate. We also believe there is utility in examining some of the common miscomprehensions and misconceptions of debate and, importantly, what happens when genuine debate is stifled, subdued or, worse still, subjugated by autocratic, unilateral posturing.

The nature and forms of debate in our contemporary society

As stated above, it is inaccurate to suggest that there is only one form of debate. Therefore, in attempting to understand more about debate, perhaps the most appropriate way to start would be to offer a definition and follow this with a number of descriptions of the more common forms. The *Oxford Concise English Dictionary* (1991, p 182) states that 'debate' is both a noun and a verb.

The noun 'debate' has two definitions/senses:

'1. *argument, argumentation,* **debate** – *(a discussion in which reasons are advanced for and against some proposition or proposal; "the argument over foreign aid goes on and on")*
2. **debate***, disputation, public debate – (the formal presentation of and opposition to a stated proposition (usually followed by a vote))'*

The verb 'debate' has four definitions/senses:

'1. **debate** – *(argue with one another; "We debated the question of abortion"; "John debated with Mary")*
2. *consider,* **debate***, moot, turn over, deliberate – (think about carefully; weigh; "They considered the possibility of a strike"; "Turn the proposal over in your mind")*
3. **debate***, deliberate – (discuss the pros and cons of an issue)*
4. *argue, contend,* **debate***, fence – (have an argument about something)'*

To expand upon these rather unidirectional definitions, we have selected four of the more common (and popular) forms of debate from those listed on the wikipedia.org website. These are termed:

- Lincoln–Douglas debate
- Policy debate
- Parliamentary debate
- Karl Popper debate.

(recovered 2005 http://en.wikipedia.org/wiki/Debate)

Lincoln–Douglas debates

The Lincoln–Douglas form of debate is modelled after the famous debates between the historical American politicians, Abraham Lincoln and Stephen Douglas. Debates following this form are most often referred to as 'values debates'. The resultant focus of the debate is the competing values that the debaters purport are inherent in the proposition or motion (whatever that may be). Commonly used 'political' examples of such debate include:

'The public's right to know always supersedes the political party or candidate's right to privacy.'

'A criminal justice (or correctional) system should be more concerned with rehabilitation of the prisoners as a means to discourage recidivism, rather than punishment to appease the moral outcry of society at the heinous nature of the crime.'

whereas some examples of more substantive P/MH nursing Lincoln–Douglas (i.e. value driven) debates might include:

'The person's inalienable human rights (e.g. right to freedom of choice and self-determination) should always take precedent over the prescribed 'treatment' regime.'

'The public's right to make informed choices to maintain their own safety always supersedes the individual's right to privacy.'

(The reader can locate such Lincoln–Douglas 'values' debates either as the titled focus of a debate in this book, or as one element of debate subsumed within a larger debate. The editors wish to point out that the inclusion of these value statements as examples in no way indicates that they either do or do not endorse and support such positions.)

In Lincoln–Douglas debates, the protagonists are expected to argue on the basis of the underlying principles of their side of the resolution (the motion). Importantly, it needs to be noted that, despite advocating poignantly for their side of the resolution, they have no associated responsibility for the practical applications of their position. Again, drawing on a 'political' example, a debater argues that

'Government should provide for the needs of the poor.'

Having proffered this broad philosophical case for this government obligation, there is no associated requirement to demonstrate or prove the effectiveness of any particular government programme. In summary, the Wikipedia.org website purports that Lincoln–Douglas debates most commonly pivot on the ideas, values and spirit governing the political, economic, social, moral and aesthetic positions we hold.

Policy debates

While Lincoln–Douglas debates can focus on values, policy debate focuses on the practical implementation of these positions. Again, to draw upon a 'political' example:

'Governments should provide 'public' jobs to the unemployed.'

whereas some examples of more substantive P/MH nursing policy (i.e. driven by pragmatism) debates might include:

'The entry requirements for P/MH nursing programmes should be reduced.'

'P/MH nursing should be amalgamated with and subsumed within existing generic nursing programmes or generic healthcare worker education programmes.'

While few insightful analysts would have difficulty in seeing the 'values' implicit or inherent in these motions, within a 'policy' debate, the emphasis is placed on the practical reasons for endorsing and advocating for these policies. In essence, the debater proposes a specific policy that, arguably, will enable the identified goal to be achieved; further, it will enable this goal to be achieved in a more efficient and effective manner than any counter-proposal. For example, with respect to the first motion, the debater recognises that the unemployed are a burden on the economic resources of the society (and government). Creating jobs for such individuals will not only reduce the demands made on the budget resulting from unemployment benefits, but will simultaneously create more 'taxpayers' and thus more revenue for the government. If these previously unemployed people are then employed in public sector jobs, they can also contribute to the improved well-being of the society by providing additional public sector services. With regard to the second and third motions, the debater recognises that society faces a shortage of P/MH nurses. At the same time, the number of 'traditional' would-be applicants is diminishing. Accordingly, the policies offered represent a number of practically driven solutions to increase the number of P/MH nursing graduates. In policy debates, the 'opposition' can construct a range of arguments to refute the proposal. They can argue that change is neither needed nor desirable, that is, the status quo is sufficient to deal with the problem. Alternatively, the opponent can critique the plan itself and subsequently argue that the proposed plan is a bad plan, demonstrating that its disadvantages outweigh its advantages. Instead, the opponent may opt for a different tactic and offer up a 'better' plan for addressing the issue. While evidence in Lincoln–Douglas debate is philosophical and literary, the Wikipedia.org website purports that evidence in policy debate is practical and statistical.

Parliamentary debates

Parliamentary debate is, perhaps not surprisingly, modelled on the British Houses of Parliament. These debates usually take the form of teams of debaters, where one team represents the Government and the other Her Majesty's Loyal Opposition. (Anyone who has recently attended some of the European Psychiatric/Mental Health nursing conferences will be familiar with this form of debate, having witnessed some titanic struggles as debaters 'play out' key issues facing European P/MH nurses.) An individual, referred to as 'The Speaker of the House' officiates and carries out the official duties; the 'Speaker' needs to remain neutral and impartial in all debates. During the debates, remarks from both 'sides of the house' have to be directed to him or her as 'Mr Speaker' or 'Madam Speaker'. Most often, the team on each 'side of the house' has (at least) two designated debaters, but this does not rule out contributions to the debate emanating from other members of the team. On the Government team, there will usually be a 'Prime Minister' and a Member of the Government (often a member of cabinet related to the particular focus of the debate – for example, health-related matters, including P/MH nursing, will often involve the Health Secretary). On the Opposition team, there will usually be a 'Leader of the Opposition' and a Member of the Opposition (often a member of the 'Shadow' cabinet related to the particular focus of the debate – continuing the example mentioned above, this debater would be the Shadow Health Secretary). In these forms of debate, the 'Government' has the primary responsibility for defining the terms of the resolution (the motion). Furthermore, there must be a clear logical relationship between the topic and the definition.

Unlike the Lincoln–Douglas or policy debate forms, the Wikipedia.org website purports that parliamentary debaters have more freedom to offer both practical and philosophical arguments for their side (thus a mixture of Lincoln–Douglas and policy debate). Another important difference in this form of debate is that, in addition to constructive and rebuttal speeches, debaters can also raise 'Points of Order, Privilege and Information'. These are debater-driven interruptions that highlight erroneous claims and/or breaches of etiquette, and thus widen the participatory nature of the debate in that these 'Points of Order' can be raised by any member of the debating team. Finally, parliamentary debaters are allowed to 'heckle' one another. As with 'Points of Order', these can be 'offered' by any member of the debate team. A good heckle has been described as a short, witty and relevant comment that challenges some aspect of the opponent's case and simultaneously, and importantly, entertains the audience (Huber 1964).

Karl Popper debates

The Karl Popper form of debate (eponymously named after the philosopher and political scientist) is perhaps the most common form taught at many seats of higher education. Here it is recognised that debating is a skill – an important skill in modern democratic society and, more specifically, within the academe. Indeed, many international debating competitions now exist and use this approach. This form of debate has been linked back to The Oxford Union, where the oldest debate form had its origin. According to the Wikipedia.org website, the most popular form of debate in universities (and the international debating competitions) today is the Karl Popper debate. Participants in the debate are usually arranged into two teams, each consisting of three members. These two teams then offer opposing positions, arguments and views on and around an issue that is vital for the contemporary world – although, it is not without a sense of irony that we note that deciding what issues are vital for the contemporary world is, in and of itself, a matter of debate. Most often, one team, referred to as the 'affirmative' team, is charged with constructing an argument that supports the motion (or thesis). The other team, referred to as the 'negative' team, is then charged with refuting the motion. Once the debate begins, the speakers are not to be interrupted, but time is usually allocated after the speech for members of the opposite team to question them. In this Popperian form of debate, both the teams are aware of the issue or motion that is to be debated, and each is given time to prepare their arguments. Most often, whether the team adopts the 'affirmative' or 'negative' view is determined by chance (e.g. draw lots), immediately prior to the debate; accordingly, both teams have to prepare both 'yes' and 'no' arguments. As a result, this approach to debate is deemed to offer participants the opportunity consider an issue 'from both sides', arguably increasing participants' awareness of the complex and convoluted nature of issues rather than polarising and entrenching one-sided, dogmatic opinions.

The facilitative and developmental value of debate: debate as an education and learning medium

While one could argue that debate has more immediate relevance to certain subjects and substantive areas than to others, the adaptability of debate means it is a pedagogical tool that should not be overlooked, irrespective of one's particular subject area. Debate as a facilitative medium has utility in any discipline or subject where there are opposing ideas, situations or examples. We will not belabour the obvious value of the use of debate in the domain of care of the person with mental health problems (and P/MH nursing can be subsumed within this more capacious term). This is perhaps especially the case given that P/MH nursing has often been described as a 'broad church', a discipline exemplified at least in part by its acceptance and embracing of ambiguity (Cutcliffe & Goward 2000), and by the various hitherto unresolved contentious issues. (The ten debates contained in this book represent only the 'tip of the iceberg' – just a selection of the many practical, educational, philosophical, ethical, epistemological and political issues that exist within the formal area of care of the person with mental health problems.) In addition, it has long been recognised that P/MH operate both within a *micro* and a *macro* context of care (see, for example, Cutcliffe & Hannigan 2001) – the *micro* context being concerned with individuals, intrapersonal and interpersonal relationships and dynamics, the *macro* context being concerned with issues broader than the individual person, such as families, communities, environments and even political climates. Clear and palpable examples of this *macro* context of care include the advocacy role of the P/MH nurse (UKCC 1998) and the sometimes neglected role of lobbying or petitioning on behalf of one's clients. Both professional duties have obvious congruence with the process (and skills) of debating – of forming and presenting convincing, cogent and compelling arguments. Accordingly, it appears as though P/MH nursing could be regarded as one of those subjects or areas that have an immediate relevance with and utility for debate. Further, it is incumbent upon P/MH nursing educationalists to prepare these nurses for this lobbying role and to equip them with skills necessary to do so (Cutcliffe & Hannigan 2001). Given that engaging in debating offers the possibility to develop different 'technical skills' as well as personal expertise, it is worth considering what some of these skills might be:

- Oral communication
- Structuring and argument
- Logical and analytical thinking and teamwork
- Information gathering (sometimes given the misnomer of 'research skills')
- Interpreting the response and reception of one's audience.

(list adapted from http://www.walesdebate.org.uk)

Oral communication

Through the processes of preparing and engaging in debate, debaters learn to translate ideas and thoughts into persuasive verbal arguments, which then have to be articulated through speech. Success, it is suggested, begets success, thus the debaters' levels of confidence can be enhanced through encouragement and support, and by means of achieving success in competition. Delivering and engaging in debate often gives rise to a love of language; an interest in words and good debate can develop appropriate and optimal use of words and phrases. Debating also allows and facilitates the presenting of information in an engaging and entertaining style, and thus debaters learn how to hold the attention of their intended 'audience'.

Structuring an argument

Constructing and engaging in debate relies upon certain skills, namely: the ability to identify the relevant arguments, the selection of congruent and compelling examples to substantiate one's point, and sequencing one's argument in a logical, cohesive structure that is followed as it is explained. Debaters learn to introduce the subject matter and provide a clear objective to be proved. They learn to draw upon various sources of 'evidence' in order to proffer supporting arguments backed by clear and understandable examples. In addition to the usefulness of these skills within the context of debate, they are clearly transferable to and can be effective in written 'academic' work such as discursive pieces, reports and opinion pieces.

Logical and analytical thinking and teamwork

In order to be successful, there is a clear requirement for debaters to construct logical and cogent arguments. This is a specific skill and, as with other skills, requires practice to perfect. While it can be argued that some people have a predisposition towards logical and analytical thinking, engaging in debate is one way to develop and enhance such skills. Furthermore, if the debate is using a team format (e.g. Popperian) then these logical 'chains of reasoning' and lines of argument need to be evident in the material presented by each debater. Not only that, but debaters need to learn to support one another, to augment the argument presented by a team member, and to do so effectively requires debaters to learn to work cooperatively with one another.

Information gathering

Almost inevitably, the focus or substance of the debate will require the debaters to undertake a detailed a thorough search for pertinent information and evidence. As it would be inaccurate to describe this activity as 'research' (as established definitions of research each refer to the *generation* of knowledge rather than simply finding existing knowledge), we have termed it 'information gathering'. A thorough debate is a well prepared debate; a well prepared debate is a well informed debate. Accordingly, it behoves each debater to undertake some (a lot of?) background preparation in order to know the subject, and be able to view the concept from a number of different perspectives.

Reading one's audience

Any public 'live' or interactive activity in which one has to convince the spectators, participants or voters will have an inherent element of 'reading the audience', and hopefully of 'connecting' with them. Accordingly, tailoring the content, pace and tone of the presentation(s) to the particular nuances of that audience is a prerequisite for 'reaching' and influencing them, and is thus an important skill. Furthermore, in order to sense whether the debate is 'reaching' and convincing the audience, the debater will need to operate with a sense of duality, in much the same way as a P/MH nurse has to be both totally 'in the moment' with a client and yet simultaneously monitoring the client's experience; the debater gains a sense of how the argument is 'going over', whether it needs to be adjusted, pitched in a different way or couched using alternative language. It is suggested that effective debaters deliver a presentation at the right level with clarity and an awareness of 'where' the audience is located

The development of attitudes and values: personal, social and citizenship-related skills

According to the Welsh Debate Federation (http://www.walesdebate.org.uk), in addition to the skills listed above, engaging in debate allows the participants to develop their attitudes and values. These authors declare that debate encourages a greater understanding of contemporary society at the local, national and international level. Through examining and discussing issues in detail, and from a range of perspectives and viewpoints, our knowledge of the systems and structures that influence our lives is enhanced. An interesting element of the value of debate, and perhaps an element that is not emphasised sufficiently, is that of considering and subsequently saying something that can be, potentially, unpopular or marginal but which might encourage the broadening of viewpoints (World Debate Organisation, http://debate.uvm.edu/wdo.html). We will return to this crucial issue later in the chapter. Lastly, the experience of expressing ideas and constructing an argument can lead to a much deeper understanding of underlying issues and areas of disagreement. Deeper understanding should, logically, lead to more fully informed decisions. The Welsh Debate Federation describes how engaging in debate influences some of the key attitudinal and value-related developments, including the following:

Personal and social education skills gained through debating

Debators gain and refine the ability to:

- Listen attentively in different situations and respond appropriately
- Communicate confidently one's feelings and views and maintain with conviction a personal standpoint
- Appreciate and critically evaluate others' viewpoints and messages from the media
- Make moral judgements and resolve moral issues and dilemmas
- Work independently and cooperatively
- Make reasoned judgements
- Take part in debates and vote on issues
- Make decisions and choices effectively
- Talk for a range of purposes, including: explanation, description, narration, exploration, hypothesis, analysis, discussion, argument and persuasion
- Talk in a range of contexts, adapting presentations to different audiences and situations, especially those that are formal.

Citizenship-related skills gained through debating

Debators also gain and refine the ability to:

- Think about topical political, spiritual, moral, social and cultural issues, problems and events by analysing information and its sources, including ICT-based sources
- Justify orally and in writing a personal opinion about such issues, problems or events
- Contribute to group and exploratory class discussions, and take part in debates
- Use their imagination to consider other people's experiences and be able to think about, express and explain views that are not their own
- Negotiate, decide and take part responsibly in both school and community-based activities
- Reflect on the process of participation.

(adapted from http://www.walesdebate.org.uk)

Having identified the nature and value of debate, it is now necessary to consider whether or not P/MH nurses should be, or are, involved in debate.

Sources of knowledge and ignorance: the function of debate in psychiatric/mental health nursing

Anyone who has studied the history of P/MH nursing will recognise that our discipline rarely stands still. Within P/MH nursing, change would appear – ironically – to be the one thing that doesn't change. While recognising that change can take many forms, we believe that informed change is prefaced by debate. Indeed, much of the relevant 'change management' literature and practice development literature (Lewin 1951, Bailey & Whale 1996, Kitson et al 1996, Ward et al 1998, Cutcliffe et al 1998) refers to the necessity of consultation, discussion and debate before initiating any substantive change. Change for change's sake is thus something to be shunned; yet change that brings about beneficial outcomes should be embraced. Another illuminating 'finding' that arises from a study of the history of P/MH nursing is that of the amount, magnitude and frequency of wide-scale, sweeping changes that have occurred; our history is replete with such transformations. Yet a parallel finding is that, often, these changes were not prefaced by wide-scale debate, and in some cases debate of any kind was noticeably absent (see, for example, Barker & Buchanan-Barker's insightful 2005 paper). Encouragingly, this trend appears to be changing, given the recent evidence of protracted and thorough debating of certain key issues (see some of the debates in this book). This contemporary trend is all the more encouraging when we consider a number of factors:

1 P/MH nursing and care of the person with mental health problems are formal areas that are synonymous with ambiguity and uncertainty (Cutcliffe & Goward 2000). Thus, issues need to be discussed and debated in order that they can be better understood.
2 The discipline of P/MH nursing has been described as a 'broad church' – a discipline that can encompass a wide variety of views, types of evidence and subsequent positions. Thus, there is a clear need to engage in debate in order that one can navigate one's way through the range of views and opinions.
3 P/MH nurses are proud of their advocacy role and thus the need to argue on behalf of (and with) service users (UKCC 1998).
4 P/MH nurses have been described as rhetoricians (Tilley 1997) – people who form arguments and engage in debate.

Debate as the *raison d'être* of academic disciplines

These points warrant further examination. As stated above, our discipline of P/MH nursing has often been described as a 'broad church', meaning that it has many and varied responsibilities, each with their attendant views and opinions. For some, the intellectual freedom that this conceptualisation brings is emancipatory as it offers up the chance to locate oneself within, and hopefully contribute to, one or more of the various discourses that are encompassed within this capacious domain. For some others, the absence or limited availability of clearly demarcated 'legitimate' topics and substantive issues will be a deterrent, needing, as some people do, the sense of safety that comes from knowing what one needs to know. As P/MH nurse academics, we are heartened to see that we have arenas (analogous to those of the Ancient Greeks – for example, the commentary sections included within some P/MH nursing journals, scheduled protected sessions at various P/MH nursing and related conferences) dedicated to facilitating debate; this speaks well of our discipline. We view these as ideal forums for engaging in what is, arguably, the *raison d'être* of any bona fide academic discipline, namely – debate. Genuine debate, without defaulting to personal attack or 'carping on', is not something to be feared, shunned or avoided. It is through activities such as debate that knowledge, perspectives and, ultimately, practice can be critiqued, considered and enhanced. Perhaps one of the most beneficial aspects of these established 'arenas' for debate is that they provide the ideal medium for challenging contemporary orthodoxies and hegemonies. While there is recent evidence of more P/MH nurses making use of these arenas, we are still relatively silent in comparison with other related professions or disciplines (Barker & Buchanan-Barker 2005). There is a great deal more debate for P/MH nurses to engage in.

Now, it is not without a distinct sense of irony that one recognises that in our post-September 11 world, one of the most pervasive orthodoxies is the shift from journalism (synonymous with freedom of speech and the expression of a variety of conflicting opinions) to 'jingoism' (synonymous with touting the often government-endorsed policy, opinion or view). We view this as ironic in that such jingoism is often in response to a perceived threat, be it rational or otherwise; it is inevitably introduced and engineered to 'browbeat' and suppress any opposing views; this strikes us as being diametrically opposed to debate. Unfortunately, there is even evidence of this phenomenon within some P/MH nursing literature. Clarke (2001, p 465), for example, has drawn attention to the practice of some P/MH nursing writers to eschew debate and critique. He stated:

'A typical ploy amongst certain nurse writers . . . is their tendency to dismiss criticism rather than engage in it. Rather than argue with critics, such

critics are deemed not to be saying very much because they are fundamentally misguided or else rooted in the past.'

It strikes us as a little surprising that a discipline that prides itself on 'advocacy of the oppressed' has, perhaps more so in our past, sometimes little to say in the face of sweeping changes, massive policy 'U' turns and 'developments' that threaten the nature of P/MH nursing itself. Further, although not strictly a finding from an empirical study, it has been suggested (Tilley 1997, Cutcliffe & Hannigan 2001, Ward 2005) that one of the defining characteristics of P/MH nurses is their willingness to speak out, to make arguments and (where appropriate) to challenge the 'status quo'. Accordingly, as editors, we join with others (e.g. Rolfe 2000, Clarke 2001, Barker & Buchanan-Barker 2005) in urging more P/MH nurses to enter into debate and live up to the defining characteristics.

Polemic, orthodoxies and hegemonies

These defining characteristics are something to be proud of. It is worth taking a moment to consider where we would be if it were not for some people – then considered heretics and now regarded as 'visionaries' – who were willing to challenge the dominant orthodoxies and hegemonies of their time. Imagine where we would be if Copernicus and Galileo had not challenged the hegemony espoused by the ecclesiastical authority of a geocentric solar system and in place suggested a heliocentric system. Similarly, imagine where we would be if Columbus had not challenged the then hegemony of a 'flat earth' and insisted on his odyssey to the 'far east'. However, should P/MH nurses collectively become complacent and cease from constructing polemic, and desist from challenging contemporary orthodoxies and hegemonies in our discipline, let us take a brief saunter 'down memory lane'. One of the editors has written previously that:

'Developments that were espoused to be evidence of progress in mental health care include: wide scale and long term prescription of phenothiazine medication; the creation and introduction of minor tranquillisers such as diazepam; "aversion therapy" to "treat" homosexuals; and preventing parents from staying with their hospitalised children. Yet, with hindsight we can see that each of these developments appears to have resulted in more harm than good for clients (and nurses). Long term use of relatively high doses of some phenothiazines has not only caused people to endure years of severely debilitating side effects, but caused some individuals to become so severely handicapped by these side effects that they are now registered disabled, and in some cases seeking compensation from the prescribers. The widespread use of minor tranquillisers brought about some short term relief and then created a far greater problem than it was meant to remedy; some clients reporting more severe symptoms than they experienced prior to taking the

medication, this is in addition to the issue of creating widespread dependency (Neal 1992). With the benefits of hindsight, "aversion therapy" can be seen for what it was, the abuse of a then marginalised group in society (Platzer & Sandford 1998). Also, the psychological harm that was caused to children as a result of forced separation from their parents during hospitalisation is now, fortunately, consigned to history.'

(Cutcliffe 2002, p 374)

Thus, as a discipline, we need but look around us to see the current 'panacea', the latest mental health care policy directive, the contemporary orthodoxy driving 'care' of the person with mental health problems, and each of these should be scrutinised, critiqued and subsequently debated. If this brief saunter down memory lane tells us anything, it is that, when faced with possible change, the absence of debate does not lead to prudent decisions, advances in mental health care or positive outcomes for people with mental health problems. Accepting this argument, it is worth considering why some people eschew debate.

Some of the miscomprehensions and misconceptions of debate

In his thoughtful and insightful 2000 paper, Rolfe identified five reasons why many P/MH nurses do not engage in formal, written debate. These were summarised as: the authority of the text, the threat of critique, the restrictions of form and content, the conventions of critique and perception of the time lag in getting published. Each of these reasons has 'spontaneous validity' for the editors, but we believe the list is incomplete. As an addendum to Rolfe's list we offer the following (and hope other authors will add more).

Debate and critique are confused with personal attack

We suspect that some aspirant debators will have experienced cutting and defamatory remarks masquerading as review or critique comments, just as we have. Therefore, we would empathise with potential debators who are discouraged by the thought of receiving such comments. Further we would (if somewhat arrogantly) like to remind reviewers, commentators and debators that each of these activities offers an opportunity for learning and development, and they should not be taken as a chance for personal attack, carping or 'getting even'. Engaging in debate is not to provide an opportunity for 'pay back' or revenge; one can be passionate without being personal!

Debate is analogous to dissent

Debate and disagreement are sometimes, mistakenly, assumed to mean the same as dissent. This is a problematic and inaccurate transposition.

Although the meanings of the words have some similarity, a closer examination of these meanings illustrates critically important differences, particularly in the connotations that the words have. Dissent has been associated with giving rise to discord – and discord means strife, lack of harmony and has obvious negative connotations. In addition to the meanings we have previously presented on pages 2–3, it is worth noting that debate has synonyms such as consider, deliberate, reflect, cogitate (Oxford English Thesaurus 1991), all of which lack the negative connotations of dissent. Thus, to engage in debate is not necessarily to practise dissent: debate is facilitative and constructive, whereas dissent is disabling and destructive.

Debating is procrastinating

Though similar to other misconceptions and myths we have described, this is slightly different in that it is often seen by those junior to an individual as a way of delaying decision-making, and to a certain degree being weak and without courage. There is a possibility that within a leadership scenario this may actually be the case, but in reality accurate decision-making demands a clear understanding of a situation, its motives, outcomes and implications, and this can often best be achieved by debating – albeit sometimes debating with oneself – the nature of the problem in hand. Failure to communicate these activities to others can certainly result in misunderstandings, but all too often others are wary of anything that might suggest a difference of opinion. Decisions are the result of discussion (or debate) which in themselves are located within a social setting, and represent the nature of the culture in which they function. As the famous pioneer, anthropologist and psychiatrist W H R Rivers (1922) once suggested, culture does not evolve, it diffuses, and similarly debated outcomes grow from their source. Debating, even with oneself, is a far better way of making decisions than simply doing what others would like you to do. It just takes longer!

Debate indicates indecisiveness and thus a weaker, lesser discipline. It indicates that you are less sure, less certain, and that is something to be avoided. A willingness to hear other opinions perhaps indicates a lack of conviction on your own

For some, these statements will have some spontaneous validity and meaning. Further, it is not difficult to locate examples of this view within recent history. Drawing on the domain of politics to provide compelling examples, we draw attention to the early 1980s political scene in Britain and the post-September 11 scene in the USA. Many political commentators bemoaned the loss of 'government by cabinet' following the Margaret Thatcher government of the early 1980s. It is recorded that debate was regarded as dissent; that the cabinet had to present (invent?) a public perception of harmony, agreement and unanimity throughout the entire cabinet (and entire party for that matter). Then, following the tragic and nefarious attacks on September 11, an unfortunate product of this disaster was the quelling of any 'anti-government' sentiment or expression. Indeed, opinions expressed that were contrary to the government-endorsed position resulted in people being branded as 'unpatriotic' (for an excellent commentary on these matters, see Vidal 2002). The irony of the United States' 1st amendment notwithstanding, and leaving aside the legacy of this encroachment still enacted in the Patriot Act, it is reasonable to suggest that such developments did little to encourage debate.

We return to the question: does engaging in debate, hearing another's opinion (and evidence), mean that we have less certainty and, subsequently, less conviction of our own views? We sincerely hope so!

As we become more experienced and seasoned as academics, the one thing we are more and more certain of (paradoxically) is how uncertain most matters are and how uncertain we are. The one thing we are certain of is how uncertain most things are. The more we learn and know, the more aware we are of how much we don't know – how much more there is to know – and this leads, logically, to a position of uncertainty. We wish to remain open to new findings, alternative views and, above all, to avoid the arrogance of (misplaced and premature) certainty. Before we draw this chapter to a close, it is worth having one more reminder of what happens when we become certain.

The state of the 'science': the misplaced confidence at the end of the 19th century

If we can draw on the state of the science in a related field (physics) as a means to urge a moment of pause before making the same epistemological mistakes in nursing science, we would like to take the reader back to the end of the 19th century. During such times, the scientific academe was content, believing that the study of physics was nearly completed: all of the big questions had been answered and there were no more key discoveries to unearth. The quantum physicist Alistair Rae (1994) summarises the somewhat premature and misplaced epistemological confidence when he points out that the scientific academe of this time believed that the basic fundamental principles governing the behaviour of the physical universe were known.

Crichton (1999) illustrates that, despite the discovery of a few hitherto unexplained phenomena (for instance, Roentgen's discovery of rays that could pass through flesh, Becquerel's accidental finding that something released from uranium ore interfered with photographic plates and, not least, the detection of the electron in 1897), the academe remained calm and assured of their convictions. Such new phenomena would, no doubt, be explained by existing theory (Feynman 1965). The relationship between scientists and the phenomena they study, it seems, appears to be one personified by irony. No sooner are such grand claims made than 'nature' reveals the next layer of her secrets and the epistemological overconfidence is shown as arrogant and misguided. Within five years of these discoveries, this complacent view of the world was completely overturned. Crichton (1999, p ix) states that the established sense of certainty was dashed and this produced:

'. . . an entirely new conception of the universe and entirely new technologies that would transform daily life in the twentieth century in unimaginable ways.'

The problem with certainty

Just imagine some of the immense discoveries and achievements that have occurred during the last century. We have travelled to and returned from the moon (and have now, by and large, lost interest in this – amazing!), created the ability (and weapons) to completely destroy our planet, broken the sound barrier and passed the very limits of our solar system (the helio-pause). At the opposite end of the 'scale' continuum, we now have the ability to view individual atoms, to look inside a person's brain and watch organic processes as they occur (e.g. positron emission tomography), have created the technology to communicate with someone on the other side of the world – almost instantaneously – by means of devices that are smaller than a postage stamp. As Crichton (1999) points out, if you had made any of these claims to a physicist at the end of the 19th century, you would have been declared 'mad'. These discoveries, developments and technologies were not even predicted because the then hegemonic certainty within scientific theory viewed such 'nonsense' as impossible.

This sense of certainty exists for some in P/MH nursing. Dr Liam Clarke (1999) highlighted how such people believe they have the answers to most of the big questions in P/MH nursing (and health care for that matter). They believe the physical sciences offer up the answers or are on the cusp of solving whatever remains. For others (the editors included) the searching for the answers in P/MH nursing (and health care) has only just begun. Currently, we stand on the brink of the latest wave of discoveries that will move care of the mental health person, for some, beyond any 'reasonable doubt' into the 'Shangri-La' of certainty. Brain imaging, selective serotonin reuptake inhibitors, the so-called 'new antipsychotics', the isolation of genes 'responsible' for mental health problems – each makes its own contribution to the pervasive sense of certainty. If these discoveries can indeed relieve suffering, improve lives, inspire hope, add meaning, help with recovery or even cure, we will be among the first applauding. But let's remember the danger of certainty; let's not repeat the mistakes of our 19th century physics colleagues and, especially, let's not minimise the value of debate in face of this pervasive and perpetual search for certainty.

Accordingly, it behoves each one of us to face up to the need to navigate our way through the various positions – to critique, debate and question these in order to find our own views; to align ourselves with evidence-based positions (in whatever form this evidence takes – the sense of irony arising from the protracted debate concerning the nature of evidence is not lost on the editors), and thus be in the best position possible to provide the best care possible for the clients we work alongside; to be in the most informed positions possible for our students and less experienced colleagues we work with; and to construct reasoned, cogent arguments for when we act in the full role of P/MH.

We look forward to debating the issues raised in this book and many more (hopefully) with you in the future.

Acknowledgements

Part of this chapter has been reproduced from Cutcliffe (2005), with the kind permission of Blackwell Science.

References

Barker P, Buchanan-Barker P 2005 Still invisible after all these years: mental health nursing on the margins. Journal of Psychiatric and Mental Health Nursing 12:252–256.

Biley A, Whale Z 1996 Feminist approaches to change and nursing development. Journal of Clinical Nursing 5:159–163.

Clarke L 1999 Commentary to 'The last wave? Promoting growth and development in community psychiatric and mental health nursing'. In: Barker P 1999 The philosophy and practice of psychiatric nursing. Churchill Livingstone, Edinburgh, p 75–76.

Clarke L 2001 Doubts and certainties in the nursing profession: a commentary. Journal of Psychiatric and Mental Health Nursing 8:465–469.

Crichton M 1999 Timeline. Random House, New York.

Cutcliffe J R 2002 The beguiling effects of nurse prescribing in mental health nursing: re-examining the debate. Journal of Psychiatric and Mental Health Nursing 9(3):369–375.

Cutcliffe J R 2005 A few comments on the Commentary Section: editorial guidance for authors. Journal of Psychiatric and Mental Health Nursing 10:502–505

Cutcliffe J R, Goward P 2000 Mental health nurses and qualitative research methods: a mutual attraction? Journal of Advanced Nursing 31(3):590–598.

Cutcliffe J R, Hannigan B 2001 Mass media, monsters and mental health: a need for increased lobbying. Journal of Psychiatric and Mental Health Nursing 8(4):315–322.

Cutcliffe J R, Jackson A, Ward M F, Cannon B, Titchen A 1998 Practice development in mental health nursing. Mental Health Practice 2(4):27–31.

Feynman R 1965 The character of physical law. MIT Press, Cambridge.

Huber R B 1964 Influencing through argument. David McKay, New York.

Kitson A, Ahmed L A, Harvey G, Seers K, Thompson D R 1996 From research to practice: one organizational method for promoting research based practice. Journal of Advanced Nursing 23:430–440.

Lewin K 1951 Field theory in social science. Harper Row, New York.

Neal M J 1992 Medical pharmacology at a glance, 2nd edn. Blackwell Science, Oxford.

Oxford Concise English Dictionary 1991 Oxford University Press, Oxford.

Oxford English Thesaurus 1991 Oxford University Press, Oxford.

Platzer H, Sandford T 1998 A shocking legacy. Mental Health Practice 1(5):6–7.

Rae A 1994 Quantum physics: illusion or reality? Cambridge University Press, Cambridge.

Rivers W H R 1922 History of ethnology: helps for students of history, no. 48. Society for Promoting Christian Knowledge. Macmillan, New York.

Rolfe G 2000 Write now! Journal of Psychiatric and Mental Health Nursing 7:469–470.

Tilley S 1997 Conclusion. In: Tilley S, ed. The mental health nurse: views of practice and education. Blackwell Science, London, p 203–210.

UKCC 1998 Guidelines for mental health and learning disabilities nursing. United Kingdom Central Council for Nursing and Midwifery, London.

Vidal G 2002 Dreaming war: blood for oil and the Cheney–Bush junta. Thunders Mouth Press, New York.

Ward M 2005 Clinical governance and nurse leadership. In: James A, Worroll A, Kendall T, eds. Clinical governance in mental health and learning disability services. Gaskill & Royal College of Psychiatrists, London, Ch 20 p 297–308.

Ward M, Titchen A, Morell C, McCormack B, Kitson B 1998 Using a supervisory framework to support and evaluate a multi project practice development programme. Journal of Clinical Nursing 7:29–36.

"

What's in a name? Are we 'psychiatric' or 'mental health' nurses?

CHAPTER 2

The case for 'psychiatric' nurses

Phyllis du Mont

CHAPTER 3

The case for 'mental health' nurses

Mary Chambers

Commentary

John Collins

"

Editorial

On the face of it this might seem like the least consequential of all the debates within this book. After all, most psychiatric/mental health (P/MH) nurses know what they do, and whether they are called one thing or another does not really matter to them. However, if that is true, why do there appear to be two separate groups of nurses who, while apparently carrying out the same clinical actions, prefix their nursing denomination with a completely different title? Is this merely sociolinguistics or is there a more significant reason for this situation?

Certainly the assumption that all P/MH nurses do the same job is patently false, and when one considers the huge breadth of clinical and other responsibilities contained in the discipline this is hardly surprising. Additionally, there seems to be a divide in different parts of the world, with nurses in the USA adopting the *psychiatric* form and the UK the *mental health* one (and this applies right across the board from Australia and New Zealand, up through Japan, across Asia and the Middle East, through Europe and over the Atlantic to Northern as well as Southern America – in each nation it is either *mental health* or *psychiatric* nursing). The titles of the respective P/MH nursing research journals of those different countries also reflect this trend. The situation is so confusing outside our discipline that, on more than one occasion, the Editors have heard people refer to *psychiatric* and *mental health* nurses as being two separate disciplines, with patients in particular presupposing that they are seeing one or the other (but not both).

There is, of course, an historical influence. Brimblecombe (2005) described the work of the attendant/nurse in the late Victorian era in a hospital near London. What was interesting was that he showed how the medical superintendents (who ran the hospitals and controlled every aspect of the treatment process) were later called psychiatrists, while the male attendants were later addressed as psychiatric nurses. By association, the relative nursing speciality was titled in accordance with the discipline to which the nurses had total accountability.

This remained the case right up till the mid-1980s, when the term *mental health* (as opposed to mental illness) began to be used in relation to care services (thus apparently reducing the stigma associated with the word psychiatry). By association nurses began to be addressed as *mental health* nurses. It could, therefore, be argued that the only reason why UK based P/MH nurses in particular have the title they do is because they have been given it by someone else! And, just to complicate matters further, if they were trained in the period leading up to the nurse education reforms of the 1990s they would have received the official qualification of 'registered mental nurse', even though they were referred to as psychiatric nurses! Confused? You should be. We wonder how the comparable names have developed in other countries. The question is whether or not the two titles imply the same clinical roles and responsibilities or if they relate to two clearly distinct specialities, one having more to do with the observation and assessment of care processes (*psychiatric*) and the other taking a leading role in interventionist activities and thus promoting health (*mental health*). Most probably, nurses will inevitably cling to their chosen disciplinary denomination irrespective of what their governing bodies decree, but the real issue is whether or not their job title describes the job they do. Is there any justification for changing from a *psychiatric* to a *mental health* nurse, and, significantly, can you be both? This is, therefore, the right debate to lead with in this book and in many ways sets the scene for what follows.

Reference

Brimblecombe N 2005 Asylum nursing in the UK at the end of the Victorian era: Hill End Asylum. Journal of Psychiatric and Mental Health Nursing 12(1):57–63.

Phyllis du Mont

The case for 'psychiatric' nurses

Introduction

Are we psychiatric nurses? Or is it important that we be known as psychiatric/mental health (P/MH) nurses? The name of our speciality is intimately tied to philosophical debates about our ontology and to scientific advances in our understanding of psychiatric disorders. Moreover, it is obvious, but critical, to note that all this takes place in a particular social and historical context. It is my contention that the term 'psychiatric mental health nursing' is deeply redundant and inadvertently connotes the existence of a mind–body dichotomy. The science of *nursing* inherently encompasses health promotion and the prevention of illness (both disease and suffering). The promotion of mental health is integral to, and inseparable from, the promotion of health.

Although it may seem so self-evident as to be trivial to observe, nursing rejects the Cartesian mind–body separation. We cannot claim to have successfully articulated a coherent synthesis of the inevitably subjective experience of the mind with the objective third person observations of behaviour and physiology. However, the essential nature of the person as an irreducible whole, continuously interacting with the environment, is a core assumption of nursing. Nurses who have a particular interest in the assessment and treatment of individuals suffering from thought disorders, impulse control disorders and dys-regulation of mood can best be described as specialising in the care of patients with psychiatric disorders. Therefore, the most appropriate name for our field of interest and area of expertise is psychiatric nursing.

Our discipline is in the midst of what could be termed a multilevel identity crisis. The titles that we have become accustomed to may no longer serve us well. For instance, in the USA controversy continues regarding the most appropriate title and role boundaries for the advanced practice nurses who care for individuals experiencing, or at risk for, mental illness. Although many clinical nurse specialists (CNSs) in P/MH nursing have chosen to limit their practice to psychotherapy, most state nurse practice acts now permit the CNS to obtain prescriptive privileges. Since 1999, nurses have another pathway to advanced education and certification in the care of persons with psychiatric disorders. A nurse can now choose to seek education and certification as a psychiatric nurse practitioner (NP). In theory, the CNS role emphasises psychotherapeutic modalities, case management and consultation, whereas the newly formalized NP role emphasises diagnostic evaluation, brief focused therapies and psychopharmacological interventions. However, in practice, there may be significant overlap and blurred boundaries between these roles. This lack of a clear difference has prompted some nurses to call for the merger of the CNS/NP role. Conversely, other nurses have vehemently supported the preservation of both options.

Even more fundamental is the question of how to describe our speciality practice. There is a certain appeal to the simpler, shorter term: psychiatric nurse. But the term psychiatric/mental health nurse originally came from a conscious decision to emphasise the expansion of the practice of psychiatric nursing to include both inpatient and community-based care. As we sought to establish the unique contribution of nursing within a crowded field of mental health disciplines, inclusion of the term 'mental health' was thought to signify the unique nursing emphasis on health promotion and disease prevention. This health promotion role was an addition to the earlier, singular emphasis on the treatment of mental illness.

Today, it is quite common to see the terms 'psychiatric nursing' and 'psychiatric/mental health nursing' used interchangeably, even by the same author within the same article. Is this distinction a stylistic matter or a substantive issue? As the precise use of language is a hallmark of science and of the professions, developing an answer to this question deserves our attention. To avoid confusing our colleagues and clients, we should attempt to reach a consensus about our name.

Each nurse may have a personal preference about what to call our speciality. This preference may be based on habit, familiarity, tradition or even idiosyncratic word associations. In order to arrive at a considered and logical conclusion about the best words to describe ourselves, it would first be useful to consider the historical evolution of nursing and our speciality. Additionally, it is important to speculate carefully about the future of the profession and consider whether our name is consistent with that vision.

Locating ourselves in our history

For more than 100 years, the nursing discipline has played a significant role in the care and treatment of individuals with psychiatric problems. As early as 1882 in the USA, nurses could seek formal instruction to care for the mentally ill in a specialised school of nursing at McLean Psychiatric Asylum in Massachusetts. Linda Richards, the first trained nurse in the USA, spent much of her career (at the turn of the 20th century) educating nurses to work with the mentally ill. She stated: *'It stands to reason that the mentally sick should be at least as well cared for as the physically sick'* (Doone 1984, p 51). By 1946, when the National Institute of Mental Health (NIMH) was created, psychiatric nursing was recognised as one of four core disciplines involved in the direct treatment of persons with mental illness (along with social work, psychology and psychiatry).

In the mid 20th century, federal support stimulated the development of graduate level psychiatric nursing programmes. At Rutgers, one of five original programmes, Hildegard Peplau created an enduring model for advanced practice nursing. Heavily influenced by interpersonal psychology, Peplau hypothesised that psychiatric problems represent an arrest in ego development that leaves the person unable to deal with the anxieties of interpersonal relationships and the developmental tasks of life. According to this view, healthy development of the personality is fostered by age-appropriate interpersonal relationships (both within the family and with peers). Disruptions in interpersonal relationships produce psychopathology. Therapeutic change was assumed to occur as a result of enhanced developmental growth (Peplau 1989). Peplau (1952) proposed that the nursing intervention to achieve such change is psychotherapeutic interpersonal interaction, sometimes called the 'corrective experience' (Yuen 1986, Beeber 1989, Peplau 1992). The pivotal nature of the nurse–client relationship remains a key tenet of psychosocial nursing today.

Although it is clear that the psychiatric clinical nurse specialist (CNS) role evolved out of those early graduate programmes, no consensus as to name or title accompanied the change in role (from staff nurse to nurse psychotherapist). Many factors contributed to this state of affairs, but fear that psychiatrists would oppose the new role was an important constraint. In fact, reading the recollections of Peplau, it is very clear that nurses interested in acquiring advanced psychotherapeutic skills felt the need to avoid coming to the attention of organised psychiatry. Peplau said: *'My interest was not to make so many waves that we would get enormous resistance ... it would be better to sort of play this subtle game of calling it something that wouldn't raise any hackles'* (Spray 1999, p 28). Because of this constraint, nurses tended to minimise the extent to which their graduate education focused on the acquisition and use of advanced psychotherapeutic techniques. That which is not named loses visibility, and during this era the invisibility of the nature of the advanced practice role was an advantage for survival.

At the same time, the entire system of care for the management of psychiatric problems was coming under intense scrutiny. With few somatic treatments of clear effectiveness, the institutionalization of the chronically and severely mentally ill person seldom produced any clear-cut individual benefit. Conditions were often dehumanising. It was not difficult to conclude that these institutions continued to exist not because of the good that they achieved for individual patients, but instead because they protected society from the distress and inconvenience of dealing with troubled or eccentric people.

The anti-establishment sentiments that flourished during the Vietnam War era led to a critical re-examination of many social institutions. By the early sixties, critical analysis of the mental health care system had already begun to fuel a movement rejecting traditional psychiatry. R D Laing (1960), who espoused an existential humanistic view, and Thomas Szasz (1962), who emphasised the oppressed social status of psychiatric patients, were major figures in the emergence of the antipsychiatry movement. Mainstream psychiatry was characterised as a mechanism for social control, and the very existence of mental illness was questioned. Instead, it was postulated that the fault lay in rigid societal norms that demanded conformity and the preservation of the status quo. In academia, nurses participated in these scholarly debates; however, in a very real way, staff nurses and nursing attendants remained responsible for implementing the treatment plans devised by psychiatry. The adoption of the person-centred psychology of Carl Rogers (1961) allowed nursing to claim to offer a less coercive, less paternalistic mode of treatment than psychiatry. But as Hopton (1997) has observed, there are obvious and unaddressed ironies inherent in the claim to practise person-centred psychology within a mental health system that routinely accepted involuntary confinement and forced medication as appropriate responses to mental distress.

At that time, somatic treatments under the auspices of psychiatry rarely led to the remission of disease or the relief of suffering. The available psychopharmacological agents had limited efficacy and were frequently associated with intolerable adverse effects. The use of high-dose neuroleptic medications was the norm. These agents potentially reduced the disruptive and intrusive behavioural manifestations of severe mental illness. This docility was achieved at the cost of new learning and the burden of stigmatising movement disorders. The results of the indiscriminate application of electroconvulsive therapy (ECT) and primitive psychosurgical techniques revolted many observers. The mechanism of action for psychotropic drugs, ECT and/or psychosurgery was unexplained. Theoretical models of the mind in psychiatry and in allied mental health disciplines offered psychodynamic and interpersonal explanations for the aetiology of mental disorders. Psychiatric nurses, social workers, and psychologists all began to suggest that the treatment of mental illness needed to come out of the 'house of medicine'. Indeed, some psychiatrists also endorsed this view. In this context, psychosocial interventions were perceived as humane, respectful and far more congruent with the caring ethos of nursing.

At the undergraduate level, psychosocial skills and considerations remained a key focus of nursing, with the graduate education of P/MH nurses targeting attainment of the knowledge and skills needed in psychotherapy. Nurses pursued training and supervision in a dizzying array of choices from the diverse universe of psychotherapeutic modalities. Clinical nurse specialists became psychoanalysts, marriage counsellors, hypnotists, psychotherapists, behavioural therapists, and group therapists, among many other sets of training and designations. Most of these clinicians still considered themselves to be nurses, but clearly the daily practice of these providers often had more in common with social workers, counsellors and psychologists.

Increasingly, pathophysiology was considered irrelevant to the practice of P/MH nursing. Many P/MH nursing programmes did not require graduate level pathophysiology, physical assessment or pharmacology coursework. This emphasis on psychosocial skills and knowledge significantly weakened nursing's claims to a holistic or even biopsychosocial perspective. Accordingly, it became more difficult to articulate the unique domain of P/MH nursing among the core mental health disciplines. In addition to the critical assessment of the mental health care delivery system by academia, patient and family advocates embarked upon a campaign for reform. Confinement to a psychiatric facility began to be conceptualised as a potential violation of the patient's autonomy. This new respect for patient autonomy supplanted the paternalistic viewpoint that 'professionals always know best' in the process of deciding among treatment options. It became commonplace to assert that psychiatric patients have a fundamental right to receive treatment in the least restrictive environment. This trend, coupled with the widespread use of major tranquillizers (which decreased disruptive behaviours) allowed the community mental health centre model of care to emerge.

It can be seen that changes in the role and preparation of the P/MH nurse occurred in the context of a rapidly changing system for the provision of services. Large state psychiatric hospitals drastically cut the number of inpatient beds. Graduates of the federally funded masters programmes found employment in the newly mandated community mental health centres. As these nurses left the 'house of medicine' there was a desire to distance themselves from the stagnation and hopelessness perceived to exist within mainstream psychiatry. As a result, the term psychiatric nursing seemed an inadequate description of the speciality. Furthermore, the word 'psychiatric' could be seen as a borrowed word representing a borrowed knowledge base. In order to emphasise that their unique domain also encompassed the prevention of mental illness and the promotion of mental health, psychiatric nurses added the term 'mental health'. Thus, the accepted title became 'psychiatric/mental health nursing'. Although this is a somewhat awkward constellation of words, it was deliberately chosen to serve this purpose. The promise of the community mental health centre model was never fully realised. Politically, there was a failure to recognise that full implementation of this model would require significant funding. Advocates of patient autonomy had genuinely altruistic goals but little understanding of the profound ways in which mental illness can limit the individual's ability to create safe living arrangements. The high incidence of mental illness among the homeless and imprisoned is a continued legacy of deinstitutionalization.

The emergence of the 'brain'

With the advantage of hindsight, we now know what could not have been anticipated during the seventies and eighties. Neuropsychiatric research was poised to achieve unprecedented advances. It is only in the very recent past that so much scientific knowledge about cellular and molecular biology has come about. In a recent third edition of his textbook on cell and molecular biology, Gerald Karp (2000) listed the Nobel prizes awarded for research in cell and molecular biology since 1958. The award for discovering the primary structure of proteins was given only in 1958; the prize for discovering the ionic basis of nerve membrane potentials in 1963; for discovering the structure and function of the internal components of cells in 1974; and the prize for elucidating the factors that affect nerve growth in 1986; for the discovery and function of GTP-binding (G) proteins in 1994; for clarification of the Na^+/K^+-ATPase mechanism of ATP synthesis in 1997; and the award for the understanding of synaptic transmission and signal transduction was given in 2000. Although we had some limited empirical evidence to support the use of psychotropic drugs at the midpoint of the last century, our knowledge base and understanding of their basic functions is a new and evolving field.

The psychiatry of the last century could be termed 'brainless' in so much as it focused exclusively on matters of the mind. Conversely, there is concern that the psychiatry of this century risks becoming 'mindless' if it overemphasises biology at the cost of failing to consider psychosocial influences. Psychiatric nursing science is not synonymous with psychiatry (and it should be observed that psychiatry is not synonymous with molecular neurophysiology). There are shared domains of interest and an intertwined development and history. Moreover, both disciplines have had to integrate the breakthroughs of the neuroscience knowledge explosion with the day to day tasks of diagnosing and treating individuals experiencing mental distress.

Some neuropsychiatric breakthroughs have had an incredibly rapid impact on the ways in which individuals receive treatment for mental distress. The development of selective serotonin reuptake inhibitors (SSRIs) precipitated profound changes in the delivery of mental health services. The health care delivery system is still reacting to the implications of these changes, and it is impossible at this juncture to foresee the ultimate and largely unintended consequences these medications have wrought. It is critical for the future of psychiatric nursing that we consider their impact.

Primary care providers (PCPs) had never been comfortable treating thought disorders, and the management of antipsychotic medications was certainly something that most PCPs would not assume. Prior to the advent of SSRIs, the medication choices for the treatment of depression were relatively effective, but for a variety of reasons had poor patient acceptance. The anticholinergic and histaminic side-effects associated with tricyclic antidepressants (TCAs) were problematic. Dry mouth, orthostatic symptoms, drowsiness, and perhaps most burdensome, weight gain were commonly experienced. Providers had other concerns. Although psychiatrists routinely used the medications at effective doses, this knowledge did not seem to be widely appreciated by PCPs. Surveys of PCPs revealed that they routinely prescribed subtherapeutic doses. Thus, although the TCAs had the potential to be effective, the many patients suffering from depression who sought treatment in primary care did not receive enough medication for relief of symptoms. The reticence of PCPs to utilise effective dosing schedules may have been related to the fact that the medications were well known to be very dangerous in overdose. The other class of effective antidepressants, the monoamine oxidase inhibitors (MAOIs), have hazardous interactions with foods, drinks, and other drugs. Many PCPs would not consider managing the complexities of these potentially deleterious interactions. Furthermore, the rather indiscriminate use of benzodiazepines without full appreciation of their potential for abuse had convinced many PCPs that psychotropic medications were a rather *last resort* intervention best handled by someone else, namely psychiatrists.

When SSRIs were first introduced, many PCPs found that patient acceptance of this approach was high. In fact, as the lay press picked up on the perceived benefits of the medication, many providers found themselves fielding patient inquiries about the medication. Not unexpectedly, the drug companies supported primary care physician education efforts regarding the potential benefits of the drug as well as its ease of prescribing. As the drug became an accepted tool for treating depression in primary care, an unforeseen consequence arose. That is, primary care nurse practitioners with prescriptive privileges began to treat many clients suffering from depressive disorders. So, at the moment when psychopharmacological treatment of depression became a favoured treatment for depression, it was our primary care nurse colleagues who were most often called upon to give it. Most clinical nurse specialists in psychiatric mental health nursing had become highly skilled in psychodynamic talk therapies, and had not sought expertise in psychopharmacology, a modality some saw as often ineffective and potentially harmful. However, a re-evaluation would become necessary as additional psychoactive drugs became available and the explosion of neuropsychiatric discoveries continued.

Who will treat persons suffering from mental distress? Within nursing, these changes led to many such persons being treated in their primary care practice by primary care physicians and nurse practitioners. However, these individuals are unable to combine psychopharmacological treatment with psychotherapy. And although it is true that in many areas there are few providers who could see patients for appropriate adjunctive psychotherapy, another issue can be raised. Does the patient expectation that a *pill* should be sufficient increase the barrier and perhaps even the stigma associated with entering into psychotherapy? In the mind of the lay public (and even PCPs), if a patient fails to respond adequately to a pharmacological approach does that mean that they are *sicker*? Should a patient who is reluctant to take medication be regarded as 'more difficult'? Although this change has increased patient access to pharmacological treatments, it may tend to decrease access to non-pharmacological treatments.

Some have expressed concern that there has been a subtle devaluing of our speciality since more easily prescribed treatments have become available. It is extremely important to note that even the best statistics on patient response to medication must concede that a sizeable subset of patients do not respond, and that many respond but do not attain remission (Stahl 2000). As a speciality within our discipline, we need to respond to these concerns.

In response, P/MH nurse clinicians began to try and acquire knowledge and skills regarding the prescription of psychotropic drugs. It seemed absurd that fellow nurses with far less understanding of the Diagnostic and Statistical Manual of Mental Disorders (DSM) criteria and psychiatric assessment and care would enter this arena and we would not. As new nurses (disconcertingly few) entered the speciality area at the advanced practice level, and as established nurse specialists worked to integrate this knowledge into their practice, it became clear that perhaps we had 'thrown out the baby with the bath water' when we moved so completely away from psychiatry and our physiological foundations. People are, after all, embedded inseparably in a body. Although there has been controversy and fear regarding the changes, many psychiatric nurses accept the need for change. Most states in the USA now have some provision for qualified psychiatric nurses to seek prescriptive privileges. Nurses who choose not to do so will still play an important role in the provision of services and in shaping our research and education. But the future of the nursing role in the treatment of individuals suffering from psychiatric disorders depends upon integration of the physiological with the psychological. There is really nothing new in that statement, but reiterating it lays the foundation for my assertion that we would be best served by calling ourselves *'psychiatric nurses'*.

If we believe that nursing has at its core a commitment to health promotion and disease prevention, then there is no need to state that we are in the business of mental health. As nurses who choose to work with individuals suffering from mental distress and mental disorders, what else could we propose to do? If we believe that mental distress is a manifestation of the unique biological individual inextricably situated in a particular environment, we cannot avoid the need for expertise in both somatic and psychosocial assessments and interventions. The word *'psychiatric'* is widely recognised as encompassing the domain and range of client problems we wish to address. Psychiatric nursing is a succinct, clear and appropriate term for our speciality and will serve us well.

References

Beeber L S 1989 Enacting corrective interpersonal experiences with the depressed client: an intervention model. Archives of Psychiatric Nursing 3(4):211–217.

Doone M E 1984 At least as well cared for . . . Linda Richards and the mentally ill. Image Journal of Nursing Scholarship 16(2):51–56.

Hopton J 1997 Towards a critical theory of mental health nursing. Journal of Advanced Nursing 25(3):1365–1378.

Karp G C 2000 Cell and molecular biology: concepts and experiments, 3rd edn. John Wiley, Chichester.

Laing R D 1960 The divided self. Tavistock Press, London.

Peplau H E 1952 Interpersonal relations in nursing. Putnum, New York.

Peplau H E 1989 Tools and tasks outline. In: O'Toole A W, Welt S R, eds. Interpersonal theory in nursing practice: selected works of Hildegard E. Peplau. Springer, New York, p 31–41.

Peplau H E 1992 Interpersonal relations: a theoretical framework for application in nursing practice. Nursing Science Quarterly 5(1):13–18.

Rogers C 1961 On becoming a person. Houghton Mifflin, Boston.

Spray S L 1999 The evolution of the psychiatric mental health clinical specialist: an interview with Hildegard E. Peplau. Perspectives in Psychiatric Care 35(3):27–29.

Stahl S 2000 Essential psychopharmacology: neuroscientific basis and clinical applications, 2nd edn. Cambridge University Press, Cambridge.

Szasz T 1962 The myth of mental illness. Secker & Warburg, London.

Yuen F K 1986 The nurse–client relationship: a mutual learning experience. Journal of Advanced Nursing 11(5):529–533.

Mary Chambers

The case for 'mental health' nurses

Introduction

When asked to write this chapter I considered it to be both an honour and a challenge. Having the opportunity to explore the difference/s (if any) between psychiatric and mental health nursing was exciting. To do so as part of a text concentrating on other key debates within nursing and health care was a great opportunity, allowing me to explore some of the key issues surrounding psychiatric/mental health nursing, and my long association with nursing allows me to bring a reflective and critical approach to the debate.

There was an appeal about having the chance to determine, (unequivocally, if possible) that a difference did exist between the roles and functions of the psychiatric nurse and those of the mental health nurse. I was reasonably confident that it would be possible to show a clear distinction between the core values and principles of each. Additionally, I was hopeful that contemporary nursing literature would be sufficiently robust in terms of the distinction between psychiatric and mental health nursing to support my viewpoint. Also, I anticipated that 21st century mental health nursing would emerge as being substantially different from that of 20th century psychiatric nursing. Finally, I had hoped that evidence, either robust empirical or anecdotal, would be available to authenticate the change of title from psychiatric nurse to that of mental health nurse. However, on exploring the literature it would seem that there is relatively little discussion around the nature of mental health nursing. Most consideration appears to focus on psychiatric nursing, with some tentative remarks about mental health nursing. There are some exceptions, for example Watkins (2002), but as far as could be ascertained there is limited in-depth exploration of what the difference(s) might be. Ideologically, it would not be unreasonable to assume, given the differentiation in title and consequently orientation (that is, one has a focus on illness, the other on health), that corresponding differences and distinctions would exist regarding roles and functions.

The literature would suggest that the terms psychiatric and/or mental health nursing are often used interchangeably. Which descriptor is used then appears to be a feature (or manifestation) of personal preference rather than any professional directive. Yet individual preference cannot account for all the variation in usage; the choice of descriptor is also influenced by the overarching educational and professional policies. In the UK, for example, the preparation of nurses for working with those experiencing mental illness or mental health problems comes within the mental health branch of the Diploma in Higher Education or Bachelor of Nursing Science programme. Completion of either programme allows the individual to become registered as a mental health nurse. In Canada, however, the four westernmost provinces each have entry level programmes that allow a person to engage on a psychiatric-specific nursing programme and subsequently register as a psychiatric nurse (Cutcliffe 2003a).

Using the terms interchangeably or linking them is not just the preserve of individuals (e.g. *The Journal of Psychiatric and Mental Health Nursing*). This could be perceived as a catch-all, and therefore both professionally and politically correct. Or might it be that in terms of roles and functions there is no actual or perceived difference and that the use of the different titles is merely cosmetic? Or could it be that when combined the words give a more helpful meaning to both professional and user groups?

Alternatively, how confusing must it be for those outside the discipline when concepts of both health and illness are combined in the title of a professional group? This leads to other questions, such as: Do we as P/MH nurses know what our core values, roles and functions are? What is our key orientation and philosophy? Some of this will be discussed later when considering education, training and socialization processes. This chapter will offer a brief overview of the history of P/MH nursing in the UK, followed by discussion of the nature of mental illness and mental health. This will lead to consideration of the perceived roles and functions of the mental health nurse and debate as to the purpose, if any, of changing the name from psychiatric nurse to that of mental health nurse, if practice is no different. Throughout, the discussion elements of a public health agenda and the principles of postmodernism will be used to illustrate particular points.

Given that nursing inevitably involves caring with/for people who access and avail themselves of this service, one should also consider the views of its users. Consequently, important questions emanating from service users might include the following:

- How do users and carers perceive the difference in title in terms of the roles and functions of the nurse?
- Is a title useful with respect to understanding what nurses do?
- What are user and carer expectations and how are they realised?

Of course, the main question would be whether or not those same users and carers actually cared about the prefix to the name of the nurse with whom they were working.

The euphemism of mental health

From examining aspects of the literature it is difficult to determine what the key elements of mental health nursing are. Most of the discussion pertains to psychiatric nursing. For example, in Tilley et al (1997), the title of the text is 'The mental health nurse: views of practice and education', yet some chapters refer only to psychiatric nursing. This same predicament is highlighted by another text, also edited by Tilley et al (2005), entitled 'Psychiatric and mental health nursing; the field of knowledge'. As is evident, the title of this book includes both descriptors. Of this text, it is worth noting the considerable contribution of service users; also that the book is dedicated to the life of Professor Annie Altschul. Annie, who gave so much of herself to psychiatric nursing, categorically refused to accept the title of mental health nurse for a variety of reasons. For example, she claimed that, like most others, she didn't know what mental health meant. With respect to P/MH nursing, nursing interventions are required only when health breaks down. Annie resented the idea that nurses would interfere in her life when she was well. She further resented as a '. . . *taxpayer, training and employing nurses to administer to the healthy when so much suffering should be alleviated'* (Tilley et al 2005, p 13).

Changing circumstances

According to Peplau (1994), throughout its history P/MH nursing has been modified in response to changing circumstances. The desire of some to be known as mental health rather than psychiatric nurses could be considered an example of circumstances driven by a professional, political and social agenda. Peplau parallels the changes in psychiatric nursing with those of psychiatric care in general. She comments on the movement from jails to asylums to mental hospitals. A further stage in the changing circumstances has been the drive towards care in the community.

Similar parallels could be drawn around the changes of term, from attendant to psychiatric nurse to mental health nurse, and their use in this field. However, to wholly accept these parallels (certainly the former, with the implication that mental health nursing and community care were inextricably linked), other changes would need to be obvious. For example, evidence of a significant ideological and societal shift with respect to mental illness and those experiencing it should be apparent. Also, evidence of a change in attitude towards those working with and caring for individuals in mental illness would be required. If stigma were removed, and there was a general acceptance that mental illness was no different from any other illness, then the parallels could be considered as more accurate.

To change the title from psychiatric nurse to mental health nurse requires a more fundamental professional ideological shift than is currently evident. For example, there needs to be a movement away from pathology and medicine to health, lifestyle and health promotion embedded within a humanistic philosophy, grounded in hope and the principles of recovery. Societal change would be necessary with attitudes moving from stigmatization to acceptance and support. Enhanced partnership working across a wider range of professional groups to promote and maintain health would be required. The nature of the relationship between health care professionals and others who help those experiencing mental illness would also need to change.

A brief history of psychiatric nursing in the UK

Many accounts have been given of the development of psychiatric nursing in the UK (see particularly Nolan 1993, Brimblecombe 2005). Having a history suggests something 'worthwhile' and as Nolan (1993) suggests, confirms the legitimacy of the service one provides. All historical accounts begin by describing the position or plight of those experiencing mental illness and how, at least from the 12th century onwards, the asylum was perceived to provide a place of refuge and safety as well as control. During the 17th century there was the beginning of an understanding of the nature and care of those experiencing mental illness and of the status of the asylum, pioneered in France by Pinel and in England by Tuke. Both men wanted changes in the treatment of those experiencing mental illness. In England, Tuke set about revolutionising the system to a more humane regime, founding the Retreat at York in 1792. This change could be considered as the start of the Moral Treatment movement, of which education was an important part.

Those attendants who cared for the mentally ill at York were given limited instruction. However, as far as can be established, this education or training was non-systematic. The first systematic approach to training was conducted in Scotland in the early 1850s and set the trend for others to follow, such as the attendants at the Surrey Lunatic Asylum. It was this training, together with other programmes in similar organisations, that provided the first courses of instruction for attendants, and graduates of these could be considered the first psychiatric nurses.

The first register for attendants was established in 1890, some half-century or more after the introduction of training. The education and training of those who care for the mentally ill, particularly nurses, has been, and continues to be, surrounded by both controversy and criticism, while being frequently subjected to change.

Most authors who have considered the education of those first called attendants and latterly P/MH nurses have commented on the contribution of doctors in general and psychiatrists in particular to that process. It is accepted that in the early years doctors provided instruction for attendants. This set the scene for their continued involvement in the education not only of attendants but also of nurses. This early engagement, together with the 'medicalisation of madness', suggested a legitimate role for medicine, and therefore doctors, in the education of psychiatric nurses.

The nursing discipline allowed, and to some extent promoted, this situation for a number of reasons. First, there were few if any nurses with the appropriate educational background, knowledge and/or skills to be able to make a significant contribution to peer education. Second, medicine was seen as an established profession, perceived as being at the top of the health care hierarchy; therefore its involvement in nurse education was considered not only as essential in terms of knowledge but also as adding a degree of acceptance and scientific value to nursing. Third, the involvement of doctors in the education of nurses could be construed as an attempt at bridging the gap between the two. In reality, such involvement promoted the hierarchical divide, reinforced the position of subservience, did nothing to advance professionalism in nursing and contributed nothing towards removing the stigma associated with mental illness. Today the role of medicine in the education of nurses is greatly diminished and in most universities is nonexistent, at least at undergraduate level. However, the legacy of the hierarchy lives on.

Socialization of mental health nurses

Cutcliffe (2003b) chronicles a number of key reports regarding nurse education and highlights the most significant recommendations emanating from them. Outlined are issues around the nature and content of the curriculum, where P/MH education is best located (including linkage with institutions of higher education), the merits or otherwise of the apprenticeship model, as well as the demarcation between general and psychiatric nursing. Brimblecombe (2005), when considering the role of the asylum attendant/nurse in the Victorian era, quotes Wood (1902), who reported a hospital superintendent as having stated that general-trained nurses described asylum attendant/nurses as 'the scum of the earth'.

In spite of the attitude of 'superiority' of the general nurse over the psychiatric nurse, the initial education and training of psychiatric nurses mirrored that of general nurses. Attempts were made at creating a distinction between the two; for example, the UK government's ministerial review of psychiatric nursing in 1968 suggested that psychiatric nurses should acquire skills in psychotherapy (Norman 2005). Other attempts to widen the demarcation between the two areas included the introduction of aspects of sociology into the 1974 psychiatric nursing syllabus and a greater emphasis placed on interpersonal skills and self awareness in that of 1982.

Any further attempts at promoting and advancing demarcation were thwarted, at least in the UK, by the introduction in the early 1990s of Project 2000, which saw the beginning of a common foundation programme that all nursing students shared, based on the belief that all branches of nursing have much in common. Project 2000-based curricula were introduced when nurse education was integrated into higher education, which was considered by many to be a positive step forward, but led to a certain irony. On the one hand, the move from education in colleges of nursing to a university was aimed at elevating the status of nursing, making it more attractive to potential recruits. On the other hand, as far as psychiatric nursing was concerned, it lost its title when it became one of the four branches of nursing and was labelled mental health nursing. Also, as psychiatric nursing had previously gained ground in separating itself from general nursing, the introduction of Project 2000 could be viewed as retrograde, given that in the 1960s general nurses and psychiatric nurses had to take the same common examination at the end of the first year of training. So 30 years later, mental health nursing was back to the same position. More recently, professional concerns were raised about the level of competency of newly qualified nurses. These anxieties led to another review of nurse education, culminating in the Fitness for Practice report (UKCC 1999). The impact of this report has yet to be fully realised.

Socialisation is considered the process whereby an individual is introduced to and assimilated into the beliefs, values, attitudes, knowledge and skills of a particular professional group. It is essential to the development of professional competencies and to the longevity and advancement of a profession. The experiences undergone during this period can determine the future contribution individuals make to their respective professions. A major part of the socialisation process is the education and learning experience driven by the validated curriculum. If a significant shift from psychiatric nursing to mental health nursing has/had taken place, the expectation would be that the curriculum would demonstrate a marked change both in terms of content and teaching methodology. The new curriculum would be heavily influenced by a humanistic, recovery, partnership perspective, oriented towards health rather than illness. Emphasis would be placed on the unity of physical, mental, social and spiritual health, together constituting a sense of well-being at different levels. Users and carers would feature highly in the development, delivery and evaluation of the curricula and many universities have adopted this philosophy, for example that described by Masters et al (2002).

Expert knowledge

Within the curricula the importance of users' stories and their expert knowledge would be acknowledged as a source of learning and wisdom and of equal importance to propositional knowledge. To this end importance would be placed on the use of language, labelling, context, and the reality of user and carer experience. Greater credence would be given to postmodernist thinking and philosophy, existentialism and humanism, with emphasis placed on promoting hope, optimism, recovery, healthy lifestyle, health promotion and prevention of mental illness. Social, political and economic influences and the impact of these on mental illness in terms of removing stigma, promoting education and employment and social inclusion would be a priority, equipping students with the social and interactive skills for effective engagement and also the knowledge and skills necessary to challenge and promote mental health and destigmatise mental illness within the wider political and social framework.

Achieving these objectives requires different forms of knowledge beyond that of the process of illness and disease (physical or psychopathological) and necessitates a variety of skills, including cognitive, behavioural, social and emotional, that make up the 'know-how' for working with those in emotional and psychological pain. The understanding of physical health issues including diet, exercise, hygiene, the environment, housing and employment requires greater emphasis. This suggests not only therapeutic skills and knowledge but also the expertise necessary for working in partnership, such as negotiation and lobbying.

Finding curricula in UK universities which embrace all of the above, although not impossible, may be difficult, as many still retain a strong illness perspective. Although the latter cannot be ignored, its position needs to be reviewed if curricula aspire to a greater emphasis on social and public health, in keeping with the role of a mental health nurse. The overall philosophy and content of curricula will be influenced by the orientation of those engaged in their development. Currently, there is little consistency in the key orientations and philosophies that drive the curricula and consequently the socialization process. Some practitioners and educators are aiming towards positive mental health, but others retain the dominant philosophy of medicine and illness. Fortunately, there is recognition that many individuals and institutions have moved or are moving towards a more challenging, proactive, inclusive approach, as described by Forrest & Masters (2005).

Mental health and illness a continuum

There have been discussions and theories as to what constitutes mental health and/or mental illness over centuries, across disciplines and cultures (Casey & Long 2003). It is often recognised that mental health and mental illness are part of a continuum. An acceptable, agreed conclusion as to what is mental health, and by contrast what is mental illness, is necessary in order to explore the differences that might exist between psychiatric and mental health nursing. If a clearer understanding is established, this may lead to a more comprehensive definition of what is mental health nursing. However, as Altschul (1997) pointed out, there is not even consensus with respect to our understanding of mental illness.

Fontaine (2003) states that cultures, families and individuals often define mental illness as behaviours, feelings or ways of thinking that are unusual to them or not easily understood by them. Cultural perceptions determine how people with mental health problems are stigmatised and treated, often with negative stereotypical attitudes preventing individuals from seeking help early. It is recognised that mental health and illness are part of a continuum. Individuals move interactively across this continuum. There is no universal definition of what is normal or abnormal and in this context what constitutes mental health or mental illness? Not everyone develops a mental illness; neither can everyone be described as mentally healthy all the time. Depending on a variety of circumstances, individuals move along the continuum from health to illness and may stop at key points for varying lengths of time influenced by culture, individual characteristics and family, societal beliefs and values. It is at these stopping off points in the life of an individual that health care professionals may become involved.

Positive mental health is not just the absence of mental illness. It is about a positive feeling of wellness, something that is difficult to articulate fully and accurately. For example, how can anyone categorically state, 'I am fully and completely mentally well'? Do we know exactly what this means? How would we recognise it? What parameters would be used to assess it? Broad measures such as Quality of Life, depression and anxiety could be helpful. However, does the absence of depression, anxiety or any other 'state' as measured at a given point in time signify complete mental health? More significantly for this debate, how does this relate to mental health nursing?

The need for political influence

As already stated, the curricula changes introduced as part of Project 2000 brought about the demise of the title of psychiatric nurse. However, a number of nurses still retain psychiatric nurse as part of their title. There is a suggestion that changing the title has been simply cosmetic and a fashion statement and therefore largely meaningless. Adding meaning to the change cannot be done in isolation, but needs to be part of a wider societal, political and professional change. This change cannot happen by the efforts of individual nurses, users, carers, individual institutions or professional groups.

Changes are more likely to happen if supported by Government exercising political influence such as that expressed by the US Surgeon General's report (Department of Health & Human Services 1999). This report makes reference to the burden of mental illness and lack of appreciation of how much of a burden it places on individuals and society as a whole. It also appeals for a greater public health perspective in our understanding of mental illness. The need for health education and promotion, leading to a reduction in the stigma associated with mental illness is emphasised.

In 2004 the UK government (Department of Health 2004) published a 5-year update on the progress made with the National Service Framework for Mental Health (NSF). This strategic initiative set out five national standards for mental health, each supported by evidence and examples of good practice. The first standard was devoted to mental health promotion, reducing discrimination and stigma and enhancing social inclusion. This document gave a well balanced account of the achievements to date but it also suggested that changing societal attitudes is extremely difficult and presents a long-term challenge.

As well as government and professional bodies influencing public perceptions of mental health and illness, charitable organisations also have a role. For example, the Mental Health Foundation (England) published a document entitled 'Bright futures' (Kay 1999). This emphasised the importance of promoting the mental health of children and adolescents through providing professional support for families during pregnancy, through childhood and beyond.

Reports, inquiries and similar government initiatives are important, as they provide context, direction and ambition. However, of themselves they cannot bring about change. This can only happen when there is societal, community and professional action as a result. Initiatives such as the NSF demonstrate how progress can be achieved when there is sustained effort through local champions working in partnership across a range of organisations, engaging with users and carers.

Of particular relevance to this chapter is the view that much has changed about specialist mental health services, such as emphasis on patient choice, workforce skills, chronic disease management and public health. Also, that emphasis has moved from specialist mental health services to the mental health and wellbeing of the community as a whole. Traditionally much of nurse education has been aimed at preparing individuals for specialist mental health services. Now this is changing, preparation needs to focus on inventiveness and creativity in terms of how nursing can facilitate and promote mental health at a community-wide level as well as attending to the needs of those requiring specialist mental health services. Although governments can develop policy and monitor its progress, it is up to the professionals, users and carers involved on a daily basis to make change happen, and their work must be correctly reflected in their working title.

Influences of postmodernism

Postmodernism and its philosophy have been gaining in popularity in mental health nursing. It provides a different way of looking at what is regarded as 'reality' and to some extent provides a basis for the shift in title away from psychiatric nurse. If it is acknowledged that psychiatric nursing is the handmaiden of psychiatry and that psychiatry is biologically and scientifically based, it is therefore considered to be based on 'truth'. Mental health nursing could alternatively be considered as almost the opposite; consequently its 'truth' will have a different basis and a very different version of reality. Stevenson (1996) proposes that postmodernism defies absolute definition because it entails an idea that the words we use to describe something are inextricable from the context. Williams (1996) sees it as a different way of viewing the world and of constructing reality. As such it has much to add to our understanding of mental illness and its reality. Williams believes that while '. . . modernism considers reality to be objective, postmodernism considers reality to be subjective, not fixed or true and immutable, consequently cannot be imposed' (p 270). It is not universal and can therefore have a variety of meanings depending on context.

These same principles relate to mental health and illness as both are, for the most part, subjective, phenomenological experiences. Despite various attempts at gaining an understanding of mental illness and the desire for generalisation and extrapolation, each individual's experiences is unique. Because of this uniqueness, experience cannot be quantified in a standardised fashion, however much medicine and other health care professionals would wish to do so. The process of reducing individual experiences to global, generalisable phenomena undervalues their uniqueness and diminishes what they are: something which is particular to an individual. Although attempts are constantly made to gain a greater understanding of mental illness through the use of 'scientific' studies, the realisation of its uniqueness cannot be established in this way. Such studies do have a role to play in mental health research, but they are not the only approach.

In terms of nursing, in attempting to understand the nature of the lived experience of those encountering mental illness, the act of committing the experience of the individual into text form limits its meaning; consequently part of the meaning is lost. Also, by converting the language into text we are controlling the nature of the language and the text, as well as the context of the experience. Consequently text will never be able to convey the 'true' lived experience of those experiencing mental illness, because the experience as represented is only as good as the language used to describe it. This will result in some of the meaning being lost.

Mental health nurses want to know and understand more about their work and to do this they need to know and understand more about the experiences of users and carers. This is not a knowledge that can be accumulated through 'scientific' experimentation, but rather from an exploration of users' experience, their own experiences and the sharing of those experiences. Exploring and disentangling the intricate nature of interactions, feelings and perceptions is more likely to provide the information necessary to understand the complex world of mental health and illness, to arrive at a position of knowledge.

Meaning behind the change of title

The change of title from psychiatric to mental health nursing could be explored from a number of different perspectives and raise a number of questions about the professional status of P/MH nursing. What was the driving force behind the change in title – was there one other than cosmetic?

It could be perceived as an attempt to normalise or destigmatise mental illness and therefore make it easier for professionals to interact more equitably with the general public. Could it be that mental health gives the impression of a holistic approach to the understanding and treatment of mental illness? Might mental health give the impression of less reliance on the medical model by placing emphasis on health rather than illness, thus interpreting it as a lifestyle issue rather than illness or disease?

Using the term mental health conveys an impression of a positive approach to life, of autonomy, independence, self-management and control. Conveyed within the concept of health is the notion of managing self and illness, such that a key role of nursing would be to work in partnership with users and carers to give them the skills to take control of their lives. Also inherent within this philosophy is the view that individuals are well informed, therefore they can exploit life chances and make life choices. However, at times of mental illness there is often little opportunity to exploit life chances and indeed such chances may be denied.

The title of mental health nurse could be viewed as an attempt to shed the shackles of medicine and make nursing a more independent profession. However, some would argue that this is not possible given the nature of mental illness and the need for medical intervention, hence any ambition to be independent of medicine is nothing less than a romantic notion; medicine equals prescription and as Clarke (1999) asks, on what grounds would a nurse not implement a medical prescription; and given that medical training confers the authority to determine treatments, in what circumstances would such treatment be modified by nurses?

Would the focus on health convey the impression of a different type of nurse when compared with the psychiatric nurse? For some the latter conveys warmth, caring and understanding. The term psychiatric nurse conveys the essence of the caring qualities long associated with nursing. Again, this is open to debate, given the levels of reported abuse experienced by patients in mental hospitals during the 1960s and 1970s, and earlier (Barker & Whitehill 1997).

Mental health nursing – aspiration or reality

At the end of this discussion, and if accepting the positions offered as to the nature of mental health nursing, it must be concluded that to embrace the title and what it represents remains more an aspiration than a reality. Modern curricula value something other than mere science and, by default, psychiatry. Those nurses who follow these curricula cannot, therefore, legitimately be classified as psychiatric nurses. Similarly, postmodernism suggests a contemporary view of mental illness that encompasses so much more than the fields of medicine and physicality. From this it logically follows that those nurses working with the mentally ill should, at the very least, be called 'mental illness nurses' or even 'nurses of the mentally ill'. However, we have also seen that the influence of the sufferers of mental illness and their carers is slowly closing the gap associated with professional power bases and so is becoming the driving force behind modern mental health care services. If language be the product of this social context, it can also be the medium through which this context is developed. In so far as nurses aspire to being in the vanguard of such changes it makes far more sense that they reflect the coming of the new era by adopting a title more befitting their future role within it: mental health nurse.

References

Altschul A 1997 A personal view of psychiatric nursing. In: Tilley S, ed. The mental health nurse: views of practice and education. Blackwell Science, Oxford, p 1–14.

Barker P, Whitehill I 1997 The craft of care: towards collaborative caring in psychiatric nursing. In: Tilley S, ed. The mental health nurse: views of practice and education. Blackwell Science, Oxford, p 15–27.

Brimblecombe N 2005 Asylum nursing in the UK at the end of the Victorian era: Hill End Asylum. Journal of Psychiatric and Mental Health Nursing 13:57–63.

Casey B, Long A 2003 Meanings of madness: a literature review. Journal of Psychiatric and Mental Health Nursing 10:89–99.

Clarke L 1999 Challenging ideas in psychiatric nursing. Routledge, London.

Cutcliffe J R 2003a The differences and commonalities between United Kingdom and Canadian psychiatric/mental health nursing: a personal reflection. Journal of Psychiatric and Mental Health Nursing 10:255–257.

Cutcliffe J R 2003b A historical overview of psychiatric/mental health nurse education in the United Kingdom: going round in circles or on the straight and narrow? Nurse Education Today 23(5):338–346.

Department of Health 2004 National service framework for mental health – five years on. Department of Health, London.

Department of Health & Human Services 1999 Mental health: a report of the surgeon general. National Institute of Mental Health, Pittsburgh.

Fontaine K 2003 Mental health nursing. Prentice Hall, New Jersey.

Forrest S, Masters H 2005 Shaping pre-registration mental health nursing education through user and carer involvement in curriculum design and delivery. In: Tilley S, ed. Psychiatric and mental health nursing; the field of knowledge. Blackwell Science, Oxford, p 101–113.

Kay H 1999 Bright futures – promoting children and young people's health. The Mental Health Foundation, London.

Masters H, Forrest S, Harley A, Hunter M, Brown N, Risk I 2002 Involving service users and carers in curriculum development: moving beyond 'classroom' involvement. Journal of Psychiatric and Mental Health Nursing 9:309–316.

Nolan P 1993 A history of mental health nursing. Chapman & Hall, London.

Norman I 2005 Models of mental health nursing education: findings from a case study. In: Tilley S, ed. Psychiatric and mental health nursing; the field of knowledge. Blackwell Science, Oxford, p 129–150.

Peplau H E 1994 Psychiatric mental health nursing: challenge and change. Journal of Psychiatric and Mental Health Nursing 1:3–7.

Stevenson C 1996 Tao, social constructionism and psychiatric nursing practice and research. Journal of Psychiatric and Mental Health Nursing 3:217–224.

Tilley S, ed. 1997 The mental health nurse: views of practice and education. Blackwell Science, Oxford.

Tilley S, ed. 2005 Psychiatric and mental health nursing; the field of knowledge. Blackwell Science, Oxford.

UKCC 1999 Fitness for practice. United Kingdom Central Council for Nursing, Midwifery and Health Visiting, London.

Watkins P 2002 Mental health nursing: the art of compassionate care. Butterworth Heinemann, Oxford.

Williams R 1996 From modernism to postmodernism: the implications for nurse therapist interventions. Clinical Notice Board. Journal of Psychiatric and Mental Health Nursing 3:269–271.

Wood T O 1902 The future of asylum nurses (letter). Asylum News 6:127.

Commentary

John Collins

'Naming a nurse is a difficult matter'   (with apologies to T S Eliot)

In the previous two papers, Chambers and du Mont have argued, both from different positions and from different nations, that the terms 'psychiatric nursing' and 'mental health nursing' are redundant. Although I have taken the same position on this issue in the distant past, my arguments were, at that time, considerably at variance with those of Chambers and du Mont. My position was not whether the occupation in which I found myself should properly be called 'psychiatric nursing' or 'mental health nursing', but whether it should be called 'nursing' at all. In the years that have followed, the urgency of this question gave way to questions about what we do and why we do it. Returning to it again after so many years is rather like waking the proverbial sleeping dog. Given that I had not resolved the issue for myself when I left it, reconsidering it now may provoke the same thoughts and feelings which I left behind some years ago. Nevertheless, I continue to have a strong interest in this debate. Chambers and du Mont have raised issues which appear germane to the present interests of a P/MH nurse. In writing this commentary, it is not my goal to resolve this debate; rather, you may find me 'pouring more oil on the fire'.

The authors' context

In the case of Chambers, the current backdrop to the issue of a name – 'psychiatric nurse' or 'mental health nurse' – can be located in recent experience in the UK where 'registered mental nurses' have been eliminated and have become a 'mental health' side speciality of an entry-level generic nursing programme. Similar changes of title or name have occurred previously in the history of P/MH nursing; 'asylum attendants' have, over the course of a century, gradually and reluctantly become incorporated into mainstream nursing. Chambers' paper demonstrates that there is still an ongoing concern in the UK with whether the title 'mental health nurse' is truly representative of the services provided by the discipline, or if it would be more appropriate to resurrect the name and category, 'psychiatric nurse'. In contrast, du Mont's paper demonstrates that, for American psychiatric nurses, issues of name are simply not relevant. They have been longer and more thoroughly consumed by general nursing. Without entry-level psychiatric nurses, their 'issues' range around what kind of nursing specialist will do the prescribing for psychiatric patients.

The chapters by du Mont and Chambers both appear to accept the notion that psychiatric nursing is, indeed, nursing. They do not appear to present discussion or argument in relation to this part of the title, though this obviously has relevance for the 'psychiatric' and 'mental health' parts of the titles. Rather, in deference to nursing's holistic philosophy, both seem to accept – or at least acknowledge – the view that the term 'mental health nursing' implies ideas of illness prevention, whereas the term 'psychiatric nursing' implies treatment of illness. In doing so they set what I consider to be a narrow plane for the exploration and discussion of the title. From that point forward, the thinking about title is reduced to two parallel, yet similar, arguments. In fairness to the authors, perhaps this was set in motion by the invitation from the editors? Nevertheless, I would contend that the 'nurse' part of the title is as much to do with the perceptions of the 'psychiatric' or 'mental health' parts of the title that the authors debate. I will say more about this later in the commentary.

At this juncture, let me return to the issue of the historical development of the discipline and the impact this had on its naming. Both authors in this debate have referred to historical development in their arguments. A review of the history of psychiatric nursing shows that, though 'asylum attendants' had been around for a significant period of time, general nursing came into existence before psychiatric nursing and thus had more influence on the development and trends of nursing overall.

The British experience

Cutcliffe (2003) and Nolan (1997) pinpoint the first documented training of psychiatric attendants at the York Retreat sometime after its founding in 1796. The first systematic course of instruction began at Crichton Royal Hospital in Scotland in 1851 (Collins 1995, Cutcliffe 2003). From these Scottish roots, the British Medico-Psychological Association (MPA) (later the Royal College of Psychiatrists) published the first textbook in 1885, and initiated the first universally examined course of instruction for asylum attendants in 1890. The first examinations took place in 1891 and the registry of 'Attendants on the Insane' was opened in 1892 (Harcourt Williams 2001). It was not until 1923 that 'attendants' were officially declared 'nurses' by the MPA (Harcourt Williams 2001). By then, Britain's first nursing registers had been established for 2 years. A similar trend occurred in those countries which took up or developed similar versions of the psychiatric nursing programme. Australia, South Africa, Canada and Denmark directly imported the programme in various forms, and training in the USA was probably influenced by it also (Harcourt Williams 2001). Indeed, an American edition of the handbook was considered in 1892 and 1906 when the American Medico-Psychological Association appointed its first committee on training schools for psychiatric nurses (Church 1986).

The North American experience

In the USA and Canada, the 'attendant' epithet lived on. Goffman (1961), for example, uses the term to describe untrained staff in charge of psychiatric hospital patients. The term continues to be used for the same purpose in some parts of the USA and Canada. In these countries, the 'nurses' working in psychiatric hospitals were general nurses. In 1896, general nurses in those countries began organising in the form of a single association, the Nurses' Associated Alumnae of the United States and Canada. The association formed common cause with British general nurses in 1899 to form the International Council of Nurses (American Nurses Association 1996a).

By 1903, general nurses were being licensed and regulated in North Carolina, New York, New Jersey and Virginia (American Nurses Association 1996b). In Canada, the first apprenticeship training of general nurses was imported from France in 1639. Following upon the British trend initiated by Nightingale and transported to the colonies (Godden 2001), nursing apprenticeships did not arrive in (English) Ontario until 1874 (Canadian Museum of Civilization Corporation 2004). General nurses in Manitoba were given self-governing registration in 1913 and those in Ontario were granted registration in 1922 (Tipliski 2004). Some North American jurisdictions also began standardised training of 'asylum attendants' but, where it happened, it was some two decades later than in Britain. By then, general nurses were already organising themselves for self-regulation. These 'mental nurses' were being trained under the control of the asylums' medical superintendents and, for a brief period after general nurse registration, they were accepted into the fraternity of general nurses. By the mid 1930s, however, entry level training programmes for mental nurses began to be subsumed into general nurse training (Tipliski 2004). General nurses began to take the view that psychiatric nursing could no longer be regarded as 'separate and distinct' from general nursing.

Even as general nurses began to assert their authority over asylum nurses and attendants elsewhere in North America, the Canadian Province of Manitoba was reversing the trend. In 1921 it had initiated an entry level programme in psychiatric nursing. Within 10 years, the four westernmost provinces had all started such training programmes.

By 1948, legislation was being introduced in the Province of Saskatchewan to give registration and autonomy to psychiatric nurses. The Act was, in part, the result of political efforts by the asylum attendants themselves (Tiplinski 2004). Similar legislation slowly followed in the other western provinces. By then, however, even in the jurisdictions with entry-level psychiatric nurses, general nurses were an established fixture, both in psychiatric hospitals and in general hospital psychiatric units.

It is evident, then, that general nurses had established their power base before psychiatric nurses managed to do so. This state of affairs allowed general nursing theory to have a major impact on psychiatric nursing. Thus, the two authors in this debate find themselves discussing the issue of title from a nursing theory perspective. They claim that the evolving philosophy of nursing has placed emphasis on a nursing rather than a medical model. Nursing has laid claim to the domain of health promotion and disease prevention (as well as addressing illness). It is from this evolution that both authors see the shifting emphasis on to 'mental health nursing', with one claiming that this does not necessitate a change of title from 'psychiatric nurse' and the other exploring reasons to support the shift. Du Mont states that nursing has long rejected the medical model approach.

Perhaps the more significant issue, still unresolved, is whether 'nurse' represents the intentions of the discipline? As I have noted above, in both Canada and the UK, asylum attendants and entry-level psychiatric nurses resisted incorporation into the body of general nursing. Indeed, they appear to have seen themselves as possessing different and more appropriate skills than general nurses (Dooley 2004).

The effects of eliminating entry-level psychiatric nurses

It might even be argued that the practice of psychiatric nurse specialists in the USA (see Ch. 2) may be more similar to present-day psychiatrists than to the attendants of old. In Britain and western Canada, which still have entry-level psychiatric nurses, 'psychiatric nursing' remains quite differentiated from medical practice. It may also indicate a refusal to recognise that psychiatric nurses and general nurses are, indeed, different 'breeds' (Norman 1998, cited in Cutcliffe 2005).

That general nurses might not find appeal in psychiatric nursing is not surprising. The jobs have quite different characteristics (Cutcliffe 2003) and the amount of training in psychiatry and mental health received by entry-level general nurses is small and diminishing (Poster 2004). The history and form of psychiatric nursing in, at least, the USA, Canada and the UK illustrates the problem. In jurisdictions, such as the UK and western Canada, where psychiatric nursing has remained a distinct, entry-level job, those jurisdictions have, in the past, retained a relatively committed workforce. In jurisdictions such as the USA and Eastern Canada, the workforce has been subject to the vagaries of the general nursing market.

This problem does not appear to be a simple 'market' problem, however. As psychiatric nursing moves closer to 'nursing', the more problems it appears to have in recruitment. The UK, while retaining mental health nursing as a separate discipline, has brought mental health nursing students into a common entry point with general nurses. Mental health nursing has shown a consistently lower student uptake than general (adult) nursing (Buchan & Seccombe 2004), although vacancies have remained consistently higher (Workforce Review Team 2004) and the relative proportion of such nurses has dropped (Genkeer et al 2003). Vacancies remain higher despite what appears to be a lower rate of turnover (Genkeer et al 2003). The problem has been dramatically recreated in the Canadian Province of Saskatchewan where new psychiatric nurse registrations have virtually stopped (Registered Psychiatric Nurses Association of Saskatchewan 2000). Accordingly, the issue might be, should we abandon 'nursing' as a means of approaching work with mentally distressed people?

Conclusion

The debate presented by the authors in these chapters covers a lot of ground, but seems to go nowhere. As Chambers pointed out (Ch. 3), they are going 'in circles'. In the final analysis, both find no substantive reason at this time to change the title 'psychiatric nurse'. Could this be due to the fact that they should have debated the complete title and not just that piece describing the form of nursing? After all, neither 'psychiatric' nor 'mental health' nursing has thrived as a 'nursing' occupation. Perhaps we should not be engaging in a debate about whether we are 'psychiatric nurses' or 'mental health nurses'. Maybe it is finally time for psychiatric nursing to grow out of its adolescence, differentiate itself from its parents, and consider an autonomous life, free from the influences of the 'medical father' and the 'nursing mother'? Now may be the time to consider expanding on the debate about whether 'psychiatric nurses' are 'nurses' at all?

References

American Nurses Association 1996a 1900s: the tasks of the first decade. Online. Available: http://www.ana.org/centenn/cent1900.htm accessed 2005.

American Nurses Association 1996b In the beginning. Online. Available: http://nursingworld.org/centenn/centbegn.htm accessed 2005.

Buchan J, Seccombe I 2004 Fragile future? A review of the UK nursing labour market in 2003. Royal College of Nursing, London.

Canadian Museum of Civilization Corporation 2004 A brief history of nursing in Canada from the establishment of New France to the present civilization. Online. Available: http://www.civilization.ca/tresors/nursing/nchis01e.html 11 June 2004

Church O 1986 From custody to community in psychiatric nursing. Nursing Research 36(1):48–55.

Collins J 1995 The context for psychiatric nursing. In: The update/refresher program in psychiatric nursing – module 1. International School of Nursing and Health Studies, Port Coquitlam.

Cutcliffe J 2003 A historical overview of psychiatric/mental health nursing education in the United Kingdom: going around in circles or on the straight and narrow? Nurse Education Today 23:338–346.

Cutcliffe J 2005 A rose by any other name: specialism, generalism and the diminution of psychiatric/mental health nursing. Keynote address: Psychiatric Nurse Educators of Western Canada Conference.

Dooley C 2004 'They gave their care, but we gave loving care': defining and defending boundaries of skill and craft in the nursing service of a Manitoba mental hospital during the Great Depression. Canadian Bulletin of Medical History 21(2):229–251.

Genkeer L, Gough P, Finlayson B 2003 London's mental health workforce. King's Fund, London.

Godden J 2001 'Like a possession of the devil'. The diffusion of Nightingale nursing and Anglo-Australian relations. International History of Nursing Journal 6(2):52–58.

Goffman E 1961 Asylums: essays on the social situation of mental patients and other inmates. Anchor, New York.

Harcourt Williams M 2001 The College archives: an outline of the history of the examination for mental nurses organized by the (Royal) Medico-Psychological Association. Royal College of Psychiatrists:London. Online. Available: http://www.rcpsych.ac.uk/college/archives/nursing/nursinghist. htm accessed 2005

Nolan P 1997 A history of mental health nursing. Chapman Hall, London.

Norman I J 1998 The changing emphasis of mental health and learning disability nurse education in the UK and ideal models of its future development. Journal of Psychiatric and Mental Health Nursing 5:41–51.

Poster E C 2004 Psychiatric nursing at risk: the new NCLEX-RN test plan. Journal of Child and Adolescent Psychiatry 17(2):47–48.

Registered Psychiatric Nurses Association of Saskatchewan 2000 Psychiatric nursing education: a program for Saskatchewan. Online. Available: http://www.rpnas.com/public/pdfs/education/education_brief.pdf accessed 2005.

Tipliski V M 2004 Parting at the crossroads: the emergence of education for psychiatric nursing in three Canadian provinces 1905–1955. Canadian Bulletin of Medical History 21(2):253–279.

Workforce Review Team 2004 Workforce planning for allied health professionals, nurses and midwives and healthcare scientists: recommendations of the Workforce Numbers Advisory Board. Department of Health, London.

"

Reconciliatory or recalcitrant: should psychiatric/mental health nursing strive for independence from or be closely allied to psychiatric medicine?

CHAPTER 4

Psychiatry and psychiatric nursing in the New World Order

Peter Morrall

CHAPTER 5

Declaring conceptual independence from obsolete professional affiliations

Liam Clarke

Commentary

Jon Allen

"

Editorial

Said of two mutually exclusive alternatives: *'A door must either be shut or open'* (according to Samuel Goldsmith in 1762). The notion of absolutes has been with us for a great many years. Yet, compromising clinical roles is something that psychiatric/mental health (P/MH) nurses have done over the years, usually as a response to the demands of medical colleagues or politicians. This has meant that, in some cases, the growth and development of nursing has been stunted because of other agendas. However, there is no denying that, as a key partner of psychiatry, P/MH nursing has gained professional credibility and, in many cases, a sense of direction and purpose. True, much of this has been steered by political priorities, but, notwithstanding the fact that psychiatry is a far more political animal than P/MH nursing, working in tandem with, and as a partner to, the medical profession has brought considerable gain to P/MH nursing and those who suffer mental health problems.

Key to this success is the focus of the medical approach to care delivery, namely its central functions of observation and diagnosis but, except in the case of those psychiatrists who are trained as psychotherapists, little in the way of actual hands-on intervention. However, partnerships, like all relationships, are not without their problems, and that between nursing and medicine in mental health care is a classic case in point. Yes, medicine and medical staff work as members of multidisciplinary teams and have a huge influence over the decisions made about the therapeutic processes. As such, seldom do they walk in the footsteps of nurses, and rightly so, because it is not their professional responsibility to do so. In truth, much of the work of psychiatry is restricted to the domains of diagnosis and treatments, located mainly within the realms of chemical prescribing, electroconvulsive therapy (ECT) and other forms of physical treatments. And this is undoubtedly where the two disciplines walk separate paths and, it would seem, specifically as a consequence of the nature of chemical interventions. We know that, over time, the use of psychopharmacological agents will alter gene transcription and translation, and that, as a consequence, molecular neurobiological processes, especially in the developing brain, may be influenced, even inducing molecular alterations. Chemical interventions are therefore capable of changing gene expressions. We also know that nurses take an active part in the monitoring of these chemicals, and for some the potential consequences of this association are a burden they are not prepared to accept.

While there are many related, and sometimes apparently unrelated, parts to this debate, it seems to boil down to whether or not you believe that mental health problems or mental 'illness' has a biological aetiology, which in turn is based on your understanding of the appropriate literature supporting the two camps and, even further back along this chain of consequence, whether you support the notion of human or non-human interventions. This is essentially the nursing versus medicine debate, and is reflected here as an allegiance between the two disciplines. What the reader must do is decide whether it is acceptable to see things as two separate camps, as Samuel Goldsmith would undoubtedly have done (albeit 250 years ago), or whether or not psychiatry exists upon a continuum with medicine at the one end and nursing at the other. Where you see yourself on this line may well determine your understanding of the debate and, ultimately, whether P/MH nursing stands as a separate discipline or as working with medicine in its more focused areas of responsibility. Has nursing developed its own ego problem or should it really be able to achieve all its professional aspirations? Is it able, capable or prepared to do all these things? This debate should at least open the door!

Peter Morrall

Psychiatry and psychiatric nursing in the New World Order

Introduction

Despite the ritualised complaining from the pseudo-intellectual and occupationally insecure malcontents of psychiatric nursing, this discipline is historically, contemporaneously and prospectively adjoined to psychiatric medicine. To argue, as I do here, that (psychiatric) nursing is not a discrete discipline, but is, and should be, closely allied to (psychiatric) medicine, is to state the obvious both empirically (psychiatric nursing and medicine share concepts and practices, and day-to-day existences) and ethically (a dissolution of the coalition has not been sanctioned by mental health care consumers). The *contra* position is the aspirational *gratis dictum* of the self-aggrandising psychiatric nursing practitioner, manager and academic, searching unconsciously or manifestly for a *raison d'être* beyond that which is realistic.

P/MH nursing malcontents suffer two interlinked and vacillating psychological pathologies: inferiority and superiority complexes. The inferiority complex element has come about through the working class cultural heritage of psychiatric nursing, resulting in an 'us and them' view of the world, and/or scholastic and employment failure or lack of opportunity (P/MH nursing being a default occupation). Moreover, training to be a P/MH nurse and working within the mental health field foments gender-role dissonance (male P/MH nurses are uncomfortable with the 'femaleness' of nursing and a disproportionate number of the malcontents are men). The superiority complex has been engendered through: unviable career expectations as a consequence of exposure to university education (and the amassing of 'add-on' qualifications);

exposure to, but gross misunderstanding of, the disparate antipsychiatry positions of the 1970s; a mere 'topsoil' excavation of Foucault's knowledge-archaeology; working alongside psychiatrists and discovering that a minority seem clinically ineffective, or even dangerous, but a denial of the reality that doctors are recruited from academic high achievers and that medical education is arduous (and that some nurses are also asinine); becoming indoctrinated with the 'politically correct' mantra emanating from established enclaves of some disaffected P/MH nurses that psychiatrists are 'the enemy' from whom both nurses, patients and society must be protected; and finally, the general demise of deference and undermining of such 'truth' as medical science within postmodern society.

Feelings of inferiority and superiority lead to resentment and hostility, or unmerited arrogance and disparagement towards those 'colleagues' who are perceived to be more privileged – in particular psychiatrists, but also psychologists and occupational therapists. This can lead to role deviancy (for example, subtle non-cooperation with 'privileged' colleagues in clinical situations; antagonism to all things medical in the nursing press; the perverse reaction I have witnessed from an audience of nurses at a conference on mental health practice when the speaker, a professor of psychiatric nursing, mentioned the term 'psychiatrist' – booing!). The projection of psychiatric nursing as a discrete discipline is, therefore, mere naive propaganda for an unobtainable occupational goal. Whilst there is the possibility for occupational advancement towards separatism in the postmodern consumerist marketplace (through, for example, epistemological bifurcation between P/MH nursing and psychiatry; the 'nursification' of presently medicalised practices), there are insurmountable counterposing structural constraints. These obstacles are (1) the historical connection with psychiatry; (2) the continued dominance of the medical profession in the health system; and (3) most significantly, the social control function of psychiatry and P/MH nursing in the *New World Order*.

History

The origins of P/MH nursing can be traced to the keeper of the various types of mainly private or charity 'houses' in which a minority of 'mad' people lived (most residing with their families or wandering the countryside) up until the middle of the 19th century. In the UK, the Poor Law Amendment Act 1834 and the Lunacy Act 1845 heralded in the beginning of 'Victorian Asylumdom', whereby local authorities were obliged to undertake formidable (economically and architecturally) public building programmes to house the 'mad' (Morrall 1998).

Asylumdom was a system of segregating the 'mad' into a centralised and unitary form of 'human warehouse' away from the rest of the community and other 'deviant' populations such as criminals and the poor (Foucault 1971, Scull 1993). Asylumdom also enabled the medical profession and the forerunners to P/MH nursing to emerge as legitimate 'surveyors' of the 'mad'. That is, the medical profession was not instrumental in the creation of the asylum movement (doctors were brought in as local notables to advise and administrate these institutions), but capitalised on a captive population on whom it could experiment with and develop methods of treatment (Porter 2002). By the time the Lunacy Act 1890 was instituted, the profession of medicine had monopolised the market with regard to the care of the 'mad'. Madness, essentially a cultural identity signifying a taboo status, became redefined as the medical category of mental illness. There was, through asylumdom, a thorough medicalisation of socially unacceptable behaviours and thoughts. Moreover, doctors were able to medicalise the custodians of the mad institutions.

After 1845, the keeper changed into the 'attendant'. The attendants were responsible for the general upkeep of the new institutions for the insane, but were to become 'the medical superintendent's servants'. The principal responsibility of the attendant was to obey the orders of the medical superintendent and those of other medical staff associated with the asylum. The creation of a Register for Attendants under the 1890 Act is the beginning of the formal recognition of the title *psychiatric nursing* (Nolan 1993). Reflecting the relationship between doctors and their assistants in other areas of medical practice, female attendants became known as 'nurses'. The title 'mental nurse' was introduced in the General Council's Supplementary Register for Mental Nurses of 1923 (Nolan 1993).

The geographical isolation of the asylum, managerial control and epistemological supremacy of the medical profession, and the social class divide between doctors (upper middle class) and nurses (lower working class, if not underclass), determined that the *psychiatric nurse* conducted the 'dirty work' of psychiatry, and of local authorities as well as the State – cleaning floors and toilets, inmates' bodies and minds, and society. Asylum medical superintendents were omnipotent. The working and personal lives of the attendants and nursing staff were monitored closely by doctors and other staff elevated to supervisory roles. Conformity was expected, and non-conformists could be dismissed instantly for relatively trivial rule-breaking (for example, intemperance, licentiousness and disobedience). Such all-encompassing influence over nurses by doctors was maintained throughout the 19th and much of the 20th century. Mental hospitals in the 1970s still operated with a hierarchy headed by the medical superintendent. Any gains made by *mental health nursing* to assert itself as a discrete discipline were undermined in the 1930s and 1940s when more physical treatments (for example, psychosurgery and insulin therapy) were introduced. In the 1940s and 1950s, the discovery of effective psychotropic drugs, stabilising such conditions as manic-depression and schizophrenia, reaffirmed the biomedical base for the treatment of mental illness. This had the consequence of focusing nursing practice on pharmaceutical routines and rituals, instigated by medical practitioners, with the *mental health nurse* organised as the 'therapeutic technician' to the psychiatrist. The 'drug round' became the most important task in the nurse's working day, symbolising the hallowed mystique of the medical profession.

By the 1980s, nurse training covered social and psychological factors in the causation and treatment of mental distress, together with (that is, not replacing) traditional medical approaches. However, since then there has been a further revolutionary period in psychopharmacology. The medical profession has an expanding arsenal of psychotropic drugs, particularly to provide treatment for mood disorders and schizophrenia, and the function of *psychiatric/mental health nurses* as managers of medicines has been magnified not diminished.

In the 1950s the community aspect of nursing began, centring on helping discharged patients to survive in the community, an essential part of which was ensuring that medication was taken as instructed by the psychiatrist. As the discharged and non-institutionalised proportion of mentally ill people has grown, so have the numbers of community P/MH nurses and the scope of their practice beyond that of managing medication for psychiatrists. Moreover, autonomous practice has been much sought after by P/MH nurses working wholly in the community, as a discrete entity within P/MH nursing rather than as part of the overall discipline. However, this has been a failed occupational project if measured by how far removed community P/MH nursing is from the domination of psychiatry. Although the delivery of talking therapies and even drug treatments may involve a degree of discretion by community P/MH nurses, most of their work remains concerned with communicating with psychiatrists and immersed in the medical discourse (Fakhoury 2000). Furthermore, since the public, media and political outcry about dangerous mentally disordered people living in the community, the medical and social control aspects of the community-based nurse's role have been accentuated (Morrall 2000, 2002).

Dominance

Medicine is a profession – nursing is not. Professions have autonomy and dominance: doctors still have a relatively high level of clinical independence, whereas nurses (still) have a relatively low level of clinical independence; doctors remain authoritative in the division of labour within the health system, whereas nurses are positioned as challengers to, not victors over, that authority. Psychiatrists are doctors, and P/MH nurses are nurses. *Ipso facto*, P/MH nursing is reliant on and beholden to psychiatric medicine (Morrall 1998, 2001). Psychiatry is itself not wholly dependent upon some stereotypical notion of 'the' medical model based solely on pharmacology, electroplexy and psychosurgery. Psychiatry is, and always has been, more eclectic than such a simplistic characterisation. Alongside the drugs, shocks and incisions, the full range of talking therapies (from psychoanalysis to cognitive behaviourism) are indulged in by many psychiatrists either directly or through referrals to psychologists, community P/MH nurses, nurse therapists and consultant nurses. Consequently, when nurses use these non-physical methods of treatment, they are not stepping outside of standard psychiatric aetiological explanations or treatments.

Psychiatry and general practice today are fortified by an effervescent pharmacological industry, sophisticated neurological diagnostic technology, finely tuned brain surgery, and research coupling genetic mutations with depression, Alzheimer's senility, alcoholism and schizophrenia. Juxtaposed with these biomedical approaches is the wider use of counselling and psychotherapy, as the market for mental illness expands.

Tactically astute, the profession of medicine first ridicules threats to its dominance from other disciplines or epistemologies (for example, by claiming that if a health product or technique has not been scientifically assessed then it should not be available), but, if this fails, it then envelopes the challenger. In general practice, alternative medicine has becomes complementary medicine. In surgery, acupuncture becomes a passable procedure. In psychiatry, humanistic counselling and social therapy are not only tolerated but instigated as legitimate psychological remedies by medical practitioners. What psychiatric medicine and general practice, aided and abetted by institutional and community P/MH nursing, have accomplished is a prolific and holistic medicalisation and psychiatrisation of everyday life and problems of living. Although there are competing 'truths' concerning how we should live our lives (from aromatherapy and herbalism to new-age spirituality and Buddhism), we still rely heavily in Western society on medical concepts, diagnoses and treatment. Far from psychiatric medicine becoming weakened, it is pervasive.

What, then, might psychiatry's rebellious progeny, *psychiatric nursing*, offer society and the health consumer as an alternative if it could (which is extremely unlikely) de-psychiatrise? What epistemology, discourse, technology and practice could be proffered by the malcontents of P/MH nursing that have not already been, or would be, discredited or adopted by psychiatry? Medical hegemony is rife. Medical ideas and technologies shape perceptions of what is normal and acceptable for somatic and psychological health. Nursing, whilst at times antagonistic to the influence of the profession of medicine in what it considers to be its own sphere of work, reproduces medical ways of perceiving psychological and physical dysfunction. Nurses may object to the paternalistic and patronising ways of their medical colleagues, but essentially embrace and reproduce the medical discourse.

Management, budgetary and regulatory restraints have not substantially undermined the foundations of medicine. The profession is wounded, perhaps seriously. It has lost a proportion of its autonomy and dominance, but is not on an occupational life-support machine. In the UK medicine has suffered: (a) public humiliation about the incompetence of doctors following the Bristol Royal Infirmary scandal (storing body parts of deceased child patients for research, without telling or seeking permission from their parents); and (b) political intimidation as successive governments have tried to 'rein in' the profession, one of its members being found Britain's most prolific serial killer (Harold Shipman) and a record number of doctors banned from practising as a consequence of serious misconduct (Laurance 2003). However, the medical imagination is formidable, medical indoctrination impassable and, with convalescence, the profession's prognosis is good to excellent.

For sure, within the UK setting nursing has improved its occupational status, and continues to do so. Nurses prescribe a number of medications, 'triage' patients, assist surgeons with minor operations, lead some hospital and community-based units, are at the forefront of primary care and at times, in well delineated circumstances, practise autonomously. Indeed, there appears to be a political commitment to extend further the clinical work that may be carried out by nurses, for example in surgery, accident and emergency departments. Moreover, role-blurring between nurses and doctors has been official government policy. However, most of these embellishments to the nurse's role are indicative of medical intrusion into nursing. Nurses are performing as junior doctors rather than as professionalised nurses. It is the author's opinion that doctors are passing on (as they always have done) areas of their work they no longer wish to do themselves because more prestigious tasks are available, there is a shortage of doctors, and junior doctors have reduced their working hours. Furthermore, just as there are forces at work to reduce the strength of the medical profession, there are counterposing processes in the practice of nursing that have contributed to its failure to professionalise. For example, the creation of Primary Care Trusts in the UK National Health Service means that general practitioners will command huge health budgets, becoming the employers of large numbers of nurses.

Two final salient points can be made that indicate the persevering authority of the medical profession over nurses and the health care system within the UK (similar situations exist in most other countries): (1) doctors are responsible ultimately for the diagnosis, treatment, admission and discharge of 'their' patients in most clinical situations, and therefore wield much influence over nursing practice; (2) both general practitioners and medical consultants were awarded a huge increase in salary during 2003 – the earning capacity of the medical profession is indicative of an ascendant occupational status, with dominance over nursing reaffirmed.

Social control

It is axiomatic that every form of human society indulges in social regulation. Without order of one sort or another there is no society. Order is maintained through the socialising and coercive actions of many agencies (for example, the family, law, government, the church, schools and the health services). Agencies and agents of social control assist in the preservation of behaviours and thoughts acceptable to the values of a society and/or those with power in that society. Much of this assistance is indirect and unpremeditated. Moreover, the power that a social agency and agent has to enact control can also be 'enjoyed' for its own sake (Foucault 1974). That is, rather than serving the State in ways that are either immediate or easily discernible, control can be exercised for the benefit of the institution and its operatives. For example, access to the 'sick role' is controlled by medical practitioners on behalf of the State, but is also indicative of the power of the individual doctor to make clinical judgements. Police officers repress social unrest and criminality for the State, but also as a salaried and pensioned career. Furthermore, the dissemination of power throughout society, at the level of organisations, groups and interpersonal communication, assuages and dissipates State control.

Social control by and on behalf of the State does not necessarily result in rigid social systems. Societies are liable to internal change, for example as a result of alterations in the status and influence of various groups. Moreover, external pressures, as a consequence of the globalisation of technologies, media and economies, may cause prolonged periods of turmoil in the cultural practices of a society. However, the foundations of most societies, including those of human society as a collectivity, are intrinsically adaptable and durable. The structural fabric of a society is at risk of dramatic mutation or total disintegration only when facing extraordinary circumstances such as civil war, invasion by a foreign power or financial collapse. In liberal-democratic societies a free press, lobby and pressure groups, judicial and civil appeal processes, and the ballot box, whilst partisan to the *status quo*, oblige rulers to temper conspicuous control. In totalitarian societies, by definition, there are either no, or minimal, checks on the State or the dictator's sovereignty and injunctions. Objection can come only from underground or extrinsic dissident groups and from 'world opinion' (leading perhaps to economic sanctions or military intervention). Liberal democracies engage in elaborate systems of control. Oligarchies and despots indulge in naked (that is, crude, cruel and clear) control.

From asylumdom onwards, psychiatry and P/MH nursing have collaborated in the governance of the mentally disordered on behalf of the State and 'enjoy' (in the Foucauldian sense) doing so. Psychiatrists and P/MH nurses collaborate in medicalising (and thereby controlling) a loose array and growing number of socially discordant behaviours under the deviant rubric of 'mental disorder'. Throughout the world, coercion is an indelible part of medical and nursing practice in the mental health field (Morrall & Hazelton 2003). Naked control includes enforced admission and treatment, physical and chemical restraint, and seclusion. Disguised coercion operates through the 'therapeutic relationship' developed between the nurse and the psychiatric patient. Nurses regulate behaviour through their 'empathic' relationships with patients. The intimate association that occurs between nurses and patients in the institution or in the community, whilst appearing magnanimous and 'person centred', functions as a virulent instrument of control.

Post-liberal social control

In mature liberal democracies there has been a major shift in social control measures. The social contract between the State and citizen has been reconfigured, focusing on rights and responsibilities. The citizen and representative collectivities (for example, trade unions and lobby groups) have demanded from, or been awarded by, the State privileges such as employment protection, consumer charters, human rights and decentralised authority. Social inclusion, however, carries with it the obligation to participate in community and political affairs. The principles of the free market (no social responsibility, only self-responsibility) and socialism (no self-responsibility, only social responsibility) have been synthesised into the 'Third Way', or what has become rebranded as 'progressive governance' (Giddens 2000, Blair 2001, Editorial 2003).

Under such political conditions, with an expanding and exacting citizenship, the system of social control has to accommodate and vitalise the active and 'free' citizen, and denigrate far more robustly the deviant (Rose 2000). Social control in post-liberal society becomes increasingly sophisticated and ubiquitous, but also naked.

Self-regulation is at the sophisticated core of social control in post-liberal society. 'Good citizens' have the responsibility of shaping and adhering to *their* world, a message that the State and its synergic organisations instil through a plethora of policies across all areas of civil life. Failed citizens, spoiled citizens, rebellious citizens, or those in the underclass of non-citizenship, pose an unparalleled threat to civil constancy and become susceptible to the concomitant discourse of risk thinking, risk management, and the technologies of risk assessment and control. Defaulting on the self-regulatory responsibilities of the revamped social contract invites literal or virtual social confinement. Paedophiles, recidivists (adult criminals, young offenders, prostitutes, drunks, litter louts, noisy neighbours), the severely mentally ill and psychopaths are demonised and marginalised.

In the UK, the criminal justice system is being 'modernised' to deal with these 'dangerous classes'. The following four examples are indicative of this shift:

1 Mandatory life sentences for second serious violent or sexual offences (for example, attempted murder, soliciting murder, rape)
2 The removal of the right to be tried by jury for certain criminal offences (for example, intricate fraud)
3 Police registers of sex offenders (anyone convicted of a serious sex offence – particularly against children – must submit name and current address to the local police)
4 Electronic monitoring ('tagging'), 'voice verification' call systems, home detention orders and nighttime curfews for adults and young offenders serving community sentences or released on licence.

With regard to the mentally disordered, the following developments have run parallel to those in criminal justice:

- The extension of supervision registers for most/all severely mentally ill people living in the community
- (Proposed) Compulsory detention of people with personality disorder without trial and without a crime having been committed
- (Proposed) Re-calling to the psychiatric institution of severely mentally ill people living in the community for compulsory treatment
- Development of the 'electronic panopticon' (i.e. microphone and video surveillance within psychiatric institutions)
- The extensive appliance of 'assertive outreach' whereby the 'social space' between the psychiatric institution and the community is supervised
- (Proposed) Victims of mentally disordered offending entitled to information about the offender's release
- Increasing numbers of involuntary admissions, and a decreasing number of those admissions discharged
- Escalating use of seclusion and restraint in psychiatric institutions
- The building of more inpatient accommodation.

A move away from the 1960s liberalism in the mental health system (with an emphasis on community-based facilities) into the post-liberal era was stimulated by the public, media and political attention given to murders committed by the mentally disordered (Morrall 2000, 2002). In post-liberal society, psychiatrists and P/MH nurses (many of whom unwillingly) have become the manufacturers and purveyors of the discourse of risk, and inextricably engaged in the 'politics' of risk (Gray et al 2002, Peay 2003). Risk assessment tools are generated, and risk assessment is conducted with a growing proportion of the mentally disordered population. This function extends to 'administering the marginalia' within the psychiatric institution as well as in the community (Rose 2000). Patients are 'surveyed' (that is, 'observed' and 'assessed') and, if found not to be compliant (repudiating their responsibility to be a self-governing citizen), they are 'disciplined'. This discipline may be meted out surreptitiously during talking therapy, or nakedly through obligatory treatment and confinement. Post-liberalism, however, has to be placed in the wider context of an immense mutation in social control where 'risk' is assessed and tackled globally. This is the New World Order.

New World Order

To understand this in relation to mental health care one has to explore the wider issue. The world is in a mess. Sub-Saharan Africa is characterised by relative and absolute poverty, genocidal warfare, AIDS epidemics, a life expectancy half of that of the West, huge social disparity between those in power and the vast majority of the population, and not just economic underdevelopment but de-development. Parts of South and Central America are economically unstable, and made perilous by murderous drug barons, political zealots and opportunistic kidnappers. The Middle East is embroiled in a tit-for-tat cycle of suicide bombing and state-sponsored homicide. India and Pakistan, both nuclear powers, disagree violently over Kashmir. Iran and North Korea are playing cat-and-mouse with the USA over their nuclear capability. Russia has a fiscal crisis, a life expectancy dropping dramatically, a rebellion in Chechnya, an embedded and audacious Mafia, and far too much vodka. China is socially paradoxical – ideologically communist but joining global capitalism through Hong Kong, 'special economic zones' and membership of the World Trade Organisation. The West (the USA, much of Europe, Australasia, Japan) is divided internally over protectionist economics and international politics. It is also faced with mass movements of impoverished people from the non-developed world searching for 'crumbs off the rich man's table', and the growing menace of terrorism after the 11 September 2001 bombing of the Twin Towers in New York. In response, the West is fortifying its borders to maintain its liberal-democratic (and economically advantageous) lifestyle founded on unfair trade regulations with the developing world.

Following the demise of the USSR, the USA is the only superpower. It has economic influence and military potential way beyond that of any of its State (The Russian Federation; Peoples' Republic of China) or super-State (for example, European Union, African Union, Association of South East Asian Nations, Andrean Pact, Organisation of Petroleum Exporting Countries) competitors. A doctrine of neoconservatism has been promulgated to support this New World Order of US supremacy. Specifically, signatories of The Project for a New American Century (PNAC), a group set up in 1997 including Dick Cheney (Vice President in the Bush Government) and Donald Rumsfeld (Defense Secretary in the Bush Government), declare (PNAC 2003):

'The history of the 20th century should have taught us that it is important to shape circumstances before crises emerge, and to meet threats before they become dire. The history of this century should have taught us to embrace the cause of American leadership. Our aim is to remind Americans of these lessons and to draw their consequences for today. Here are four consequences:

- *we need to increase defense spending significantly if we are to carry out our global responsibilities today and modernise our armed forces for the future;*
- *we need to strengthen our ties to democratic allies and to challenge regimes hostile to our interests and values;*
- *we need to promote the cause of political and economic freedom abroad;*
- *we need to accept responsibility for America's unique role in preserving and extending an international order friendly to our security, our prosperity, and our principles.'*

Robert Kagan (2003), however, argues that Europe and America view the world and its problems differently, owing to their respective histories and present influence globally. Europe has a tendency to support international agreements to resolve disputes within and between nations, and consequently spends a minimal proportion of its gross national product on armaments and armies. The USA, on the other hand, is willing to embark on, and pay for, the direct policing of the world and to carry this out unilaterally if necessary. This divergent world view has been all too evident in the case of the 2003 Iraqi War, when major European countries (specifically, France and Germany) disagreed vehemently with the USA over the 'liberation' of Iraq. The European exception, however, is the UK (along with Spain). The UK, because of its 'special relationship' historically, culturally and economically with the USA, and its fluctuating commitment to European unity, gave allegiance to the USA. Kagan points out, however, the main reason that France and Germany can opt out of *Machpolitik* (political persuasion through military might) is because the USA accepts this task and has, since World War 2, protected Europe. That is, France and Germany can enjoy its 'postmodern paradise' of liberalism, peace and diplomacy, and be critical of *Machpoltik*, only because the USA is there to act militarily.

Britain has been willing to indulge in a double standard: liberalism at home but *Machpolitik* abroad. However, even at home there is a double standard: liberalism has turned into post-liberalism. The New

World Order, initiated by the USA and supported by the UK, its 'special ally', is responding to a perceived threat to its dominance through measures (internment, economic sanctions and military invasions) that are intended forcibly to pacify 'evil axis' countries. Within many Western societies, but especially the USA and the UK, this atmosphere of 'toe the line or else' is reflected in the post-liberal policy of 'rights and responsibilities'. A direct link between the threat of (external) terrorism and (internal) social deviance is made overt. In these extracts from a speech by the British Home Secretary, delivered in New York, the connection of terrorist acts (the bombing of the Twin Towers) with 'antisocial behaviour' (for example, truancy, making a noise, dropping litter) are made explicit. Moreover, the Home Secretary made plain the move to a post-liberal governance and New World Order with the contention that (Western) freedom and democracy depend upon rights *and* responsibilities, security, stability and national/international control (Blunkett 2003):

'Those of a liberal political bent have not always accepted that security and freedom go hand in hand

'. . . The relationship between security and freedom is an issue pertinent to new international threats and also to our community life. Crime and anti-social behaviour destroy communities . . . [W]e have to ensure that people are safe and feel safe.

'. . . [T]errorists and terrorist acts cannot be escaped by any of us. They have engaged with us and therefore it is a necessity for new forms of engagement by us, which cross national boundaries.

'. . . [I]nsecurity, and the fear it brings, require humanity to share the task of providing international order and security.'

For reasons of security, freedoms are removed. For example, in the USA (both within its borders and in Guantanamo Bay, Cuba) and other Western countries such as the UK, Australia and Spain, emergency legislation has resulted in long-term or indefinite detention without trial or criminal charges for suspected terrorists (Norton-Taylor 2002, Valley 2003). Moreover, part of this (internal) post-liberal control is the surveillance and supervision of the 'mad' by psychiatry and P/MH nursing.

Conclusion

Post-liberal social control is now enacted in a style reminiscent of the Stasi era (the infamous Ministerium für Staatssicherheit in socialist East Germany) or as was predicted by George Orwell (Stuart 2003):

'Baxter, 42, is [litter] enforcement officer for Southwark Council in south London. His devotion to duty has seen him armed with a camera and

dictaphone when shopping with his daughter in case he spots any offenders. Such is his influence that, at the age of six, she grassed up her uncle for flinging a cigarette butt out of his car window, correctly identifying it as an 'enviro-crime'.

'. . . If he's on a dog fouling sting in the park, Baxter will don shades, combats and a baseball cap in order to blend in . . . Offenders who incur a fixed penalty and refuse to give their name and address are followed in relays back to their home or care by the undercover officers and then traced through records.

'. . . Baxter reveals another tactic up his anti-littering sleeve: Bin It to Win It. This campaign, which he devised himself, involves him stalking the streets armed with a klaxon and megaphone, and rewarding people who use the litter bins with a golden envelope containing £10 . . . It is questionable, however, as to how effective the campaign is. Baxter doesn't promote it, for fear of children hanging around litter bins waiting for the 'bald man' with the megaphone to appear.'

Surveillance is pervasive (monitoring not just deviants but all citizens), informants are omnipresent, and compliance to the New World Order mandatory. Am I suggesting that the future of the P/MH nurse is one with the nurse patrolling the streets on the lookout for any signs of 'madness', armed with a risk assessment form instead of camera and dictaphone, a syringe of medication instead of a fixed penalty, or a counselling intervention by megaphone positively reinforcing acceptable behaviour? Oh, if only it were possible to have this naked social control delivered with such focused commitment and role clarity! Can it be imagined, P/MH nursing with a patent mission and demonstrable practices? Nurses knowing what their job is about and given licence to carry it out?

No, of course this is self-parody!

What I am pointing out is that psychiatrists and P/MH nurses share a history, and a discourse. A fundamental constituent of this history and discourse is social control. Rather than complaining about the reality of their ties with, and the dominance by, psychiatry, the malcontents in P/MH nursing would be better occupied working with their medical allies to define the parameters of their social control role in the New World Order.

References

Blair T 2001 Third Way, Phase 2. Prospect Magazine. Online. Available: http://prospect-magazine.co.uk/highlights/opinion_blair_mar01/index. html

Blunkett D 2003 Securing our freedom; balancing security and liberty post 9/11. (Ref. 101/2003). Home Office, London. Oneline. Available: http://index.homeoffice.gov.uk/n_story.asp?item_id=439

Editorial 2003 Fine words cannot hide the fact that Blair's Third Way has lost its direction. The Independent, 12 July.

Fakhoury W 2000 Communication and information needs of a random sample of community psychiatric nurses in the UK. Journal of Advanced Nursing 32(47):871–880.

Foucault M 1971 Madness and civilisation. Tavistock, London.

Foucault M 1974 The order of things. Tavistock, London.

Giddens A 2000 The Third Way and its critics. Polity, Cambridge.

Gray N, Laing J, Noaks L 2002 Criminal justice, mental health and the politics of risk. Cavendish, London.

Kagan R 2003 Paradise and power: America and Europe in the New World Order. Atlantic, London.

Laurance J 2003 Record number of doctors banned for serious misconduct. The Independent, 29 July.

Morrall P A 1998 Mental health nursing and social control. Whurr, London.

Morrall P A 2000 Madness and murder. Whurr, London.

Morrall P A 2001 Sociology and nursing. Routledge, London.

Morrall P A 2002 Madness, murder, and social control. Mental Health Today, 23–25 August.

Morrall P A, Hazelton M 2003 Mental health: global policies and human rights. Whurr, London.

Nolan P 1993 A history of mental health nursing. Chapman Hall, London.

Norton-Taylor R 2002 Terror crackdown 'encourage repression'. The Guardian, 17 September.

Peay J 2003 Decisions and dilemmas: working with mental health law. Hart, Oxford.

Porter R 2002 Madness: a brief history. Oxford University Press, Oxford.

Project for the American Century 2003 http://www.newamericancentury.org

Rose N 2000 Government and control. British Journal of Sociology 40(2):321–339.

Scull A T 1993 The most solitary of afflictions: madness and society in Britain, 1700–1900. Yale University Press, New Haven.

Stuart J 2003 Fighting the dirty war. The Independent Review, 4 July.

Valley P 2003 The invisible. The Independent Review, 26 June. Project for the New American Century 2003 Statement of principles. Online. Available: http://www.newamericancentury.org/statementofprinciples.htm

Liam Clarke

Declaring conceptual independence from obsolete professional affiliations

Introduction

We need to dispose quickly the question of what nursing is. We mustn't dwell on it: it's been 'done to death' over the years and we are no closer to a definition than we were fifty years ago – albeit more confused. Still, it needs examining as it bears directly on the issue of professional independence. Psychiatric/mental health nurses, after all, do claim to practise nursing and, although nurses and nursing are different topics, such claims beg the question of what exactly is being practised. In most studies, P/MH nursing is side-stepped by general nurses who see questions of definition as exclusively theirs; that which distinguishes psychiatry is ignored. Matters are not helped by P/MH nurses who are reluctant to split from their general nursing cousins. True, a minority wish to enter the ranks of the psychotherapists. Yet the identification with *nursing* – both in theory and in practice – is still strong. Therefore, before making a case for P/MH nursing (by whatever name) as an independent profession, I will examine what nursing is.

Defining things

For over thirty years countless writers have wrestled with the question of what nursing is (in professional, ethical and/or clinical terms), with the unifying goal of distinguishing it from medicine. Many of these texts are American, but are not without influence in the UK. Indeed, the movement of British nurse education into the universities – even at preregistration levels – suggests a new-found identity no longer detached from mainstream education, no longer second rate. This is not to say that it *was* second rate, merely that it had come to be persuaded thus – by an overvaulting elite (Humphreys 1996) – such that acquiring academic credentials would improve its position. In examining nursing, I will critique three constructs – caring, knowledge and language – which infused the new thinking about nursing. I will then review a recent declaration by the Royal College of Nursing (RCN On-line) in the UK as a prelude to assessing the status of P/MH nursing in particular.

Caring

To say that nursing is caring is a tautology: it adds little to discussion. Undoubtedly, 'caring' literature has produced some well intentioned rhetoric about the compassionate propensities of nurses as well as an (idyllic) concept of nursing as a 'caring profession'. This has always sounded to me as if, somehow, other (allied) professions are less caring or not caring at all. For if one supposes that all medically based professions *are* caring (and why not?), what is to be gained in calling them this? But, of course, the intention is to separate nursing out, to distil nursing as uniquely equipped, possessed of an ethical duty to care.

The weakness of this position is demonstrated by Peter Allmark (1995), who says that it is not enough to care if you do not then say what you care about. Caring, in effect, can lead to outcomes, desirable and undesirable, depending on how you evaluate its consequences. For instance, I administer a lethal substance to someone in pain because I care; equally, someone strives to keep the same person alive because *they* care. Caring, in other words, is devoid of ethical content unless the object of its attention is stated. Allmark's point is ignored in much of the 'caring' literature, although it raises issues that advocates of caring ethics should address. However, this is unlikely as the latter favour continental philosophy and not the analytical methods of post-Enlightenment Western philosophy. In place of propositions from which arguments can be mounted and conclusions drawn, 'reasoning' emerges via interactions between people governed by a (variously described) ambience of caring coupled with beliefs about holism. This orientation has produced some of the most circuitous and self-deluded writing ever, with some nurse theorists struggling to attach (to nursing) new ways of knowing and experiencing. For example, Chinn & Kramer (1999, p 52) talk of *'personal knowing in nursing'* as being *'the inner experience of becoming a whole, aware, genuine, self'*, and continue: *'One does not know about the self, one strives simply to know the self'*. While there is nothing wrong with this as such, imagining its commonsense application within treatment settings becomes difficult. That concepts of self are themselves problematic is also set aside; more strange, however, is the unworldliness of this writing, its refusal to handle knowledge in ways that can be tested and argued over. Here is another quote taken from the holistic/caring axis in nursing (Rew 1996, p 66):

'Mercury [the metallic liquid] *symbolises, for me, the unity of life that I believe is a truth in nursing. The individual drops, in constant interaction with each other, at one moment appear separate and autonomous. In the next, they collide and collude, forming communities that appear to act as a whole, then separate, once again, into dozens of singular bodies scampering across a seemingly thoughtless and impenetrable surface'.*

Because nothing is asserted here, nothing can be argued. In a way it does create theoretical distance between nursing and medicine; it certainly makes nursing *sound* different. But it is an almost incomprehensible analogy: what is it meant to be analogous to? If medicine is as much about practice as theory – it is typically practised in hospitals and treatment centres – then theories that inform its practice must 'make sense' in these settings and it seems hard to reconcile this with the anti-medical attributes of holism. (That said, consumerism and 'putting patients first' policies have created a medical version of holism or, at least, of how governments see the future of medicine.) Nevertheless, early advocates of holism, because hostile towards medicine, envisaged nursing as preventive and community based. For the moment, let's say that non-medicalised caring – compassionate, empathic, sympathetic – can be a formidable part of nursing. What is questionable is its elevation to an 'ethics of caring' which, although well intended, is but a manoeuvre to promote a separate profession. This has fostered a false consciousness about academic reputation which sits uneasily with the working lives of most nurses. Indeed, there is as much evidence that nursing, particularly in institutions, is as uncaring as it is caring (Stanley et al 1999). One contemporary study of general hospital nursing in the UK found such practices as patients being denied drinks so as to remain continent or being left in wet beds (Carsons 1996). Most humiliatingly, day clothes were put over their night clothes so as to save dressing and undressing them.

Knowledge

In trying to get beyond models and theories – which have done little more than cosmetically enhance the credibility of nursing – RJ Holden (1996) defines a nursing knowledge base by injecting a concept of non-articulation. She says that propositional knowledge can be either articulated or non-articulated. In other words, nurses draw upon science (propositional, empirical data) but then subject it to (an inherent?) non-articulated perceptual knowledge. Apparently, the non-articulated refers to 'emotional knowing', which may be similar to empathy. Holden's account is a standard tactic: formulate a multifaceted hypothesis to do with knowledge; claim that nurses tap into the variety of forms it contains (but without argumentation as to what these are); and then conclude that nursing knowledge is fundamentally a prescience that lies beyond analytical examination. What practising nurses make of this is hard to fathom; certainly, human attitudes contain elements of emotion as well as of belief and it is feasible that we come to 'know' things, especially in ambiguous and difficult situations, in terms of 'trusting our instincts'. That said, knowledge that stems from hunches (or unresearched experience) is hardly sufficient in medical contexts (though it may 'work' in counselling relationships), and nurses need more if they are to attain epistemological credibility.

The problem here lies in the difference between truth and validity: making conclusions flow from strings of premises can look impressive but is relatively easy to do if you uncritically accept the initial premises. On my desk are six texts, all of which claim to define nursing, though none of them do. What they actually do is set out initial terms or premises that are *assumed* to be true and then use these as the basis for developments, conclusions and models, logically assembled, internally coherent, semiplausible, valid, but untrue. For instance:

Premise 1:	Nursing knowledge is emotion in relation (or some other speculative, unchallengeable function).
Premise 2:	Emotion in relation consists in engaging with patients emotionally.
Premise 3:	Nurses engage with patients emotionally.
Conclusion:	Nurses possess nursing knowledge.

For nurses, the difficulty in finding a knowledge base is that it cannot have medicine because another group already has that one. In any event, the object is to distance nursing from medicine and eschew, wherever possible, too clinical an emphasis on things. Holism seemed to do the trick and became the bedrock of UK nurse education courses in the 1990s, half of which, initially, were comprised of common foundation elements supposedly relevant to all nurses (the latter driving a stake through the heart of P/MH nursing as a speciality). Matters have sobered up somewhat but the crisis of identity continues, exacerbated by current demands that nurses extend their role into areas of medical intervention, such as diagnostics and prescription, which, until now, were the antithesis of holistic nurses and their antipathologisms. No doubt some will claim that including diagnostics and prescribing is evidence of holism at work! The essence of holism, however, was its spirited defence of 'patients as persons' in opposition to the perceived reductionism of medicine. Now we face a turnaround of significant proportions and the overall effect is of confusion and disarray. At the same time, the inclusion of medical functions is but the latest in a long line of 'inclusions', a progressive assimilation of 'outside' elements in the campaign for autonomy. For example, bringing sociology into nurse education courses held out the prospect that nurses might apply its analytical tools to their own history and current operations; what happened was that sociology was trumpeted as further evidence of nursing's holistic identity, yet another push in the long struggle to establish epistemological demarcation from medicine. Such moves, however, were less genuine attempts to define authentic relationships with patients and more a bid for traditional forms of power.

Language

The question of cultural groups *controlling* language or vice versa – the latter favoured by postmodernists – is important here. Professional nurses attend sick people in treatment settings where the dominant language is medical. That a holistic/experiential language could impede medical requirements (for the same patients) is improbable. A nursing language might influence practice, but only if it did not contradict medical prescription. This is not Brown & Crawford's (1999) view: they outline a nursing language/communication system, but apart from listing 'reflection' as its integral element they remain silent. They assert that the agendas of doctors and other groups *'may not be compatible with nursing philosophies'* (p 42).

These writers want nurses to seize upon 'the power of language' so as to author human behaviour, but they omit the philosophical distinction that denotes language as referring to real objects and issues in a society and its organisations. They take it for granted that we 'shape the world around us with language'; for many nurse-philosophers this is now a truism. In fact, linguistic constructions are often a *product* of culture and hierarchical systems, for example hospitals – a point well argued by some (Etzioni 1960, Gahagan 1984). Grant (2001) shows how power is 'built into the interpersonal and material structure of organisations and its influence is reflected in the ways in which its members are socialised'. This socialisation forces an acceptance of the mores of organisations; implicitly, that organisations deploy language so as to make sense of (and account for) behaviour within their boundaries. Neither is the wearying reiteration of 'primitive doctor' versus 'enlightened nurse' all that reassuring: yet it is this, typically, that drives calls for new 'nursing languages', a perception that 'medical language' is malevolent, iatrogenic and antihuman. And all of this within an overall contextual veneer of endorsement of multidisciplinary teamwork!

These, then, are the three elements – caring, knowledge and their respective articulation – that infuse definitions of nursing as well as discussions about its probable futures. We shall see how these are further distilled into a juxtaposition of, on the one hand, science and, on the other, experience. But first. . . .

A royal detour

In 2003, the Royal College of Nursing in the UK (On-Line) announced that it had defined nursing. No more tortuous tracts from would-be international nurse-philosophers on what nursing might mean – the denizens of Cavendish Square had finally cracked it. Now a sentence could begin: 'Nursing is . . .' and end ten or fifteen words later – succinct, informative and complete. Yes? Well, not quite. Here, in fact, is what they did. Tragically, they formed a committee. Advised by the Scottish Home and Health Department (1996, p 5) that *'the responsibilities of each professional group are quite clear – except for nursing, where there is a considerable variation in perception'*, they asserted that *'nurses must articulate what they do and ensure that the quality of their service is adequately communicated to patients to whom they owe a duty of care'*. This is interesting – to embark on a definition of nursing with unsubstantiated claims about 'duty' and 'care'. Although subsequently voicing a need to avoid media stereotypes of nursing, they seemed impervious that notions of 'duty' and 'care' are the basis of such stereotypes.

In fact, the committee's views are drenched in contradictions; it acknowledges Florence Nightingale's 1859 dictum: *'The elements of nursing are all but unknown'* and that this is still the case. Although skilled nursing makes a difference, it says, it remains impossible to say just what this is; what skills, for instance, improve a patient's condition. Contrasting nursing between relatives and professionals, the committee states that differences exist here but not, interestingly, in the tasks or levels of skill involved. Rather, differences lie in such things as *'clinical judgement, diagnosis, prescription, knowledge, evaluation'* (RCN 2003, p 4). In other words, the province of medicine is now misappropriated; true, the committee also mentions ethics and accountability, where important distinctions exist between professional and lay nurses. However, the core distinctiveness of nursing, as they see it, lies pre-eminently with 'clinical judgement'. The definition they give is as follows (RCN 2003, p 3):

'The use of clinical judgement in the provision of care to enable people to improve, maintain, or recover health, to cope with health problems, and to achieve the best possible quality of life, whatever their disease or disability, until death'.

This isn't bad: the sentiments are positive, life enhancing. In fact, most people could sign up for it – including relatives – if it wasn't for the first five words. These five words smack of medicine; their usage is where areas of conflict are most likely – conflict of role, judgement and responsibility. No one could detract from the rest of the definition; it is so encompassing that denying it would be to defer from humanity.

Clinical judgement confers on nurses responsibilities for the medical status of patients that go beyond being cognisant, in scientific terms, of what one is doing (for example, inserting a catheter); the issue now is about deciding *whether or not* to insert it. The two are different: whilst nurses have over time accrued clinical skills (some nurses may be more technically equipped than some doctors), does this mean that society is now prepared to confer diagnostic or prescriptive power upon them? Perhaps. My contention is that that changes their nursing identity, requiring as it does an altered definition of who they are. This already is happening; debates in the UK about National Health Service work-forces are intensifying, and changes in the roles and demarcations of traditional disciplines are increasing. Allen (2003, p 14) submits that most change is driven by *'policy, demand, labour markets and demography'*, to which he adds shortage of doctors and increasing patient numbers. As Farmer (1995, p 793) says: *'What better way* [to cut junior doctors' hours] *than to off load the more menial medical tasks on to nurses'*.

That said, changes, when (and as) they come, will be attributed to 'putting patients first', which has, as its justifying tenet, teamwork and the blurring of responsibilities for what until recently had been clearcut. Typical is a scheme being piloted at Kingston Hospital, Surrey, UK, where generic health care workers (usually nurses) are involved in tasks previously implemented by junior doctors. Amongst these are taking patient's histories, instigating tests, such as chest X-rays, and interpreting them, performing chest physiotherapy and prescribing certain drugs. One of the scheme's first graduates, Dave Flood, says (Waters 2003, p 17):

'The training has changed my mindset and my role is different in terms of knowledge and skills. Now I definitely see myself as a healthcare practitioner and not as a nurse' (emphasis added).

What emerges from this, as an account of a similar scheme suggests, is a straightforward extension of the medical team, one reason perhaps why existing medics are not antagonistic. Says Pearce; (2003, p 16): *'Doctors think medical emergency assistants are the best thing since sliced bread'*. It's no wonder they do, as if this is not the modern equivalent of the 'nurse as handmaiden' I don't know what is. These 'nursing' activities boil down to little more than a second layer of medical practice, what Elizabeth Farmer (1995, p 793) calls a marriage of convenience, whereby doctors continue to do what they have always done, which is hand over jobs to nurses:

'The fact that these new jobs might be a bit more technical does not alter the fundamental assumption . . . that nurses . . . are there to be used'.

The RCN Committee's predilection for clinical judgement gives a blessing to these developments. But using the word nurse like this is a misnomer. What really is happening is nurses *medically* prescribing within a context of economic necessity; it also, of course, reflects a desire (for some) to leave nursing. One final point here: prescriptive responsibilities mean forfeiting the advocacy/befriending role whereby nurses act on their patient's behalf. Nurses are fully implicated in administering medication to patients. To prescribe drugs, however, alters the relationship between the prescriber and the recipient. Assuming such a responsibility changes everything, especially in the context of the legal status of the recipient and their relative willingness to cooperate.

Debate

This debate is between those who look to personal experiences as central to understanding patients' and nurses' positions and those committed to (explanatory) biological data coupled with medical or psychological treatments. I will argue that, whatever the merits of the latter, it says little about what *nursing* is (although much about what 'it' may become), because its principles and practices have evolved outside nursing. The experiential position has equal difficulty in describing nursing, but it captures something of its meaning, something perhaps unique in its ethical mandate to respond to human ills *in the first instance*, even if lacking the wherewithal to cure or assuage those ills. Having said that, *some* knowledge, over and above compassionate responding, is needed – if only to avoid injuring patients. Until recently, that knowledge was medically supervised. Even if this supervision was frequently superficial, the assumption was that nurses' medical interventions were subsidiary to their defining role of managing the basic physical and emotional needs of patients. I have indicated the sorts of problems that the experiential position elicits: it *seems* to locate nursing independently (outside medicine), but as an empathic undertaking, hardly as a profession and not fundamentally different to lay nursing. The dawning realisation of this, I believe, is now shunting nurses towards the acquisition of a sturdier medical base.

Confused?

As a generalisation, nurses are confused and, unsurprisingly, bones of irresolvable contention abound. The disjunction between the experiential and medicalist positions is formidable and as Keen (2003, p 34) notes: *'it's certainly difficult to imagine both parts of the conjoined craft surviving together'*.

Kitson (1996) observes that nursing's enduring image is of subordination to medicine: when it affects a scientific (quasi-medical) visage and sports this as 'advanced nursing practice', nurse leaders *'effectively alienate the majority of nurses who give care'* (p 1649). That (basic) care is only rarely articulated in professional or public domains; this hardly surprises as *'Nursing's persistent inability to grasp the nettle of reconciling our technical skills with our caring skills is at the heart of the matter'* (Kitson 1996, p1650).

Like Keen, Kitson ruefully suspects that these two factions will split (resulting in a new 'therapeutic' nursing), less through malevolence than through ineptitude. Parker (2002) also calls for both dimensions to combine so as to offer the best of both worlds. But why should they? What if they are logically incompatible; what if, in certain settings, one naturally takes precedence over the other – settings inhabited by sick people, for example? Kitson will have none of it (Kitson 1996, p 1651):

'The future could hold the reconciliation of our two sides. It could herald the dawn of health care systems around the world committed to promoting health and wellbeing instead of systems that treat illness'.

Naturally, these systems will be run by 'advanced practice nurses', Kitson says, 'supported by doctors, nurses and family members'. So there it is: nurses *and* advanced nurses, nurses *supported* by doctors, a world without illness – and no mention of the fact that when nurses previously practised health prevention in the UK their name (and status) was altered to health visitor!

Psychiatric/mental health nursing failures

Kitson's fusion and 'great advance' has yet to materialise; this is particularly true for P/MH nursing, where different perspectives have actually become more pronounced and with a marked absence of anything resembling a coherent strategy. Hopton (1997) traces this failure to P/MH nurses' refusal to address historical, structural or ideological problems. Specifically he lists three items: the critique of institutional care, the emergent antipsychiatry of the 1960s and 1970s, and the damning findings of government inquiries into nursing abuses across roughly the same period. P/MH nurses missed the boat of autonomous practice by failing to appreciate that antipsychiatry might have helped them develop approaches of their own. They stood by while others provided social and intellectual appraisals of institutions, failing to see connections between institutional abuses and the medicalisation of human problems. In the absence of a cohesive framework they continue to flail about, latching on to person-centredness, biological models or user movements as a means of bolstering their identity. User movements, of course, favour person-centred approaches, reserving their fire for what they see as the oppressive (detention and medication) elements of psychiatry in which nurses, of course, are implicated. Understandably, service users act from perspectives usually dependent on individual experience. This is a problem for user movements: how to critique things from outside individual experience and account for a range of perspectives – perhaps, even, those where psychiatry have 'satisfied customers'. However, it may be too early for that (still too many axes to grind), but it needs doing eventually. Or does it? It may be that users may *choose* to operate from outside psychiatric systems where, of course, they are perfectly free to say what they like. For the moment, it is premature for nurses to affiliate with user movements that, as part of psychiatric systems, proclaim assumptions based upon individual and possibly egocentric perspectives. Such perspectives are not the same thing as phenomenological accounts of distress, and so may be related to differently by psychiatric nurses.

Returning to the question of P/MH nurses not appreciating antipsychiatry, this is debatable. That movement would shortly lie in ruins anyway and one wonders how it could have influenced developments in P/MH nursing. Others, though, see things differently. Ritter (1997) states that, since the 1970s, nurses have challenged their own legitimacy, taking it as read that P/MH nursing was repressive and immoral, a central tenet of antipsychiatry. This denial of legitimacy essentially pooh-poohed the validity of treatment interventions. According to Ritter (1997, p 97):

'Until psychiatric nurses centre their activities in a legitimating moral framework any attempts by them to justify their interventions by research into effectiveness will be worthless'.

By 'legitimating moral framework' is meant close liaison with 'collaborative' medical workers, both in practice and in research. Far from ignoring antipsychiatry, says Ritter, nurses took from it, and as such played down discrete, measurable interventions, disregarding a (moral) requirement to account for their practice in evidence-based terms; in this instance, an evidence base settled on epistemological rather than experiential frameworks.

Two versions

Thus we are left with two versions of P/MH nursing. One sees nurses in collaborative research and practice, and apparently disdaining notions of separatism. This view promotes the assumption of wider medical/psychological responsibilities. An alternative view seeks independence by denying medical legitimacy in favour of concerns about the socio-political-cultural status of patients and an advocacy function that looks to their general welfare. This invites a further point about antipsychiatry. This was, at best, a philosophical exercise about the nature of mental illness, but it failed to examine its social implications. When it tried to, in the family studies of David Cooper (1972) for instance, it was always a critique of 'The Family' and never about how actual families fared within class and other demographic boundaries. If antipsychiatry threw down a gauntlet to cherished diagnostic values (and so it did, brilliantly), it did not make its criticisms relevant to everyday practice. P/MH nurses may have been affected by some of its ideas, but also instinctively recognised its antipragmatism – its basically philosophical (speculative) nature.

Insightful obeisance

I believe that P/MH nurses *do* read the changes (albeit they seldom ring them). In the case of antipsychiatry, they *did* recognise its significance, and rejected it, but not by working through antipsychiatric literature or attending conferences and seminars. No: they had *come* to psychiatry with beliefs about mental illness that stemmed from everyday socialisation. While some were fascinated with antipsychiatry, the majority continued to prop up a (broadly conceived) medical model. Some nurses have difficulty in accepting that nursing plays such a supportive role, but what they overlook is that contained within that role is an implicit acceptance of the *appropriate*ness of medical governance. The way in which this governance is played out changes: professionals are nowadays on first name terms, and general relationships display a surface collegiality. However, changes in etiquette do not reflect alterations in power relationships and, whilst devolving medical responsibilities to nurses may seem like progression, its effect will be to enmesh nurses further within medical frameworks where, ultimately, power is hierarchical and grounded in bioscientific principles. The whole thing is wrapped up in a pragmatism that is embedded in the daily practice of psychiatry: the perceived necessity of its operations in society.

Summing up

The history of nursing models is littered with discontinuity and despair at the lack of a unifying theme or cohesive strategy. If anything, what fused these models was a negative: the search for an ever-elusive nursing knowledge. Insofar as this takes a scientific turn it promotes distance between patients and nurses, whereas holism (arguably) demolishes abstract barriers, replacing them with the balm of interpersonal relationships. In effect, stalemate is reached, the irreconcilability of these approaches becoming clear in relation to nursing practice: gradually the nurse as holistic carer is giving way to the nurse as medical or psychological therapist.

The RCN committee had noted the change, but cautioned that extended roles *'fail to show the particular contribution that nursing brings'* (Royal College of Nursing 2003, p 5). They noted the confusion between extended nurses' responsibilities (into medicine) as against expansions of the *nursing* role. Quick to differentiate these, the committee compared social service staff (in caring for the elderly) and learning/mental disabilities nurses, regretting the lack of clarity of the latter's role. This is disingenuous, as anyone in the UK who recalls the Jay Committee (1979) will know. This committee investigated the appropriateness of nursing for people with learning/mental disabilities and concluded that it wasn't! If such people are by definition not ill (and they aren't), then they do not need nurses (and they don't). The Jay Committee recommended absorbing learning/mental disabilities nurses into a general social care provision. Violently rejected at the time, this has in practice come to pass, even if some of those involved obstinately cling to the title 'nurse'.

P/MH nurses link more closely to the criteria that constitute illness and thus also medicine. This is not to minimise sociological and psychological contributions to understanding mental illness, and nurses can take comfort that psychiatry has assimilated these to some extent. That said, a resurgent interest in biological aspects of behaviour has inspired a challenge to social psychiatry, a reassigning of aetiological primacy to biochemistry and genetics. This debate has implications for how P/MH nurses define themselves, as well as adding to the difficulty of nursing definitions overall. If traditional descriptions of nursing have, like the RCN Committee, indemnified nursing as synonymous with general nursing, then introducing P/MH nursing spices things up considerably. For one thing, a knowledge base, derived from psychology or the psychotherapies, is now included and *is* genuinely problematic when considered in purely medical terms. In general nursing the holistic position has to contend with the dominant language and technology of medical treatment settings and does not undermine or diminish that dominance. And, while the move to nurse prescribing in the UK extends nurses' responsibilities, this is palpably a medical and not a nursing extension; indeed, it sustains and strengthens medical frameworks. In other words, whether adopting holism or embracing prescribing, general nursing connects with, and is inescapably influenced by, medicine. In essence:

'Nursing is neither a profession nor a vocation; it is neither a science nor an art. Nursing is a job of work, the limits of which are defined largely by medicine, which at its best is carried out with competence, displays respect for persons, and aims to achieve the best possible levels of health'
(Lucas 1993, p 24)

My view is that this does not describe P/MH nursing, which differs insofar as many of its activities are not authentically medical at all. For example, cognitive therapy and other psychological interventions are not the province of psychiatry – they are psychology's children – and are practised independently of any medical model. This is the difference: unlike general nursing, adopting these practices does not require a liaison with medicine. Neither does their absorption reinforce the nursing role. For those who say that it does – that the practice of psychotherapy leaves their nursing status unaffected – my response is that they continue as P/MH nurses in that they continue to be employed as such. The typical response to *this* is that nurses bring personable qualities to bear on client relationships that are beyond the province of non-nurse therapists. But this is straightforward arrogance: there is no evidence that nurses possess inherent qualities of humanity any more than other groups or that they imbue, for instance, cognitive therapy with empathic dimensions beyond the reach of other therapists.

Finale

- For the mass of nurses, psychiatric/mental health and general, the 'job of work' quote (above) suffices.
- For general nurses who espouse holistic care, this does not represent a discrete separation from medical practice.
- For general nurses who acquire wider medical responsibilities, this also militates against a discrete discipline.
- For P/MH nurses who acquire prescriptive or diagnostic responsibilities, they too will remain locked within medical frameworks.
- The limitations of holistic practice apply to P/MH also.
- For P/MH nurses who practice psychological therapies, this can represent a separation from medicine.

However, in this case, there must and needs to be an abandonment of the nursing identity and the legendary baggage that goes with it. This is not an idea that most P/MH nurses relish, and they will continue their confused (love/hate) relationship with (and within) clinical psychiatry. Those wishing to separate might experience difficulties renegotiating their employment contract, but they could at least make a start by declaring conceptual independence from professional affiliations that are no longer as relevant as they were.

References

Allen D 2003 Wings of change. Nursing Standard 17(33):14–17.
Allmark P 1995 Can there be an ethics of caring? Journal of Medical Ethics 21:19–24.
Brown B, Crawford P 1999 Putting the debate on nursing language in context. Nursing Standard 14(1):41–43.
Carsons M 1996 An investigation of factors influencing the care older people receive in community hospitals. MPhil thesis, Anglia Polytechnic University.
Chinn P L, Kramer L K 1999 Theory and nursing: integrated knowledge development, 5th edn. Mosby, London.
Cooper D 1972 The death of the family. Penguin, Harmondsworth.

Etzioni A 1960 Interpersonal and structural factors in the study of mental hospitals. Psychiatry 23:13–22.

Farmer E 1995 Medicine and nursing. British Journal of Nursing 4(14):793–794.

Gahagan J 1984 Social interaction and its management. Methuen, London.

Grant A 2001 Psychiatric nursing and organisational power: rescuing the hidden dynamic. Journal of Psychiatric and Mental Health Nursing 8:173–188.H

Holden R J 1996 Nursing knowledge: the problem of the criterion. In: Kikuchi J F, Simmons H, Romyn D, eds. Truth in nursing inquiry. Sage, London, p 19–35.

Hopton J 1997 Towards a critical history of mental health nursing. Journal of Advanced Nursing 492–500.

Humphreys J 1996 English nurse education and the reform of the National Health Service. Journal of Educational Policy 6:644–679.

Jay Committee 1979 Report of the Committee of Enquiry into Mental Handicap Nursing (The Peggy Jay Report). HMSO, London.

Keen T 2003 Post-psychiatry: paradigm shift or wishful thinking? A speculative review of future possibles for psychiatry. Journal of Psychiatric and Mental Health Nursing 10:29–37.

Kitson A 1996 Does nursing have a future? British Medical Journal 313(7022):1647–1651.

Lucas J 1993 The nature of nursing. Health Care Analysis 1:23–25.

Parker J M 2002 The art and science of nursing. In: Daly J, Speedy S, Jackson P, Darbyshire P, eds. Contexts of nursing: an introduction. Blackwell, Oxord, p 22–35.

Pearce L 2003 Handing over. Nursing Standard 17(22):14–17.

Rew L 1996 The individual as a measure of truth. In: Kikuchi JF, Simmons H, Romyn D, eds. Truth in nursing inquiry. Sage, London, p 55–67.

Ritter S 1997 Taking stock of psychiatric nursing. In: Tilley S, ed. The mental health nurse: views of practice and education. Blackwell Science, Oxford, p 94–117.

Royal College of Nursing 2003 Defining nursing. Online. Available: www.rcn.org.uk accessed 2004

Scottish Home and Health Department 1996 The role and function of the professional nurse. HMSO, Edinburgh.

Stanley N, Manthorpe J, Penhale B, eds 1999 Institutional abuse: perspectives across the life course. Routledge, London.

Waters A 2003 First of a new breed. Nursing Standard 17(33):16–17.

Commentary

Jon Allen

In both of the preceding debates the authors, despite claiming to align themselves to different sides of this debate, appear to present challenging arguments about the inability of nursing to identify and assert a robust, discrete, professional identity based upon the usual building blocks of professional status. The first chapter provided what seemed to me a disturbingly accurate analysis of the motivations of what the author termed the 'malcontents' denial of the relationship between psychiatry and psychiatric nursing'. The subsequent analysis of the historical development of psychiatry and psychiatric nursing put nursing's difficult relationship with psychiatry and with itself into an evolutionary context. It gave some insights into how the roles that people called psychiatric nursing play out in the world of health care have, and might develop, as a response to developing health policy. The further emphasis on the socially ascribed roles and responsibilities of state-funded mental health services, and those who work within them, illustrates some of the futility of what seems a collective grandiose delusion of psychiatric nurses, namely that they have some inherent right to define for themselves an identity other than that socially ascribed. It is also clearly asserted that, although continued role developments are leading to nurses taking on more medical tasks and developing more areas of technical expertise and role autonomy, the hard reality is that real power will continue to lie in the hands of doctors.

Importantly the second chapter acknowledges that for some (most?) nurses, nursing is merely a job of work, defined by the expedients of the day. This chapter bursts open the nonsensical attempts to define nursing as having some special claim to the concept of caring, and having special abilities to handle tacit, intuitive and emotional knowledge within caring relationships. Powerfully, the author asserts that, of course, caring is not the sole province of nurses, and indeed there are many examples where nurses clearly have not shown caring characteristics. The author points to nursing academics' ability to engage in all sorts of pseudoscience and some of the poor and confusing attempts to philosophise about nursing. This author clearly identifies nursing and particularly psychiatric nursing as being beyond any meaningful definition of itself by reference solely to itself (albeit that they are supposedly arguing the discrete disciplines case). However, the argument is made that nursing does not only have to tie itself to psychiatry, but a more promising future lies in psychiatric nursing defining itself on psychotherapeutic lines, traditionally the province of psychology. The first author, however, argued that psychiatry is more eclectic and has a survival mechanism of rejecting or absorbing.

Psychotherapies have clearly been absorbed into the world of psychiatry. Between them, these chapters unpack some of the complex issues and tensions inherent in trying to define psychiatric/mental health nursing. Both ultimately assert that nursing has to be defined in relationship to another discipline (e.g. medicine) in the broadest sense, or psychology in a narrower psychotherapeutic sense.

Despite these complex issues and tensions, both chapters seem to fall into the trap that a definition of nursing as an all-embracing concept that brings coherence, unity and historical stability to all the things that nurses might find themselves doing, has to be found. The subsequent conclusion is that this cannot be done and therefore that all that can be done is to define nursing by its relationship with a 'real' discrete discipline such as medicine or psychology. However, I am sure all will agree that both debates are imperfect and still only partly define the job of work done by some nurses.

Empirically there is a discrete discipline of nursing that is not dependent on medicine or other disciplines, and can be identified as having historically stable characteristics, its own knowledge base, and so forth. However, not all nurses nurse, and not all nursing is done by those legally allowed to call themselves nurses. (I suspect this is true of medicine, in that not all diagnosis of illness and prescription of treatments is done by those legally allowed to call themselves doctors, and so on, across all professional groups.)

All disciplines are best defined by the most fundamental element of what their job role is; for example, car mechanics fix cars, and the fact that they might also provide retail services does not make this an inevitable part of defining their role as mechanics. Inevitably one has to tolerate the ambiguity that people develop competencies, abilities and responsibilities outside of traditional roles, and over time these are instituted into training and so forth; consequently the world of health care, or any other area of work, becomes messy and confusing.

The fundamental identity of nursing throughout history has been the provision of personal, 'hands on' care, doing the personal things that people cannot do for themselves because of their illness or disability, such as washing, dressing, eating, and so forth. This is most clearly expressed with the seriously ill with high levels of dependency. That this exists independently of other disciplines is self-evident through the fact that the provision of this care is not dependent on the existence of any other discipline or its knowledge base. Like all other disciplines, of course, nursing can learn and advance by means of the findings of other disciplines' research and practices. This independent role of nursing is articulated in a theoretical way in the text of nurse theorists such as Henderson (1966) and Roper (1976).

Working upwards from this fundamental defining base, one starts to be able to identify the additional tiers of work that nurses have taken on over the years. These have been driven by emergent technologies and economic and political expediencies. For example, as models of understanding particular diseases have emerged, nurses have been a useful workforce to ask for their observations in order to help diagnosis. As various physical and psychological treatments have emerged, again nurses, owing to their relative prevalence, affordability and constant presence, have been used as a workforce to provide or assist with these treatments. This process inevitably continues to develop, with a constant handing down of new roles and responsibilities from doctors and psychologists to nurses, and from nurses to health care assistants. Inevitably the more traditional, power-holding professions have led these processes. An excellent case example of this can be seen in the development of nurse behaviour therapists (Marks et al 1977).

In my opinion, the ultimate reality that psychiatric/mental health nurses have to face, along with every one else, is that in the main, and especially in most of Europe and Australasia, we are part of a state-sponsored health care system, in which people with health problems expect a range of services to be delivered, and are willing only through taxation to pay so much for such services. They expect their illnesses to be diagnosed and treated; while ill they expect to be helped, with compassion, to do the things they cannot do for themselves. They expect to be given enough information and support to manage any longer-term complications or issues arising from their illness. The workforce employed to provide these services is deployed in the light of the skills and abilities they bring, each of which has its own market value. That certain professional titles attach themselves to these various work tasks merely reflects the current division of health care labour at the primary entry points into the world of health care work. That the roles each of these professional groupings play becomes increasingly blurred, post qualification, is an inevitable consequence of how people develop in their work lives, and the practicalities of providing services where customer demand for skills outstrips an economically restricted supply.

Ultimately the real power of who decides who does what lies with the employer (the State in the above example, but equally an independent provider in other situations). Nurses, doctors and the leaders of other disciplines may seek to influence these agendas, but ultimately the employers decide. In today's National Health Service in the UK, for example, there are radical movements in role configurations and responsibilities. Ultimately all disciplines have to relate to the health and social care and treatment needs of the people using the services. What should be done to meet these needs is increasingly being determined by evidence-based guidelines and care pathways. All that will matter will be who has the skills to deliver the element of care and treatment provided most efficiently and effectively. We are already seeing, even today, that this is not always by people who call themselves *doctor* or *nurse*. The National Institute for Mental Health England (NIMHE) workforce team issued a range of guidance on new role developments, and the core competencies required of the mental health workforce (Hope 2004). This and other developments, such as the Southampton (UK) assistant mental health practitioner programme, illustrate that, as some psychiatric/mental health nursing academics sit around trying to define psychiatric/mental health nursing's place in the world of mental health work, others are getting on and just doing it!

More radical change is on our doorsteps. In the UK, the Royal College of Psychiatrists and the NIMHE have developed proposals for a radical review of the role of psychiatrists (NIMHE et al 2004). Within this document is recognition that consultants do not have to hold responsibility for all the clients seen by the teams for whom they work. In addition, there is an acceptance of the need to move away from the need to have restrictive population-based ratios per consultant psychiatrist. This heralds huge opportunities for change and challenges traditional professional demarcations. It will do this by freeing up employers' cash and allowing them to think differently about the workforce and skills they need to meet the needs of those who use their services. They will no longer be restricted to having to think in terms of *how many doctors* and *how many nurses*. The traditional professional power bases will be significantly changed, and the professional architecture of mental health care that has been built over the last 100 years will not just be given a face lift, but will be fundamentally redeveloped.

The potential impact of this one national policy change illustrates where the real power in professional relationships lies. If the political will exists to change the way we work or what we are responsible for, there is apparently little that even the most powerful of our professional groups can do to resist. The language of modernisation and the moral high ground of service user-centred services compel even the most conservative to lay aside resistance and work outside traditional demarcations. Of course, one then must ask what motivates political will to change traditional ways of working, and this inevitably brings us to service users as the emergent power-holders. So, rather than the socially policed of the first chapter in this debate, in a strange twist of fate those who use mental health services have become the puppet-masters, with an increasingly firm grasp of the mental health workforce strings – another debate for another day, I think.

References

Henderson V 1966 The nature of nursing. MacMillan, New York.

Hope H 2004 The ten essential shared capabilities – a framework for the whole of the mental health workforce. Department of Health, London.

Marks I M, Hallam R S, Connolly J, Phillpott R 1977 Nursing in behavioural psychotherapy: an advanced clinical role for nurses. Royal College of Nursing of the United Kingdom, London.

National Institute for Mental Health England, Consultative Working Party, Royal College of Psychiatrists, Department of Health 2004 New ways of working for psychiatrists in multidisciplinary and multi-agency contexts. Department of Health, London.

Roper N 1976 Clinical experience in nurse education. Churchill Livingstone, London.

Heterogeneous or homogeneous: should psychiatric/mental health nursing have a specialist or generic preparation?

CHAPTER 6

Generic nurses: the nemesis of psychiatric/mental health nursing?

John R Cutcliffe & Hugh P McKenna

CHAPTER 7

Debating the integration of psychiatric/mental health nursing content in undergraduate nursing programmes

Olive Younge & Geertje Boschma

Commentary

Stephen Tilley

Editorial

One's views, opinions and even values are likely to be influenced by one's experiences. Indeed, if one was to draw upon psychodynamic theory, then one's formative experiences have a huge influence on each of us throughout our lives. It is thus not surprising that impassioned, yet seemingly polarised, positions exist with respect to the most appropriate preparation for psychiatric/mental health nurses. Even a cursory examination of the international variety of approaches to preregistration preparation will illustrate that many different versions exist, perhaps the most notable difference being the choice between specialist or generic programmes. Accordingly, this has given rise to articulate and passionate debate, often from individuals advocating an approach to preparation that they themselves undertook. Impassioned arguments can, because of their very passionate nature, at times be lacking in supporting empirical evidence; however, we wholeheartedly welcome and embrace such arguments. For some, academic writing is synonymous with objectivity, dispassionate inquiry and balance, but the editors share Rolfe's (2000) view, that polemic writing is not only stimulating and interesting but also provokes debate.

The evidence and value of such polemic writing is brought out in both of these chapters. John Cutcliffe and Hugh McKenna use emotionally laden, challenging expressions and terms, and suggest that generic nurse preparation threatens the very essence of P/MH nursing – a polemical view if ever there was one. Similarly, Olive Younge and Geertje Boschma remind us that 'there is a place for specialisation in nursing but only after the student has a solid grounding in basic nursing, such as health promotion, basic nursing care and health assessment', quite clearly a 'one-sided' and confrontational view. Interestingly, although Steve Tilley's thoughtful commentary points out that *'each* [chapter] *adopts a position that would rule the other out'*, offering these polarised positions may, paradoxically, stimulate and provoke rather than stifle a most thorough and meaningful debate. It has been noted that nursing (as an academe) and nurses per se have, traditionally at least, been prone to soliciting balanced points of view (Clarke 2000). In so doing, it seems that nurses do not wish to be regarded as being unable to appreciate (or understand) the merits of the 'other side'. Clarke (2000) goes on to point out the crucial difference between choosing a 'side' because of the lack of *ability* to see both sides (ergo – ignorance) and because of the *willingness* to uphold certain views (purposeful choice).

There are many hitherto unanswered questions related to or arising from the debate about appropriate preparation, such as: why have these educational trajectories developed in the way they have in certain countries and differently in others? Whose interests are being served by retaining the preparation in one form or another? Which set of (or rather, whose) interests takes precedence in informing these decisions (when the interests of the workforce planners [employers] cannot be reconciled with the needs of service users)? When one begins to consider these and other important questions, the ramifications of any eventual decisions emanating from this debate begin to become clear. In essence, the ramifications include: will P/MH nurses still exist twenty years from now? As a result, we applaud the authors, irrespective of which 'side' they wish to champion, for writing passionate, compelling, polemical arguments, as these are critical debates that absolutely require such qualities and feelings.

References

Clarke L 2000 Necessary debates: the need for controversy in mental health. Journal of Psychiatric and Mental Health Nursing 7:363–370.

Rolfe G 2000 Write! now! Journal of Psychiatric and Mental Health Nursing 7:467–474.

John R Cutcliffe & Hugh P McKenna

Generic nurses: the nemesis of psychiatric/mental health nursing?

Introduction

After more than a hundred years of practice, psychiatric/mental health (P/MH) nurses around the world find themselves in a position of uncertainty. According to Duffy & Lee (1998), on the one hand these nurses are grasping the opportunity to enhance their role and develop professional autonomy, while on the other aspects of their role are being threatened by an erosion or loss of their professional status. Such a position has led some to assert that P/MH nursing is deeply immersed in a crisis of legitimacy. Several authors (Huxley 1995, Chan & Rudman 1998, Gournay 1998, Norman 1998) argue that central to this issue is the possible introduction of the generic nurse and the potential diminution or dilution that this could have on P/MH nursing. Indeed, the review of nurse education undertaken by the United Kingdom Central Council (UKCC – which has now become the Nursing and Midwifery Council) highlighted that one of the key issues it considered was whether a cross-discipline approach should be adopted. It is noteworthy that UK P/MH nursing authors appear to be the ones 'leading the charge' where this debate is concerned. This is not entirely surprising given that generic nurse preparation is the norm in some countries already, for instance North America and Australia (Gournay 1998, Norman 1998). However, the issue is not exclusive to the UK, and neither is it an 'esoteric' point: the issue is a genuine polemic with wide-reaching ramifications, particularly on future workforce structures. It is somewhat naïve, therefore, to think that considerations of future workforce structures would not have regard to the emergence (or deployment) of a generic nurse.

This is especially poignant when one factors in the current international shortage of qualified P/MH nurses. Drawing upon evidence from a country where the majority of its undergraduate (preregistration) nurse programmes follow the 'generic model' provides some compelling insights. In 1998, the education committee of the Canadian Federation of Mental Health Nurses issued a position paper (Chan et al 1998) which declared that the committee was concerned about the quantity and quality of undergraduate P/MH nurse educational preparation. Further, the evidence was that, when Canadian nursing students had an option to elect a psychiatric rotation (clinical placement), they did not do so because *'P/MH nursing is not an area in which they choose to practice in after graduation'* (p 2, original emphasis). Perhaps more worryingly, despite the claims of some universities, there is also compelling evidence that some generic nursing education models are underpinned by the belief that nursing students need not have specific clinical experiences on psychiatric placements. Such models purport that psychiatric nursing skills can be learned in any setting. This has led to the situation where, in many Canadian colleges and university schools of nursing, psychiatric or mental illness rotations are not required (Chan et al 1998). Furthermore, even when psychiatric specific clinical rotations are required, students spend a cursory amount of time on clinical placement and, instead, have a disproportionate amount of time dedicated to medical and surgical placements. For example, the current situation at a university in northern British Columbia is that undergraduate nursing students can spend as little as six days out of four years on a psychiatric clinical placement. Even then, this time is divided between various clinical placements (e.g. substance misuse, community mental health, acute inpatient psychiatry). This is by no means the only Canadian example of disproportionate underrepresentation of psychiatric nursing (both theoretical and clinical) content in generic nursing programmes. Accordingly, there is a body of evidence that indicates two things. First, even in the best case scenario, generic programmes contain little mental health nursing content. Second, some generic programmes have abandoned mental health nursing altogether – in some ways, this might be regarded as a more 'honest' position. This evidence indicates a tentative link between generic nurse preparation and a resulting national and international shortage of P/MH nurses.

That P/MH nurses should lose their specialist status (in the UK) and become generic nurses is based on the argument that there is compelling evidence to support the introduction of multiskilling and cross-training (Norman 1998). Yet opponents of such an argument maintain that there is something crucial and unique in P/MH nursing that is distinct and worth preserving (Nolan 1993). Nonetheless, the literature is, at best, unclear regarding the precise nature of this alleged uniqueness. The present authors assert that this lack of precision is one of the problems. If P/MH nurses are unable to articulate what their contribution is, and expound the nature of this uniqueness, then arguably it is more difficult to defend this distinctiveness. Accordingly, by reviewing the relevant literature, such as it is, this chapter makes some attempts to articulate and explicate the distinctiveness to which Nolan (1993) refers. Thus, we first consider whether P/MH nursing has a sense of self. Following this we describe what we understand the distinctiveness of P/MH nursing to be under the headings:

- The contribution of P/MH nurses
- The action component of P/MH nursing
- The human component of P/MH nursing
- The collaborative component of P/MH nursing.

This review is summarised by the identification of eight alleged elements of uniqueness. We then turn our attention to how the introduction of a generic nurse may affect this alleged uniqueness, and conclude by offering a brief strategy that might help preserve the uniqueness of P/MH nursing.

Does psychiatric nursing have a 'sense of self'?

To address whether or not P/MH nursing is unique, it is worth considering whether it has a sense of what it is about and what it does. Although P/MH nurses have developed some models for P/MH nursing, most available theories and models of nursing do not focus specifically on the unique context of psychiatric nursing care. Additional arguments submit that P/MH nursing does not have a clear sense of what it is about or what it does, and that P/MH nurses' own uncertainty about themselves and their skills has obstructed the freedom of being all that they can be with clients. Similarly, the range of activities that are alleged to be in clients' best interests cause many of the difficulties that P/MH nurses have in agreeing about what they do, let alone what they ought to do.

Perhaps these are some of the reasons why arguments are made for P/MH nursing to ally its training and practice with other specialities of nursing. Maybe we lack a real sense of our collective self; if so, it is worth considering why there is an absence of this sense of self. One possibility is that the world in which P/MH nurses live and work is one personified by ambiguity (Ryan 1997, Cutcliffe & Goward 2000). The terms used to describe the phenomena of mental distress are, at best, diverse: for instance, there is a lack of clarity between such terms as mental health and mental illness. Similarly, many of the processes and outcomes of mental health nursing are not wholly congruent with fixed, rigid and predictable views of the world. Much of mental health practice involves dealing with situations in which certainty does not exist, for example the problem of assessing and responding to aggressive behaviour within a context of the ambiguity of the madness/ badness divide.

Additionally, many people suffering from some form of mental health problem may not subscribe to a rigid, positivistic based approach to care, wherein diagnosis leads directly to a treatment that, in turn, has a predictable outcome. Using schizophrenia as an example, a not insignificant number of recent reviews of a large body of evidence cast considerable doubt on the reliability, the construct validity, the predictive validity and the aetiological specificity of the diagnosis of schizophrenia. If there is a significant degree of uncertainty regarding the very nature of the condition and the notion of schizophrenia is rejected as a meaningful scientific construct, then it could be regarded as somewhat inappropriate and premature to adopt a treatment paradigm that is fixed or rigid.

Furthermore, the nature of what constitutes credible and useful knowledge for practice, and the nature of evidence to underpin practice, both add to the position of uncertainty (Nolan 1993). Given the extent of the current empirical knowledge base of P/MH nursing, it is not surprising that, at times, P/MH nurses are unable to justify their practice with the kind of evidence offered by a randomised control trial of a treatment or intervention. Neither could they always underpin their practice with the evidence produced form longitudinal studies. Yet there is a well established alternative view that argues that such evidence is not the only source of valid knowledge that P/MH nurses draw upon.

It is not surprising that, in a world where ambiguity is the axiom, many nurses lack a shared vision of their uniqueness. Nonetheless, the presence of this uncertainty does not appear to be a hindrance for P/MH nursing practice. Learning to operate in a position of limited certainty is an essential part of becoming an effective P/MH nurse (Cutcliffe & Goward 2000). The skilled P/MH nurse is influenced by an unconscious perception of chaos as their guide to understanding the human condition, and as such does not necessarily seek resolution of all life's uncertainties. It is possible that this ability to survive in clinical practice without the satisfaction generated by a certainty that one is heading along clearly marked paths distinguishes P/MH nursing at its best (Cutcliffe & Goward 2000). These arguments are paradoxical: although it might be regarded as unrealistic to expect nurses who live and work in an ambiguous world to share a collective sense of self, the very fact that these nurses embrace such ambiguity may be one of their defining characteristics and, consequently, an element of their uniqueness.

The contribution of psychiatric and mental health nurses to mental health care: considering the vital service user evidence

In one of the largest UK studies of service users' ($n = 456$) appreciation of psychiatric services, Rogers et al (1993) found that, when asked who helped them the most, 32% said psychiatric nurses and only 12% said psychiatrists. Additionally, 32% reported being satisfied and 26% very satisfied with their P/MH nursing care. As there is no universally accepted definition or shared meaning of what constitutes client satisfaction, any positive findings are an indication of the clients' perception that the service has fulfilled their expectations. Clearly, for people with no previous experience of mental health services, service users are unlikely to know what to expect until they have had some experience of the service. Furthermore, it would be inaccurate to describe nurses as the only group within health care systems that has been identified as being helpful. However, the findings in the Rogers et al study, which are echoed in a substantial body of literature from studies from around the world, are difficult to ignore, and affirm what service users want from their P/MH nurses and that this help is valued.

Consequently, the next logical step would be to examine what it was about the P/MH nursing care that users found helpful. The present authors regard this as an important issue. In a study that focused on clients with enduring mental health problems and whether or not their needs were met, Cutcliffe et al (1997) found that users appeared to regard as important those nursing interventions that were concerned with providing emotional support. They also felt that P/MH nurses were particularly effective at meeting these needs. Users also identified medications and their side-effects as areas where their needs had not been met adequately. These findings are in keeping with the significant body of evidence that now exists that has focused on service user satisfaction; see, for example, the recent report by the Mental Health Foundation (2000). Each of these studies reported that users value interpersonal relationships very highly and that this is often what leads to high user satisfaction. Hence, there is a growing body of evidence suggesting that what users want from their nurses, and find helpful, is the interpersonal, empathy based, human relationship and that this is a particular, worthwhile, contribution that P/MH nurses provide.

The action component of psychiatric/mental health nursing

In 1994, the Department of Health reaffirmed what P/MH nurses should be doing, and summarised these activities (Box 6.1).

Studies focusing on this substantive issue, albeit with a recognised vintage, have differentiated the role of psychiatric nurses in different clinical settings. These roles varied from acting as intermediaries between medical and other staff on admission wards to having a significant role in treatment within therapeutic communities. Similarly, P/MH nursing staff were found to be effective at staff-initiated interactions, administration, planning, and monitoring of care and personal functions. Although the vintage of these sources must be recognised, recent research appears to indicate that these early findings remain viable.

BOX 6.1   Summary of the key elements of psychiatric nursing practice (Department of Health 1994)

- Establishing therapeutic relationships that rest in a respect for others
- Responding flexibly to changing patient needs
- Making risk assessments and judgements

Duffy & Lee (1998), for example, found that the core conditions within a contemporary trust were: assessment, care planning, providing treatment and care, psychosocial interventions and therapies, medication and injections, monitoring patients' medication and progress, referral, admissions/transfers/discharges, liaison with other staff and agencies, meetings, record-keeping and paperwork.

From the foregoing it is apparent that P/MH nursing incorporates many diverse and varied functions. This is not surprising as nursing, whatever the speciality, has a fundamental action component. In addition, P/MH nursing is not the only speciality of nursing that possesses a diverse and varied range of activities that are all encompassed under the 'banner' of nursing action. This is not to suggest that each speciality shares the same activities (although there are some activities that are common to each speciality), more that each speciality has its own wide variation of activities. It is possible that the essential differences across specialities are related to the nature of these activities. However, when Duffy & Lee's (1998) list of activities are examined, it could be argued that the only activity unique to P/MH nurses is 'psychosocial interventions and therapies'. This is not a very robust argument for maintaining the uniqueness of P/MH nurse training rather than adopting generic nurse training. The present authors contend that there are two major issues that refute this: first, Duffy & Lee's list is incomplete, and second, the activities of P/MH nursing are not limited to visible and easily articulated actions.

A core nursing activity missing from the above-mentioned list relates to the constant endeavour to preserve a sense of equilibrium between the roles of an agent of social control and a therapeutic agent (Peplau 1988). The only other speciality of nursing that deals with such a fundamental ethical dilemma and the resulting choices of action faced by P/MH nurses on a daily basis is that of the learning disability (LD) nursing. Whether they choose to be seen in this role or not, P/MH nurses occasionally have a role in exerting control over their clients. This control takes many forms, from the removal of an individual's right to freedom and self-determination (i.e. detaining the client against their will by exercising the nurses' holding power), to physically restraining a person to prevent them from harming themselves or others. LD nurses aside, no other speciality of nursing has the legally sanctioned ability to detain people against their will under the Mental Health Act. Simultaneously, nurses also have a responsibility, duty and role in establishing and maintaining therapeutic relationships with the clients over whom, ironically, they may be expected to exert their control (Peplau 1988). These nurses have to give of themselves through using themselves therapeutically. Consequently, the resulting nursing action is, in part, determined by what role the nurse needs to occupy, and making this critical decision can be regarded as not only a nursing action, but perhaps an important element of the unique function of P/MH and LD nurses.

Several authors have made reference to the invisibility of some P/MH nursing activity (Michael 1994, Altschul 1997, Chambers 1998). This is not a new perspective: more than twenty years ago Brown & Fowler (1971) referred to the work of P/MH nurses as consisting of 'high' and 'low' visibility functions. Nonetheless, Duffy & Lee's (1998) list of activities appears to be comprised of mostly high-visibility functions such as referring/admitting or discharging patients and record-keeping. These activities are in keeping with the high-visibility functions of Brown & Fowler's study in that they are tangible and most valued by nurse managers. The low-visibility functions, such as conveying warmth and empathy, are much less evident in the Duffy & Lee study. This leads the present authors to ask: is it that these functions were not taking place, or are there other explanations for this disparity? In response to this question, we believe there are alternative explanations. First, nurses may have been reluctant to report that the bulk of their time was spent engaged in intangible and invisible activity. Second, it could be that some of the invisible functions were subsumed within one or many of the more overt, tangible functions on Duffy & Lee's list (e.g. providing treatment, care and support).

Being with people who are experiencing distress, understanding and empathising with the meanings people ascribe to their particular situations, and Chambers' (1998) assertion that the primary functions of P/MH nursing are relationship building and therapeutic interventions, are further examples of invisible action. Earlier, Altschul (1997) stated that it is especially difficult to make visible what the nurse does to create a safe environment, how a therapeutic atmosphere is provided, how anxiety is calmed or how violence is prevented. Michael (1994) declared that not only are these skills of great value and need to be recognised, but P/MH nurses must articulate the value of such skills to people who do not have this understanding. While we concur with Michael's summons, we would add that this call needs to be considered within the current context of today's preoccupation with:

- The demand for evidence-based practice
- The demand for a greater emphasis on biological hypotheses concerning the origin and resolution of various forms of mental distress

- The potential failure to appreciate the human importance of anything owing to today's preoccupation with 'scientism' (Barker et al 1997, p 18).

The human component of psychiatric/mental health nursing

Hill & Michael (1996) used a phenomenological approach to uncover the 'concrete activity' of P/MH nurses. Their initial findings indicate that the core activity is working with extraordinary people within 'ordinary' relationships and in ordinary contexts. They caution that these findings offer only a tentative understanding and, consequently, psychiatric nurses have a moral and ethical duty to make every effort to define and describe such skills, no matter how difficult this may prove. Chambers (1998) made similar remarks suggesting that P/MH nurses must demonstrate ordinariness and humanness through their verbal and non-verbal behaviour. But perhaps this 'human focused' nursing is being sidelined owing to the emphasis on such things as measurable outcomes, critical pathways and explicit quality standards. If the uniqueness of P/MH nursing is not something that is easy to quantify or measure, then the current preoccupation with measurable outcomes will do little towards uncovering and defining this uniqueness.

Hill & Michael (1996) stated that the 'craft' of P/MH nursing often gets overlooked. They argued that one element of uniqueness is in the psychiatric nurse's skill in giving all types of relationship an ordinary context: this is an integral part of our craft of care and a core activity. They asserted that such nurses focus on ordinary contact that is respectful and empathic. While this could be applied to all specialities of nursing, it is behaving in this way with extraordinary people that is one of the unique aspects. Repeatedly, studies continue to indicate what service users consider to be the important aspects of their care. It is the presence of the quality of caring, the relationship established with the staff and the 'human connection' that users value the most and want from their service. However, establishing and maintaining such relationships, relationships founded on empathy and trust, with extraordinary people is not a simple process. It is important to note that the authors are not suggesting that other groups of people do not present with their own set of unique, problems and challenges (e.g. oncology clients). Yet what is evident by the very nature of the people involved, engaging with extraordinary people (Hill & Michael 1996) involves different attitudes, skills and knowledge to those needed when engaging with less extraordinary people.

As a result of a collaborative inquiry, Barker et al (1997, p 666) maintained that because P/MH nursing is concerned primarily with establishing the conditions necessary for promoting the individual's unique growth and development, *'developing a relationship with people in care must be a primary concern for all nurses, but should have a more specific concern in psychiatric nursing'.*

Similarly, Gallop (1997) is convinced that have P/MH nurses have a relationship with their clients that is qualitatively different from that of workers in other disciplines. She goes on to suggest that,

'The potential power of psychiatric nursing comes from the unique nature of the caring relationships and this uniqueness is centred on the use of empathy, whereby the nurse comes to know and understand the world of the other and to use this understanding constructively'.

However, perhaps an argument could be constructed that says this is applicable to all specialities of nursing. Surely, all nurses make some attempts to form relationships with clients? While the authors of this chapter would not dispute that some attention to relationship formation does occur in other specialities (and similarly within some generic nurse programmes), it is both the importance and significance given to this activity, and the nature of the relationships formed, that appear to be different in P/MH nursing. Contrast these arguments with other specialities of nursing where there is less evidence of emphasis on forming and maintaining relationships. That is not to say that such endeavours are not encouraged or regarded as worthwhile, but there appears to be limited argument that suggests forming and maintaining relationships is primary.

The collaborative component of psychiatric/mental health nursing

Barker (1996, p 241) has asserted that it is impossible independently to define the proper nature of nursing, as what might be needed from nurses may vary from person to person. He states that

'it can only be defined as a function of the relationship between the person with a need for nursing and a person who has met that need'.

Therefore, in order to articulate the uniqueness of P/MH nursing, there is a need to understand the client's perspective, and P/MH nurses are well placed to do so. As Nolan (1993) argued, the great strength of P/MH nurses lies in their closeness to clients. Such closeness enables the client and nurse to work together, collaboratively. Examination of the literature illustrates that both clients and practitioners have advocated the need for collaborative care. Much of the literature emanating from the service user groups frequently points to the value and rationale of P/MH nurses working in partnership with service users and carers. Such growing awareness of and the movement towards collaborative care in P/MH nursing is rooted in the reflexive and interdependent nature of the relationships between clients and practitioners (Barker et al 1997). That such 'consumers' deserve and need a voice in determining their affairs, and the resulting collaboration in care, arises as an indirect result of these relationships, which, as indicated in the previous section of this chapter, are qualitatively different from those in other specialities of nursing.

The P/MH nursing literature is replete with statements professing the necessity of 'empowering' clients (Tilley 1997), perhaps so much so that empowerment has become something of a 'buzz word'. Although the notion to empower can be seen to have an element of rhetoric, it can be located within a greater underpinning philosophy that regards clients as partners in care. Consequently, efforts to empower clients can be seen as some indication of more collaborative practices. Such collaborative care is rooted in a respect for the client's individual personhood and the beginnings of his or her search for the truth about themselves and their life experiences. Therefore, in order to explicate and further understand the uniqueness of P/MH nursing, there is a need to access clients who feel the need to be engaged in collaborative care and clients who feel the need to be empowered by entering into a partnership with their P/MH nurses. There is an urgent requirement to discover what it is in their nurses that clients feel is unique.

Generic nurses: the nemesis of psychiatric/mental health nursing?

The Collins Dictionary definition of nemesis is *'an agent of such a downfall'*. The present authors posit that the introduction of a generic nurse can be regarded as the nemesis of psychiatric/mental health nursing. Never before has the essence and truth of P/MH nursing been the focus or subject of such attenuated debate. Tilley (1997, p 204) recounted:

*'to a greater extent than before, what is true about psychiatric and mental health nursing, and **what are the rights and obligations of psychiatric and mental health nurses are in the light of this truth, contested matters'**.*

In the UK, the alleged common ground between nurses was emphasised in the common foundation programme of Project 2000 nurse training. Subsequent to this, pressure to introduce a generic nurse has increased with the development of the internal market within health care (Norman 1998). However, many leading authors within P/MH nursing would dispute this viewpoint. Altschul (1997) is convinced that people who want a career in P/MH nursing are different from those who wish to become general nurses. She goes on to state that,

'Because different people recruit themselves, psychiatric and general nursing should remain separate. Generic training does not make sense. Generic training has played havoc with social work; it could do so in nursing . . . the overlap of some elements does not justify a generic approach to nursing' (p 2).

BOX 6.2   Elements of the uniqueness of P/MH nurses

1   The acceptance and embracing of ambiguity
2   The particular health care contribution currently recognised and valued by clients
3   The constant balance of the roles of 'agent of social control' and 'therapeutic agent'
4   The often used, yet invisible and immeasurable, less tangible elements of P/MH nursing practice
5   The ability to exist in a world that is not explained and understood solely by positivistic means and methods
6   The ability to work in ordinary ways with extraordinary people
7   The human component of P/MH nursing, best seen as the craft of nursing, forming and maintaining relationships founded on empathy
8   The endeavours to form partnerships with clients and work in collaboration with clients

---

The limited body of evidence in this area is consistent in showing fundamental differences in attitude towards treatment, and these findings support Altschul's assertions regarding the greater 'liberal mindedness' of P/MH nurses. Indeed, such findings led Clarke (2000) to assert that choosing a nursing speciality is not an external, objective act but rather a reflection of a person's core values. According to these authors, generic training would at best limit and at worst prevent students from immersing themselves in the subjects and experiences that are of interest and importance to them (Altschul 1997). The present authors support this position, and add that the introduction of a generic nurse challenges the very essence of P/MH nursing. These elements of uniqueness are outlined in Box 6.2.

If training for generic nurses is introduced, it will need to include knowledge, theory, skills and interventions that equip the nurse to become fit for purpose. Most of the training will be centred on more fixed or rigid approaches to care, wherein diagnosis leads directly to a treatment that in turn has a predictable outcome, as has happened where generic nurse training has replaced P/MH nurse training, for instance in Victoria, Australia (Happell 1997). As stated above, such approaches to care are not befitting of P/MH nursing and would do much to limit or hinder such practice. It is unlikely that such irreconcilable fundamental differences can be conciliated within the same training. As Happell (1997, p 241) pointed out, the introduction of an integrated curriculum has *'seriously challenged the viability of psychiatric nursing on these courses'*.

It is already recognised that P/MH nurses make a significant contribution to care and that this care is appreciated and valued by clients. It can be regarded as somewhat inappropriate then to remove a form of nursing that is already valued and replace it with an untested form.

The more logical thing to do would be to gain a better understanding of what it is about this form of nursing that is valuable to and appreciated by clients (Chambers 1998). The subsequent dissemination of this deeper understanding may help P/MH nurses become a more effective, better equipped, caring body of people. Given the unique ethical dilemmas facing P/MH and LD nurses outlined above, and the skills required to deal with such situations, the issue of the appropriation of these skills on a generic nurse training course or programme is raised. Serious concerns about the acquisition of mental health nursing knowledge have already been raised following the introduction of the common foundation programme in Project 2000 training (Department of Health 1994). The introduction of generic training is likely to exacerbate this problem in that it is likely that these skills will be rejected in favour of more universally applicable skills, an argument supported by Chan & Rudman (1998, p 144), who point out: *'The tendency towards the majority (in nurse education) invariably produces distortion at the expense of academic rigor in the specialties'*.

Similarly, the invisible or immeasurable components of P/MH nursing practice may give way to the more overt, tangible, measurable components of practices that would be better valued in other specialities of nursing (Huxley 1995, Happell 1997, Chan & Rudman 1998, Norman 1998). Given that there is a need to begin to understand and articulate the value of these practices (Michael 1994), and such endeavour dictates the need for some inquiry into the lived experiences of these practices (Chambers 1998), difficulties arise when there is a dearth of nurses who have had these experiences. Furthermore, it is difficult to perceive what motive or incentive these individuals would have in wishing to understand and articulate any practice that is not integral to their education or training needs. As a consequence, it is possible that the invisible and immeasurable would remain unexplained, implicit and unexpressed, and as a result could become lost to future generations of P/MH nurses.

Given that an alleged element of the uniqueness of P/MH nurses is that they work with extraordinary people, this suggests that other specialities of nursing would concentrate on working with less extraordinary people. The very nature of these extraordinary people means that they present with extraordinary problems that require a specific set of attitudes, skills and knowledge; first and foremost, these people want nurses who have the personal qualities and skills to forge personal relationships (Norman 1998). Indeed, Norman (1998) is adamant that an inevitable effect of a generic nurse programme would be a dilution of mental health nurse expertise. Again, the present authors are not suggesting that working with clients who do not present with mental health problems is simple or straightforward. However, there is something qualitatively different, and hence extraordinary, about mental health problems that creates the need for a specific set of skills, attitudes and knowledge that is unique to this client group.

As alluded to above, the relationships that P/MH nurses form with their clients, compared to those in the other specialities of nursing, are qualitatively different in nature, with a particular emphasis on human interaction. This leads logically to the question: what emphasis will the human side of nursing, the craft of care, be given within generic training? In response to this question, if, as Norman (1998) asserts, generic training will be rooted in the biomedical tradition of general nurses, then the centrality of the interpersonal relationship, as championed by P/MH nurses, is unlikely to be advocated (Huxley 1995, Happell 1997, Chan & Rudman 1998). There would be little value of such an endeavour when these relationships may be inappropriate and/or surplus to requirement for the majority of clinical situations.

A further point for consideration is the nature of the person who is attracted to P/MH nursing. Altschul (1997) and Clarke (2000) have argued that different kinds of people are attracted to P/MH nursing and general nursing, a position supported by the findings of Norman (1998), who regards general and P/MH nurses as different breeds. He argued that many would-be applicants to nursing specialities are reluctant to apply for nurse training while it remains dominated by general nursing experience, a situation that would be exacerbated by the introduction of generic training. Indeed, such a development has already occurred in the USA, and consequently specialist services are rarely seen in the community services (Gournay 1998). Such arguments lead Professor Gournay to declare (p 4):

'It is clear that mental health services need specialists . . . and that we have to recognise that a creation of a generic nurse will put such people off, as they will not wish to undertake a long and arduous generic preparation in clinical areas which are of little interest . . . therefore mental health nurses must resist the move to generic preparation with their combined might'.

Conclusion

In this chapter the authors have argued that there are three steps to help preserve the uniqueness of P/MH nursing. First, there is a need to provide evidence that such uniqueness exists, which would then enable the uniqueness to be recognised and acknowledged. Second, attempts should be made to increase our knowledge of the nature of this uniqueness by explicating and articulating it, initially by the means of qualitative inquiries. Third, there is an obvious need to demonstrate the value of this uniqueness, even though this may be methodologically difficult given the often invisible and immeasurable nature of P/MH nursing. Consequently, the key to this demonstration is genuine collaboration and collated evaluative feedback from clients. Perhaps, then, the unique value of P/MH nurses would not be challenged, diminished or diluted by arguments for introducing generic training, and P/MH nurses could get on with developing ways in which they might better form partnerships with clients and work with these extraordinary people.

Acknowledgements

This chapter is based on two papers published in *Mental Health Practice* (Cutcliffe & McKenna 2000a, 2000b), which have been modified and reproduced here with the kind permission of RCN Publishing.

References

Altschul A 1997 A personal view of psychiatric nursing. In: Tilley S, ed. The mental health nurse: views of practice and education. Blackwell Science, London, p 1–14.

Barker P 1996 Chaos and the way of Zen: psychiatric nursing and the uncertainty principle. Journal of Psychiatric and Mental Health Nursing 22:316–322.

Barker P, Reynolds W, Stephenson C 1997 The human science basis of psychiatric nursing: theory and practice. Journal of Advanced Nursing 25:660–667.

Brown M, Fowler G 1971 Psychodynamic nursing: a biosocial orientation. W B Saunders, Philadelphia.

Chambers M 1998 Interpersonal mental health nursing: research issues and challenges. Journal of Psychiatric and Mental Health Nursing 5:203–211.

Chan A, Buchanan J, Forchuck C, Moore S, Wessell F 1998 Essential psychiatric/mental health nursing (PMHN) education for entry-level nursing programs in Canada. Education Committee, Canadian Federation of Mental Health Nurses, Toronto.

Chan P A, Rudman M J 1998 Paradigms for mental health nursing: fragmentation or integration? Journal of Psychiatric and Mental Health Nursing 5:143–146.

Clarke L 2000 Challenging ideas in psychiatric nursing. Routledge, London.

Cutcliffe J R, Goward P 2000 Qualitative research methods and mental health nurses: a mutual attraction? Journal of Advanced Nursing 30(3):590–598.

Cutcliffe J R, McKenna H P 2000a Generic health care workers: the nemesis of psychiatric/mental health nursing? Part One. Mental Health Practice 3(9):10–14.

Cutcliffe J R, McKenna H P 2000b Generic health care workers: the nemesis of psychiatric/mental health nursing? Part Two. Mental Health Practice 3(10):20–23.

Cutcliffe J R, Dukintis J, Carberry J et al 1997 User's views of their continuing care community psychiatric services. International Journal of Psychiatric Nursing Research 3(3):382–394.

Department of Health 1994 Working in partnership: a collaborative approach to care. Report of the mental health nursing review team. HMSO, London.

Duffy D, Lee R 1998 Mental health nursing today: ideal and reality. Mental Health Practice 1(8): 14–16.

Gallop R 1997 Caring about the client: the role of gender, empathy and power in the therapeutic process. In: Tilley S, ed. The mental health nurse: views of practice and education. Blackwell Science, Oxford, p 28–42.

Gournay K 1998 Imminent new policy issues poses fresh challenges. Mental Health Practice 1(10):4.

Happell B 1997 Psychiatric nursing in Victoria, Australia: a profession in crisis. Journal of Psychiatric and Mental Health Nursing 4:417–422.

Hill B, Michael S 1996 The human factor. Journal of Psychiatric and Mental Health Nursing 3:245–248.

Huxley P 1995 Can mental health specialism survive the NHS and community care reforms? Journal of Mental Health 4:323–327.

Mental Health Foundation 2000 Strategies for living. Mental Health Foundation, London.

Michael S 1994 Invisible skills. Journal of Psychiatric and Mental Health Nursing 1:56–57.

Nolan P 1993 A History of mental health nursing. Chapman Hall, London.

Norman I J 1998 The changing emphasis of mental health and learning disability nurse education in the UK and ideal models of its future development. Journal of Psychiatric and Mental Health Nursing 5:41–51.

Peplau H E 1988 Interpersonal relations in nursing, 2nd edn. Macmillan, London.

Rogers A, Pilgrim D, Lacey R 1993 Experiencing psychiatry: users' views of services. Macmillan/MIND, London.

Ryan D 1997 Ambiguity in nursing: the persona and the organisation as contrasting sources of meaning. In: Tilley S, ed. The mental health nurse: views of practice and education. Blackwell Science, Oxford, p 118–136.

Tilley S 1997 Conclusion. In: Tilley S, ed. The mental health nurse: views of practice and education. Blackwell Science, Oxford, p 203–210.

CHAPTER

7

Olive Younge & Geertje Boschma

Debating the integration of psychiatric/mental health nursing content in undergraduate nursing programmes

Historical perspective

Whether the educational preparation for psychiatric/mental health nurses prior to registration should follow a specialist or a generic model has been a longstanding debate in nursing. Both options exist, although in various countries the evolution of psychiatric nursing education has followed different paths. In Europe, for example, using the Netherlands and Britain as a case in point, from the onset of state registration of nursing about a century ago, a separate registration existed for psychiatric nurses, following a specialist training traditionally established in mental hospital training schools (Nolan 1993, Boschma 2003). In the USA, specialist mental hospital training in asylums ceased earlier, particularly after the Second World War, in the wake of the rise of community mental health nursing. Psychiatric mental health nursing education evolved in the USA as speciality education at Master's level, following generic integrated baccalaureate education, which also included a general introduction to psychiatric mental health nursing (Church 1985, 1987).

Canada provides another interesting example. Nationally, psychiatric nursing became integrated into generic baccalaureate programmes, which became the dominant trend as of the 1960s, gradually replacing traditional general hospital training school educational preparation. In Canada's mental hospitals, speciality training emerged as well. However, particularly in Ontario, mental hospital graduates were able to register under the generic state registrar for registered nurses (RNs), after a 6-month general hospital 'affiliation', that is, a practical training period in the general hospital. So, in eastern Canada a separate registrar for psychiatric nursing never evolved (Tipliski 2002, Cutcliffe 2003). In the western provinces of Canada, on the other hand, speciality training in mental hospitals did not bridge easily with generic hospital training schools through affiliations, and speciality mental hospital graduates remained largely separated from the larger group of graduates from baccalaureate and hospital-based programmes. In the western provinces, staffing of mental hospitals in isolated rural areas was a unique problem. Organised western nursing associations were not as open to mental nurse graduates as their eastern colleagues, and mental hospital superintendents tended to support speciality education in the post Second World War staffing shortages. Very different circumstances in western Canada resulted in a separate registrar for registered psychiatric nurses as of the 1950s (Tipliski 2002).

This complex historical situation creates a number of questions. One important one is: what do we mean when we state that psychiatric/mental health nursing is a speciality? This is a very important question, especially from an international point of view. As history makes clear, there are a number of different routes of preparation at varying educational levels, located in a number of countries and evolving in different ways. As a result, the discipline of nursing deals with a variety of practising psychiatric mental health nurses, who, depending on the route they took, have developed different understandings and loyalties towards their practice and their nursing colleagues.

Although such a pattern is common in nursing, where speciality education and splitting across educational levels has always been the practice, resulting in a wide-ranging and varied professional tapestry, it is important to be aware of this complexity and only an effort to understand the differences can adequately bridge rifts among the different groups of nurses working in this speciality area. In Canada, for example, registered psychiatric nurses (RPNs) understand themselves as being quite different from RNs specialising in mental health, following either diploma, post undergraduate diploma or an integrated baccalaureate preparation. In the USA, Masters-prepared RNs, serving as clinical nurse specialists or advanced practice nurses in the mental health field, again differ from baccalaureate-prepared generic RNs who happen to choose a career in mental health care. For example, their relation to and impact on nursing research in mental health is very different. Currently, in both Europe and North America, advanced practice nursing is a rapidly evolving and changing field, which furthers, and in some ways fuels, the debate about generic versus speciality education in nursing.

Speciality is defined by the Concise Oxford Dictionary as a *'special feature or characteristic; . . . special pursuit, product, operation, etc., thing to which a person gives special attention'* (Fowler & Fowler 1959). There is a definition for generalist in this edition of the Concise Oxford Dictionary, but in North American nursing vernacular it usually refers to basic, generic, nursing care offered in multiple settings, including the mental health field. The present authors, both nurse educators in undergradu-ate baccalaureate nursing curricula taught over four years, prefer to use the term 'integration' at the undergraduate level rather than a linear model implying movement from generalist to specialist, or beginning with a speciality and evolving in that speciality. However, other authors do refer to the term generalist, and it will be used in this chapter in that context.

Integration infers that key nursing concepts such as the promotion of health and prevention of illness are being taught in a manner that is built on sound curricular principles, whereas the term generalist infers 'basic nursing care performed at an elementary level'. It is under-stood that, within the integrated approach, beginning nursing students are introduced to the complexity of nursing care from the outset. Undergraduate nursing education viewed from a holistic perspective, encompasses education in speciality areas of psychiatric/mental health (P/MH), adult health, women's health, child and family/maternal health, critical care nursing and so forth. Knowledge in the specialities is supported from applied content areas such as pathophysiology, anatomy, physiology, pharmacology, nutrition, psychology, sociology and other liberal arts. Lastly, the discipline of nursing, regardless of speciality, is taught through assessments (health, mental status, pain, etc.), nursing process, ethics, history, legalities, critical thinking, com-munication and philosophy. The content is framed in a curriculum based on values such as primary health care, nursing theories and/or basic views of humans, health and society. At the end of the integrated undergraduate programme, nurses will have basic skills and the choice of working in a variety of areas in nursing, some of them explicitly identified as speciality areas.

There are concerns when proposing to argue integration or gener-alisation versus specialisation in nursing education. On the surface it appears simplistic and sets up a conflict whereby 'either/or' systems are chosen. If a student obtains a RN's diploma or baccalaureate in nursing degree versus a RPN (the Canadian version of registered mental health nurse) diploma, there may be a tendency to equate a superior status to more years of education and credentials. This perpetuates divisiveness and erodes professional respect among nurses. It also creates a barrier between those who have a certain educational preparation and those who do not, and, regardless of years of experience or contribution to the speciality, this barrier cannot easily be transcended. Important questions such as 'What, why, how well and where was it taught?' are equally important considerations when assessing the adequacy of an educational programme. Unfortunately these latter questions are often ignored owing to the complexities of assessing across programmes; it is simply easier to judge a programme by the credential.

Situating nursing education programmes in universities versus hos-pitals, and integrating speciality knowledge across programmes, opens the door to discussion and participation in health policy development. Currently, policy development is informed by science and research-based decisions, whether we like it or not. Traditionally nurses had difficulty contributing to these debates as they lacked adequate academic preparation to participate in the fast technological and research-based changes that characterised post Second World War health care. Through their hospital-based training, they found themselves isolated from the mainstream educational system and were not accepted as equal partners, not being 'cultured' in academic traditions. Integrated baccalaureate programmes in academic settings were in part designed to overcome this gap (McPherson 1996, Mussalem 1960, 1962, 1964). Another key point in locating nursing education programmes in a university setting means that students could have access to qualified professors and receive transferable credit for courses taken in the programme. Furthermore, their degree in nursing is recognised by other disciplines and faculties of graduate studies, allowing graduates to pursue additional degrees in law, medicine or graduate work if they so choose. Demonstrating the contribution that nurses make to health care, in any field, requires a sound curriculum that measures up to other important key players in the field such as those in occupational therapy, social work or psychology, and prepares nurses in such a way that they will be listened to.

From another perspective, the workplace must also be considered. General hospital medicine has a higher status than psychiatry as a medical field (Rosenberg 1992). To link psychiatry with mainstream medicine and overcome the isolation of mental hospitals, psychiatric clinics and departments began to be integrated into general hospitals. Mental hospital administrators have at points supported speciality education as it bound personnel to the mental hospital, whereas administrators in general hospitals have opted to support the hiring of nurses who could work in all or any speciality areas. From the perspective of general hospital administrators there was a preference for RNs with psychiatric nursing experience as they could be transferred to different areas. This consideration supports the need to staff an agency, and may or may not promote higher levels of patient care. Priorities for administrators are to ensure staffing for safe and ethical care, particularly when agencies are short staffed.

In concluding this section we are brought to another question, which we would like to discuss in greater depth in this chapter. Is the preferable route for entry into P/MH nursing practice a speciality or an integrated baccalaureate preparation? And, in relation, what are the strengths and limitations of such integrated preparation in terms of serving the complex population of people suffering from mental illness? The purpose of this chapter is to contribute to the 'speciality versus generic' discussion. It is timely to rethink the existing differential between generic and speciality preparation, in light of the demands of the broader developments in health care.

Frame of reference

This section will describe what it means to have P/MH integrated into the undergraduate nursing curriculum at the baccalaureate level. Integration of content begins with the identification of a particular curricular framework and underlying values. This is followed by identification of content areas and relevant concepts. For P/MH nursing, the first step for nurse educators is to define the terms mental health and psychiatric nursing, and to understand their historical use. Next, related concepts and interventions such as mental health promotion, wellness, stress, depression, neurobiology, systems theory or emotions are identified. Nurse educators then take and level the concepts and interventions, and determine where in the curriculum they will be addressed and by whom. The latter is an important point because P/MH concepts could be addressed through a support course such as health ethics or by nurse educators in community health, and not necessarily initially through a P/MH course. Assuming the programme lasts for four years, usually during the second or third year of the programme all students have theory and practice in a setting that may or may not be directly linked to P/MH nursing. In North America in their final year of the programme, the students may choose a preceptorship experience, that is, working along with practising nurses in P/MH nursing, whereas initial practicums are with programme-based professors. This model is different in other areas of the world; for example, in the Netherlands all baccalaureate practicums are taught by preceptors. Regardless of the location, in the final practicum the students will have P/MH nursing theory linked with practice. Settings that have been chosen by students include: drug addiction recovery, sex offender rehabilitation, specific clinics addressing conditions such as eating disorders, adolescent or general adult psychiatric programmes. Throughout their practicum experience they are expected to engage in research-based practice, write papers, and integrate theory and practice. There is an explicit expectation that fourth year students will get a broader understanding of the practice issues and health care service problems/dilemmas, so they can begin to analyse health care from a policy level. As students may choose their final clinical experience, they fan into other speciality areas such as emergency, cardiology, pediatrics or gerontology, and thus a minority enter P/MH nursing. Their selection of a practice area is based on a number of factors: career planning, a positive experience in a clinical area in previous years, wanting a unique or novel setting, self-assessment, availability of clinical sites and even proximity of a site. Regardless of the speciality area they choose, they are viewed as a graduate from a basic baccalaureate nursing programme. They cannot claim that they have speciality education or designation.

Assumptions

This section focuses on the assumptions that have been made regarding generic versus speciality preparation. When we examine our assumptions we become more aware of our thinking and behaviours. A number of assumptions underlie the values inherent in an integrated curriculum. The most obvious one is that students require a broad and holistic approach truly to understand nursing as a discipline and profession. The student learns content that can be applied to all settings and situations, and as they progress through the programme they will generalise and transfer their knowledge from one setting to the next. Curricula are structured to provide continuity, relevance and integration. The processes usually proceed from: simple to complex; normal to abnormal, health to illness, individual to family to group; and local to national to international health care systems. This means that when the concept of nurse–patient relationship is taught in the first year of the programme to a student in a community health setting, the application is simple, observable and forms one aspect of the therapeutic alliance. The concept of nurse–patient communication then evolves as the student progresses through other areas of nursing, such as caring for a critically ill child in paediatrics and then being able to interact with the family and care for their needs. In the P/MH nursing practicum the student refines their understanding of nurse–patient communication and demonstrates an ability to apply this intervention in a variety of interactions. Through difference experiences, it is argued that the student comes to understand more fully the complexity of nurse–patient communication.

The second assumption is that there is a place for specialisation in nursing but only once the student has a solid grounding in basic nursing, such as health promotion, basic nursing care and health assessment, as well as a beginning understanding of the complexity of health care service delivery. This education provides the basis upon which clinical experience in a speciality area can be built. Work experience and post diploma programmes or graduate work yielding the credential of clinical nurse specialist or advanced nursing practitioner are based on the premise that the nurse has a unique and well deserved body of knowledge in a speciality area. Specialisation is a goal to be achieved and not a beginning point in a person's career.

Limitations of speciality education

A significant advantage in using integration as a model is the understanding of the concept of holism whereby body and mind are viewed as a helix, intertwined and functioning as a system. There are numerous examples of physical illnesses coupled with mental illness: hypothyroidism and depression, hypoglycaemia and anxiety, or birth of a child and postpartum psychosis/depression. Grounding in the biological sciences also assists the nurse to understand better the mechanism of medications, neurological basis of certain illness, and the underlying pathophysiology when patients have multiple diagnoses such as pneumonia and schizophrenia. Holism is not limited to the coupling of physical and emotional disorders. It also encompasses new ways of viewing nursing, use of complementary therapies, attending to the art and science of nursing, and breaking free of practice barriers imposed by nurses themselves and other health care providers.

There are times when a speciality means a disease state or pertains to a grouping of conditions around a specific body organ such as the heart, liver or kidney, or the brain as in psychiatry. It may refer to a specific life event such as childbearing in obstetrics, or the growth and development of the child in paediatrics. Inherent in a speciality focus is that extensive and expert knowledge is required to function effectively within a speciality. However, when a new graduate begins working in a speciality they will be challenged to see broader perspectives or how their speciality fits into the landscape of nursing. The culture of a speciality is often to go deeper and not broader.

Entry into nursing education via specialisation can be stressful for the graduate. The expectations of the employing agency can place excessive demands on the graduate while not recognising the need and time for them to develop competence and confidence. Furthermore, depending on the area of employment in psychiatry, a graduate may not quickly or easily identify their limitations, expecting to have knowledge in the speciality. With the advancement of specialisation in some professions, nursing too has introduced nurse practitioner, clinical nurse specialist, advanced practitioner and nurse therapist roles, to name but a few. There appears to be a genuine confusion around role titles, definitions, boundaries and expectations (Daly & Carnwell 2003). Herein lies the problem: there is a lack of leadership and coordination among health care professionals, administrators and educators. The end result is confusion for the graduate.

The challenges

There are a number of challenges that must be considered when discussing specialisation, particularly as it relates to working in the field. Nurses who perceive themselves as specialists may also believe that they cannot fully realise their potential owing to other factors. For example, one research study found that some P/MH nursing staff did not feel they could keep abreast of new developments, interventions and lobbying for resources. Nolan et al (2002) researched a small group of mental health nurses in the USA and the UK. Although the findings cannot be generalised, the authors revealed insights about the nature and stressors of P/MH nursing. Both groups of nurses were challenged by changes in the health care system, and the US nurses specifically identified the difficulties inherent in the managed care system. The latter group also identified the need to develop competency in psycho-pharmacology. The nurses in the UK stated that they felt uncertain of their professional role, particularly when expected to engage in inter-professional collaboration, and were increasingly expected to work harder and longer with little support.

Another challenge is the dynamic and evolving nature of nursing. In fact, nursing programmes are associated with the act of change. Nurse educators are constantly examining the relevance of curricula for students, practice and society. Beech et al (2002) stated that mental health nurses feared that they would go to bed one night to awake as an endangered species and lose their identity. This fear was due to the changes being introduced into curricula and the creation of generalist courses in the UK, specifically Wales. Critics of these changes question whether there is sufficient general theoretical and clinical knowledge to develop helpful skills.

One wonders whether the quest to keep a speciality focus as entry into practice is actually the fear of change – and perhaps even extinction – rather than a curriculum that better serves the needs of society? In addition, there may be issues pertaining to loyalty and not feeling acknowledged for the experience they bring to the field. Leaders in nursing education must look at the curriculum from the perspective of how it best serves society and patient services with the objective of overcoming the fear of extinction and eliminating professional turf wars.

A third challenge is to retain what is working with what needs to be reworked or retooled. The preparation of nurses mirrors the needs of society. An enhanced care delivery system is emerging as a result of the demands of consumers, available technologies and increased health research. Cotroneo et al (2001) argue that the following are required: a generic core speciality, solid ground of evidence and best practices involving Master's students, collaboration with other professionals, complete support to students, community involvement, and balance between instructional technologies and interactive learning experiences. They state the need for a broad and multidimensional conceptual framework to support the emerging role of mental health care, includ-ing physical, mental, emotional, spiritual, relational, environmental and cultural aspects. They recommend how an existing speciality cur-riculum might be modified to be a multidimensional conceptual frame-work. They suggest a move towards an integrated curriculum at the graduate level. Their ideas are worth examining to determine how best to capitalise on the existing curricular structures and modify them to meet the needs of society. There is one caveat to the recommendations made by Cotroneo et al (2001). One of their recommendations is that graduates have prescriptive authority. To accomplish this outcome, nurses would have to have a strong foundation in the biological sciences, legalities and ethics.

Product versus process in the integrated baccalaureate programme

Cotroneo et al (2001) identified an important understanding of curriculum when they stated that teaching and learning methods must support a new curriculum. The old ways of teaching using lectures and note-taking are being replaced with problem-based learning methods or a combination of methods. Increasingly curricula are designed to teach students to question, engage in critical thinking, use evidence-based interventions and technology, and employ a problem- or inquiry-based approach to learning. Regardless of specialisation versus generalisation approaches, the methods of teaching and learning must be rethought. Hannigan et al (2001), in their research of community mental health teachers, noted that teaching is a process and that the quality of teaching based on adult learning principles is highly valued.

Dissemination of research has outstripped educators' abilities to know the latest research findings, let alone evaluate its effectiveness against basic research standards. One method of addressing this very real issue is to focus on process versus product. Process means that students are taught skills of critical thinking: how to ask certain types of question, be skeptical, examine assumptions, and consider the effects of context on thinking. Students do need basic nursing knowledge, but they also need to know how to access knowledge quickly, how to consult and work with others, and to live with the realisation that to be a nurse means to engage in lifelong learning and does not end with the completion of their undergraduate nursing education programme.

Proponents of speciality as entry to practice, as espoused by Beech et al (2002), state that a generalist curriculum will mean loss of knowledge in other speciality areas. This is true, particularly if knowledge is viewed as product and not as process. Ironically, one of the content areas that is key in the integrated curriculum is the use of technology. Knowledge in technology facilitates the process of knowledge acquisition: web searching, library work, data organisation, and so forth. Students are expected to access research papers via the web, critique them and forward them to peers. They are also expected to use technology such as PowerPoint or HyperStudio for presentations, given that nurses do health teaching and professional presentations.

Another process that is heavily stressed in an integrated undergraduate baccalaureate nursing curriculum is written and verbal communication. It could be argued that this would be part of any nursing curriculum. However, in the integrated model, students must demonstrate more evidence of learning, particularly through written communication given the organisation of the content. Students must prove that they are scholars, draw from multiple sources and correctly apply writing guidelines such as those of the Publication Manual of the American Psychological Association. Students are expected to write essays, nursing care plans and journals, and have the privilege of answering test questions through a written versus a multiple choice format. Through writing assignments, students are able to reflect, organise their thinking and demonstrate their ability to conceptualise their knowledge of a condition, event or experience. The feedback they receive on their assignments is just as critical in shaping their development as communicators. Educators, when marking assignments, focus on fairness, sufficiency of research, integration of research and thinking patterns. In the area of verbal communications, students are expected to give presentations using multiple methods: current technology, group discussion techniques, mini-lectures, etc. Their presentations are marked on content, presentation style, organisation or group participation, depending on the goals of the presentation. In seminars, students are expected to be active and to prepare fully prior to the seminar. When they contribute to the discussion topic, they are to do so in a scholarly manner. The outcome for students is full engagement in the process of learning, and in doing so becoming self-directed lifelong learners.

Personal reflections

Nurse educators in many parts of the world have wrestled with this question of specialisation as entry into nursing. We argue that baccalaureate nursing preparation in a programme that crosses over speciality fields has the greatest potential to create a route towards full participation in decision-making about health care services, and best serves the needs of society and nurses themselves. We are aware that this argument is not new, and has been debated all along, but at times of transition, in which we now again find ourselves, it may be important to recall the reasons why, as a discipline, we worked hard to establish an integrated undergraduate nursing curriculum. We need to reflect on the question, whether again as a profession, we have worked hard enough to support all nurses to enter a profession where they can contribute valuable expertise. In the Netherlands, for example, a change in the nursing education system in the mid 1990s brought to closure the separate register for psychiatric nurses that had existed for almost a hundred years, shifting this education into integrated nursing programmes as well as furthering the development of post-baccalaureate speciality education in mental health nursing. The basic consideration in making such decisions should be: how to support the best possible patient care while creating the best potential for preparing nurses who have the academic grounding to participate adequately in decision-making.

An initiative at the University of Alberta bears mentioning. Working closely in the 1990s with the Registered Psychiatric Nurses Association, Alberta Hospital – Ponoka Psychiatric Nursing Training Program and the Alberta Government, a programme was developed to allow RPNs to complete a baccalaureate nursing degree (BScN). In Alberta, RPNs did have an opportunity to obtain the credential for a RN diploma through Grant MacEwan Community College. Shortly after this initiative, the University of Alberta introduced a P/MH nursing speciality at the masters level of education, facilitating student movement from RPN to BScN to Masters in Nursing (http://www.ualberta.ca/homepage.nsf/website/History). The RPN to BScN programme strengthens the profession while bridging the gap and developing opportunities for RPNs to participate in existing academic routes. Such bridging requires strong support and acknowledgement of the expertise of all parties involved.

The challenge has been, and still is, to develop the profession of nursing and contribute to a broad range of health care services – and not just to staff an asylum, hospital or programme. An integrated baccalaureate nursing programme, grounded in an academic setting, enhances the chances that nurses can participate in service provision and day-to-day decision-making. That is not to say that such an approach also resolves the longstanding problem of how to provide the numbers of nurses needed to staff the necessary services and agencies adequately. However, further debate, critical questions and a political will are required to invest adequately in sound health care.

We would like to stress that nurses, regardless of speciality, must have career mobility, be at the same level as other health professionals and, most importantly, advance the development of the profession through innovation. They need to have the critical thinking skills to link and evaluate concepts across settings. Their allegiance would be to the profession of nursing and not just to an agency that taught them about nursing.

In summary, those invested in our discipline – from nurse educators, to professional associations to administrators – need to advocate curricula based on the needs of society. All must work together to strengthen and develop the profession of nursing. The history of nursing education in P/MH nursing has shown that this has not always been the case. Rethinking the ideas that have played an important role in creating integrated undergraduate nursing curricula can help to bridge existing chasms as well as develop an open mind to supporting nursing as an inclusive profession.

References

Beech I, Coffey M, Hannigan B 2002 The case for specialist mental health training. Nursing Times (98)15:40–41.

Boschma G 2003 The rise of mental health nursing: a history of psychiatric care in Dutch asylums, 1890–1920. Amsterdam University Press, Amsterdam.

Church O M 1985 Emergence of training programs for asylum nursing at the turn of the century. Advances in Nursing Science 7(2):35–46.

Church O M 1987 From custody to community in psychiatric nursing. Nursing Research 36(1):48–55.

Cotroneo M, Kurlowicz L, Hopkins Outlaw F, Burgess A W, Evans L K 2001 Psychiatric–mental health nursing at the interface: revisioning education for the specialty. Issues in Mental Health Nursing 22:549–569.

Cutcliffe J R 2003 The differences and commonalities between United Kingdom and Canadian psychiatric/mental health nursing: a personal reflection. Journal of Psychiatric and Mental Health Nursing 10:255–257.

Daley W, Carnwell R 2003 Nursing roles and levels of practice: a framework for differentiating between elementary, specialist and advancing nursing practice. Journal of Clinical Nursing 12:158–167.

Fowler H W, Fowler F G, eds 1959 The concise Oxford dictionary of current English, 4th edn. Clarendon Press, Oxford.

Hannigan B, Burnard P, Edwards D, Turnbull J 2001 Specialist practice for UK community mental health nurses: the 1998–99 survey of course leaders. International Journal of Nursing Studies 38:427–435.

McPherson K 1996 Bedside matters: the transformation of Canadian nursing, 1900–1990. Oxford University Press, Toronto.

Mussalem H K 1960 Spotlight on nursing education: the report of the pilot project for the evaluation of schools of nursing in Canada. Canadian Nurses Association, Ottawa.

Mussalem H K 1962 A path to quality: a plan of the development of nursing education programs within the general educational system of Canada. Canadian Nurses Association, Ottawa.

Mussalem H K 1964 Royal Commission on Health Services: nursing education in Canada. Queen's Printer, Ottawa.

Nolan P 1993 A history of mental health nursing. Chapman & Hall, London.

Nolan P, Bourke P, Doran M 2002 UK and USA clinical mental health nurse specialists' perceptions of their work. Journal of Psychiatric and Mental Health Nursing 9:293–300.

Rosenberg C E 1992 The crisis in psychiatric legitimacy. In: Rosenberg C E, ed. Explaining epidemics and other studies in the history of medicine. Cambridge University Press, Cambridge, p 245–257.

Tipliski V M 2002 Parting at the crossroads: the development of education for psychiatric nursing in three Canadian provinces, 1909–1955. Doctoral dissertation, University of Manitoba, Winnipeg.

Commentary

Stephen Tilley

Introduction

These two chapters provide much food for debate and argument. However, they are not evidently constructed as arguments with each other. The reader wanting to use them as resources for developing her or his own thinking about the merits of specialist and/or generic practitioner and education must both evaluate the claims made by each and develop a framework for relating the claims of each to those of the other. As resources for development, the chapters together are rich material.

The chapters focus on substantially different issues and construct different contexts for reading and response. In Chapter 6, the main issue is the 'uniqueness' of 'speciality' psychiatric/mental health (P/MH) nursing; the context is one in which the 'nemesis' of generic nursing threatens to dilute or displace that 'uniqueness'. Readers are invited to align with Chapter 6 in defence against attack by the nemesis. However, I argue that the nemesis is undercharacterised, leaving the requirements for a defence of specialist nursing unclear. Incidentally, Chapter 6's specialist nursing is not actually what we find in Chapter 7, which, by contrast, constructs a context of past rivalry among 'tribes' of P/MH speciality nurses, the tribes being marked by a common experience of having qualified in specific ways, and puts forward as the issue of concern that this rivalry has delayed generic nursing's contribution to the shaping of health policy and meeting society's needs. Readers are invited to defend Chapter 7 against the threat posed by those who would divert from the good of unified nursing in the interests of meeting society's health needs. But, as with the nemesis in Chapter 6, the 'tribes' are undercharacterised, and we do not know whether they are what we find in Chapter 6.

The particular problem the chapters pose – a problem to which I will return at the end of this commentary – is that the each adopts a position that would rule the other out. But first I shall try to determine whether an alternative argument might be made that takes account of the strengths and limitations of both.

Chapter 6

The main claim in Chapter 6, namely that specialist preparation should be preserved, depends on accepting two subclaims: that P/MH nursing is unique, and that it is valuable; along with the implicit principle that the loss of what is unique and valuable should be resisted – as should whatever would lead to that loss. The practical consequence of the claim is that the move to generic preparation should be resisted, specialist preparation and practice being preferable to generalist.

As reasons for accepting these claims, the authors identify eight 'elements of the uniqueness of P/MH nurses' (Box 6.2). The first move in considering the argument is to test these reasons. In my opinion, all, to varying degrees, are vulnerable to challenge owing to lack of specificity (points 1, 3, 4, 7, 8), clarity (2, 4, 5, 6) and/or evidence (2). The reasons – with my very condensed notes on problematic aspects – are:

1 *'The acceptance and embracing of ambiguity'* – This may not be unique to P/MH nurses.
2 *'The particular health care contribution currently recognised and valued by clients'* – The 'particular' aspect of this is insufficiently specified.
3 *'The constant balance of the roles of 'agent of social control' and 'therapeutic agent'*' – This is shared with some other nurses, e.g. learning disability nurses.
4 *'The often used, yet invisible and immeasurable, less tangible elements of P/MH nursing practice'* – This seems too vague a basis for justification of practice.
5 *'The ability to exist in a world that is not explained and understood solely by positivistic means and methods'* – Is the intended focus on the ontological character of the world, on the P/MH nurse's ability to exist beyond that epistemological radius, or on setting P/MH nurses apart from those who are less 'able to exist in . . .'?
6 *'The ability to work in ordinary ways with extraordinary people'* – Who the latter are is not specified clearly enough to show that other nurses do not work with extraordinary people; nor is it clear why other nurses could not learn and use 'ordinary ways'.
7 *'The human component of P/MH nursing, best seen as the craft of nursing, forming and maintaining relationships founded on empathy'* – It is not clear how this is unique to P/MH nurses.
8 *'The endeavours to form partnerships with clients and work in collaboration with clients'* – Would a key source (Peplau) not say that other nurses could/should do this too?

Further analysis of specific reasons in Chapter 6

I will now consider problems with some of these reasons, namely those concerned with:

1 The ability to survive without certainty: epistemological uncertainty, and ambiguity of role
2 Uniqueness
3 Concern with a more specific focus of the conditions in which patients live – 'trephotaxis' (Barker 1989).

The authors assert that the *'ability to survive in clinical practice without the satisfaction generated by a certainty that one is heading along clearly marked paths distinguishes P/MH nursing at its best'*. They claim that the ability to survive demonstrates adaptation to unavoidable aspects of the 'world' in which P/MH nurses work, namely ambiguity, uncertainty and chaos. This 'ambiguity' exists in two distinct spheres of experience, the philosophical and the sociological; it relates both to lack of epistemological certainty and to duality of role (control/care) in work with people with mental health problems, particularly those people subject to Mental Health Act regulations.

The relevance of the 'ambiguity' argument to the central question of 'specialist or generalist' hinges on whether the *'ability to survive in clinical practice without the satisfaction generated by a certainty that one is heading along clearly marked paths'* is *unique* to P/MH nursing. If not, this key quality might equally well be inculcated in a generalist education curriculum and programme. In fact, I do think that a case could be made that other kinds of nurses face uncertainty and a care landscape without clearly marked paths. A similar argument could be made regarding the sociological claim that the 'core activity' is 'constant endeavour to preserve a sense of equilibrium between the roles of agent of social control and a therapeutic agent'. This is true at least in some contexts, not only for P/MH nurses, but also for learning disability nurses, health visitors, district nurses and nurses caring for older persons (all of these groups have reconsidered practice in Scotland in the light of changes in the Mental Health Act Scotland 2003) – indeed, all nurses working with vulnerable persons (and that might include all nurses).

Other reasons supporting the 'uniqueness' claim are similarly vulnerable. The authors cite Barker in claiming that:

'because P/MH nursing is concerned primarily with establishing the conditions necessary for promoting the individual's unique growth and development, "developing a relationship with people in care must be a primary concern for all nurses, but should have a more specific concern in psychiatric nursing".'

In an earlier text, Barker characterised nursing generally, not P/MH nursing exclusively, as 'trephotaxis' ('concerned with the conditions . . .') (Barker 1989). Peplau, too, emphasised the centrality of interpersonal relationships in nursing generally, not P/MH nursing alone (Peplau 1952/1988). Again, one might argue that a generic nurse education programme based on Peplau's work could prepare all nurses to address the 'primary concern'.

We can turn now to another key claim, the authors' assertion that it is *'evident by the very nature of the people involved, engaging with extraordinary people* [the authors cite Hill & Michael] *involves different attitudes, skills and knowledge to those needed when engaging with less extraordinary people'*. This claim is problematic in two respects. How these people are 'extraordinary' is not spelled out in the chapter, leaving the authors open to a retort that those with whom generic nurses work are no 'less extraordinary'. The authors anticipate this retort, but fall back on assertion that the 'very nature of the people involved' substantiates their claim. If the 'extraordinary' qualities are restricted to those with mental health problems, the argument is circular. The problem of circularity applies to other reasons in the chapter. For example, the authors state:

'Therefore, in order to explicate and further understand the uniqueness of P/MH nursing, there is a need to access clients who feel the need to be engaged in collaborative care and clients who feel the need to be empowered by entering into a partnership with their P/MH nurses'.

In short, in my view, the reasons are not sufficiently strong to warrant accepting the main and subsidiary claims as stated.

An alternative, more adequate response

The above critique has been selective. I have focused, rather uncharitably, on criticisms of aspects of the argument, and not on the substantial strengths of the chapter. Nor have I addressed a potential response – that it is the constellation of reasons, rather than any taken separately or all taken together, that grounds the claim of uniqueness. But that argument is not presented in the chapter.

If we consider the eight reasons not simply as statements about P/MH nursing as-anyone-might-find-it, they may provide more sound support for the claim of 'uniqueness'. That is to say, let us imagine the authors of Chapter 6 as saying that *they* as P/MH nurses are unique for the reasons given, that *they* practice and teach and write from within experienced relationships and collaborations, without certainty. We are asked to consider them as an exemplary variety of P/MH nurse reporting on the world as they see and construct it in a particular context of socially ordered interaction. Furthermore, they are heard as saying that they are hounded by a nemesis of generic nursing that threatens their identity and, with their identity, their construction of the world and of nursing practice.

To see the issue this way has required a shift in focus on my part. When I see them not as describing P/MH nurses as abstract entities, but as situated social actors, I find that each one of their eight points makes a different kind of sense (e.g. *'The ability to exist in a world that is not explained and understood solely by positivistic means and methods'* may refer to the 'world' including the authors, who are not 'explained or understood solely' by those means). From personal experience I recognise that there is a 'version' of P/MH nurses who *have* embraced ambiguity in 'unique' ways, that is, in ways I have not found in self-representations by nurses of other sorts. These are the survivors of vociferous debates in the UK P/MH nursing literature about, for example, epistemological certainty, which were written and read as serious challenges to other P/MH nurse authors' views of reality and identity; survivors also of debates about the legitimacy of care and control in specific inpatient settings. Similarly, their views accord with those of a recognisable cohort of P/MH nurses in the UK who have asserted, in the face of potentially fatal challenges to their 'version' of nursing, the centrality of the nurse–patient relationship (Peplauvian variety). If the challenges to those of their reasons I have presented are substantial, I would judge them to be less so than challenges faced by such nurse-writers in the UK over the past decade. I can, in short, envisage – or read into the chapter – a nemesis, but a political nemesis socially and historically situated. (The nemesis would be multidisciplinary, population-serving and mental health service-delivering, emphasising 'science' rather than the 'art' of the unique variety – akin therefore to the 'generalist' figure in Chapter 7, but a mental health generalist. That said, I note also that writers over the past five years (e.g. Repper 2000, Norman 2005) have seen, or anticipated, a move towards a perspective based on 'respect' for both partners in the unique P/MH nurse–nemesis dyad.)

Chapter 7

The authors of Chapter 7 set out as context the *'complex historical situation* [that] *creates at least two interesting and compelling questions'*, the argument consisting essentially of answers to these two questions. The first question is: 'What is meant by saying that P/MH nursing is a speciality?' A history of different routes to preparation has resulted, according to these authors, in *'rifts among the different groups of nurses working in this speciality area'*. 'Rifts' are linked to a kind of tribalism based on a sense of difference and (implied) superiority of one version (based on one kind of preparation) over another. All this is regarded as problematic, compromising efforts to create an 'integrated' profession, eroding mutual respect among nurses working in different clinical fields or settings, and weakening the advance of professionalism. 'Integrated' and 'integration' are the authors' preferred terms, rather than 'generic'. 'Integration' would be better achieved by a curriculum that introduced all 'beginning' students *'to the complexity of nursing care from the outset'* via a curriculum based on *'values such as primary health care, nursing theories and/or basic views of humans, health and society'*. 'Difference' is associated also with site of preparation for practice: specialists traditionally prepared in hospitals, with horizons and status thereby limited; generic in higher education – *'equal partners* [with other professionals] . . . *"cultured" in academic traditions'*.

This sets up the second question, of the relative merits of speciality versus 'integrated baccalaureate preparation' as a 'route into P/MH nursing practice'. The comparison is set in a context, parallel to the 'historical' view above – here the context of 'broader developments in health care'. Curriculum content and structure, and practice experience, are considered in this light. Essentially, these are geared to preparing P/MH nurses to '[serve] *the complex population of people suffering from mental illness'*. The foundational elements are health promotion, basic nursing care and health assessment, as well as a beginning understanding of the complexity of health care service delivery.

The main problem with this account is that it does not formulate what P/MH nursing *is*, as distinct from nursing generally. It does not indicate what the different hospital-based versions were, nor whether or why they were inadequate for any reason other than that, by virtue of their difference, they threatened the integrity of a unitary profession.

Further critique of the argument in Chapter 7

The key charge in Chapter 7 is that maintenance of specialism might be simply defensive – *'whether the quest to keep a speciality focus as entry into practice is actually the fear of change – and perhaps even extinction – rather than a curriculum that better serves the needs of society'* – and damaging both to the specialists and to nursing generally. The positive claim of their chapter is that *'baccalaureate nursing preparation . . . has the greatest potential to create a route towards full participation in decision-making about health care services, and best serves the needs of society and nurses themselves'*.

The difficulty with this claim is that the authors fail to explain what they mean by a 'speciality focus as entry into practice' and what would be lost if this focus were displaced. The reader may say that this is surely not the authors' duty, as they are arguing against the 'speciality focus'. However, those who would reduce the variety of any species (here, of P/MH nurses) are, I think, obliged ethically to take account of the 'ecological', whole system, consequences of that reduction.

Particularly notable is the putative association of hospital-based training with speciality nursing. This is not now relevant to the UK, where 'specialist' P/MH nurses graduate as diplomates from higher education institutions (for a comparative analysis of the state of the specialist–generalist debate in the UK, see Norman 2005). In Chapter 7, 'specialists' are characterised in terms of the route to practice rather than what they value, what they claim to know, or how they practise. In short, 'specialists', one version of which we have seen portrayed in Chapter 6, are missing from Chapter 7 and its argument. Statements such as *'the concept of nurse–patient relationship is taught in the first year'* convey nothing like the sense, as in Chapter 6, of development and use of that relationship as the primary principle and medium of P/MH nursing practice.

Nor is there a clear argument in Chapter 7 about the significance of the context(s) in which P/MH nurses practise. Hospitals are cast as the environment responsible for constraining P/MH nurses as professionals. But the nexus of interests and power that shape community mental health practice, and implications for the role of community-based P/MH nurses, may be no less powerful (cf. Tilley & Ryan 2000).

An alternative, more adequate response

As with Chapter 6, the authors of Chapter 7 appear insufficiently reflexive about their role in constructing the context they present as a frame for their argument. They characterise specialists as dated, and as disrupting the advance of nursing professionalism, but do not acknowledge the limitation of this characterisation in the game of controlling the site and direction of P/MH nursing education and practice (see above, regarding the particular obligations attendant on those who would reduce variety). Again, considering their argument in light of recent UK-based arguments, I can see that if they took into account the 'other' to generic preparation they might strengthen their pitch for gaining a role in policy formation, and for meeting needs on a population (or subpopulation, e.g. 'seriously mentally ill') basis. Fuller attention to specialists' claims could help to support a more vigorous case based on the consequences of failure to attend to policy formation, and to consideration of population-based health gain.

Conclusions and suggestions for further argument

In conclusion, Chapter 6's specialists ground their claims in the P/MH nurse–'extraordinary person' relationship, and in the context of role ambiguity and epistemological uncertainty. Chapter 7's generalists/integrationists ground theirs in critique of a past which they claim has damaged P/MH nurses and nursing generally, and in appeals for nursing's greater role in decision-making about the health care service and commitment to meeting society's needs. Chapter 6 views the P/MH nurse through the eyes of an(other) on whom the nurse depends for recognition (indeed, partnership) in the dance of need-expression and response: the generalist through the lens of professionalisation and health service development. Because the authors do not construct their arguments as direct assertion–rebuttal responses to each other – because each 'misses' the other – we face a challenging task if we are to use them to inform our own thinking.

We can start work on that task by asking: 'What is at the heart of the tension between the specialist and the generic accounts?' I offer three resources for considering that question, all found in texts referred to in Chapter 6.

Resource 1

Trevor Clay, then general secretary of the Royal College of Nursing of the UK, observed in his forward to the 1988 edition of Peplau's 'Interpersonal relations in nursing' (Clay 1988: vii):

'the real reason why I believe nurses will welcome this book is that nursing in many parts of the world has lost its way with regard to the fundamentality of the nurse–patient relationship . . . We have concentrated in the last decade or so on the service of nursing – vitally important and necessary to continue so doing – but Peplau's mission is to concern herself with the art of nursing in order that it might complement and enable the service'.

In this light, we can see Chapters 6 and 7 as phases in an unacknowledged dialectic. Chapter 6 asserts as thesis the centrality of the nurse–patient relationship; Chapter 7, that of service. As neither provides an adequate account of the other, neither formulates an antithesis that might propel development of the argument. The tension recapitulates the quandary that British P/MH nurses found themselves in during the 1990s care wars (Tilley 1997): P/MH nurse 'artist' (specialist) *or* 'scientist' (generic). (By 2000, Repper and others considered this antagonism passé in the light of service users' needs for both P/MH nurse scientists and nurse artists [cf. Norman & Ryrie 2004].)

Resource 2

Desmond Ryan's analysis of the 'amphibian' P/MH nurse (Ryan 1997) provides a complementary way forward. (The authors of Chapter 6 cite Ryan [1997] as their source on ambiguity, but not on the aspect we need for the hermeneutic task.) For Ryan, ambiguity is an *essential* characteristic of the P/MH nurse (and nurses generally). This amphibian lives in two worlds simultaneously: the world of natural persons to whom the nurse is responsible (in Chapter 6, 'extraordinary persons' who articulate needs for 'care with'); and the world of artificial organisations (in Chapter 7, the profession serving the needs of society or of a specific population) to which the nurse is accountable.

Each chapter foregrounds a figure of P/MH nursing by reference to an 'other' that threatens it (generalist nemesis; rift-ridden specialists). Chapter 6 cited Ryan as a source in characterising ambiguities with which the P/MH nurse must live, and the authors indeed attended to ambiguous features of P/MH nurses' knowledge and practice more clearly than did Chapter 7. But the ambiguity of artificial organisations writ large (profession, society, population) they have not addressed. Precisely because the argument in Chapter 7 is cast in those terms, we need some further elaboration of the fundamental ambiguity, in order to appraise the potential for 'both/and', rather than 'either/or', resolution of *that* ambiguity.

Ryan offers no magic solution to the amphibian's dilemmatic task, but affirms that the best nurses, teachers, etc. avoid resolution-by-reduction to one element of their dual identity (e.g. 'warderly', 'matter teacher', 'academechanic') and instead find a 'line' that allows the integration of the two elements – in short, 'both/and' rather than 'either/or.' And so it is here: each chapter clearly 'needs' the other – some kind of 'both/and' (re)solution is necessary.

Resource 3

I offer Peplau as a third resource for a more productive argument between those committed to interpersonal relationships and the interdependence of nurse and patient in projects of development, and those committed to meeting the health needs of society and professional development. Peplau saw the interpersonal relationship as *grounded* in 'democratic method' (*'working toward consent and understanding of prevailing problems, related reality factors, and existing conditions by all participants'*; Peplau 1952/1988, p 23) – these tasks offer the authors of Chapters 6 and 7 much to work on together!

Peplau's larger argument might still prove timely for bridging too-easily-separable ways:

'Participation is required by a democratic society. When it has not been learned in earlier experiences nurses have an opportunity to facilitate learning in the present and thus to aid in the promotion of a democratic society.' (Peplau 1952/1988, p 259)

What is required, to address the dilemmatic task facing the amphibian P/MH nurse both responsible to the person and accountable to the profession and society, is fuller participation by each chapter in the 'democratic society' of argument with the other, in which each sees the other and self as fully and only one.

References

Barker P 1989 Reflections on the philosophy of caring in mental health. International Journal of Nursing Studies 26(2):131–141.

Clay T 1988 Foreword. In: Peplau H, ed. Interpersonal relations in nursing. MacMillan, Basingstoke, pp vii–viii.

Norman I 2005 Models of mental health nursing: findings from a case study. In: Tilley S, ed. Psychiatric and mental health nursing: the field of knowledge. Blackwell Publishing, Oxford, pp 129–150.

Norman I J, Ryrie I, eds 2004 The art and science of mental health nursing. Open University Press, London.

Peplau H 1952/1988 Interpersonal relations in nursing. MacMillan, Basingstoke.

Repper J 2000 Adjusting the focus of mental health nursing: incorporating service users' experiences of recovery. Journal of Mental Health 9(6):575–587.

Ryan D 1997 Ambiguity in nursing: the person and the organisation as contrasting sources of meaning. In: Tilley S, ed. The mental health nurse: views of practice and education. Blackwell Science, Oxford, p 118–136.

Tilley S 1997 Conclusion. In: Tilley S, ed. The mental health nurse: views of practice and education. Blackwell Science, Oxford, p 203–210.

Tilley S, Ryan D 2000 Reviewing the literature constructing the field: accounting for the CPN in practice and research. Journal of Mental Health 9(6):589–604.

"

Practice or theory centred: should psychiatric/mental health nursing be located within higher education and have a theory emphasis, or should it be practice oriented?

"

CHAPTER 8

The case for maintaining P/MH nurse preparation within higher education

Ben Hannigan & Michael Coffey

CHAPTER 9

Theory versus practice – gap or chasm? The preparation of practitioners: academic and practice issues

Linda Marie Lowe

Commentary

Maritta Välimäki

Editorial

The debate concerning the 'proper' or most appropriate emphasis within P/MH nurse (or any nurse) preparation will be familiar to many readers; it has been described as 'the old chestnut'. This expression usually refers to an old joke that is well known (its origin appears to be located in a near-forgotten melodrama by William Diamond, first produced in 1816), but in contemporary dialogue most often refers to an issue that is widely known, much debated and familiar. Despite the attention this debate has received, in historical and more modern extant nursing literature, it is clear that the debate is far from resolved.

Ben Hannigan and Michael Coffey (Ch. 8) draw attention to the range of clinical and analytical skills, which need to be underpinned by an advanced knowledge base, that are a prerequisite for professional competence in today's P/MH nurses. Their persuasive arguments vis-à-vis the modern day demands of P/MH nursing and mental health care per se, and the inadequacy of vocational training, are noteworthy. So too is their point regarding pragmatism, universities being institutions with a long and distinguished tradition of professional education. However, Linda Lowe (Ch. 9) reminds us that P/MH nursing is, and always has been, a practice based discipline, practice being the *raison d'être* of nursing; the alpha and the omega. Furthermore, the compelling evidence provided by Linda regarding the 'work readiness' of recent graduates, their sometimes lack of basic skills, and the various postgraduate mechanisms that have been introduced to safeguard new graduates entering practice, are very difficult to ignore. Maritta's thoughtful commentary adds a further dimension to this debate with the notion that given the very different states of P/MH nursing in various countries, it is unlikely that one model will work for everyone; it is doubtful that 'one size will fit all'.

In apparently polarised debates such as this, sometimes referred to as binary opposites (Derrida 1972), protagonists often think in terms of opposites. All things are identified in part by what they are not (the sky is dark but not bright). In addition to being binary opposites or dichotomies, Derrida illustrates how these pairs are also hierarchies. Inevitably, we ascribe ascendancy and greater value to one aspect than we do to the other. Thus, we predicate that beginnings are more important than endings, presence as better than absence and, most disturbing to Derrida, speech as more important than writing. The extant literature that refers to nurse preparation is replete with evidence of such thinking. Thus, in this context, either an emphasis on practice or on theory is ascribed the ascendancy. In his 1972 seminal work, Derrida confronts this idea and attempts to challenge and destabilise these boundaries between binary opposites. Similar challenges have been levelled in this current debate, both within this chapter and elsewhere (see Cutcliffe

2003). Contained in these challenges is the notion that theory and practice are not mutually exclusive; they are fruit from the same tree; the one cannot exist without the other. However, far from rendering this debate redundant, this position purports that the issue of finding the correct balance between theory and practice in P/MH nursing education is very much 'alive'.

References

Cutcliffe J R 2003 A historical overview of psychiatric/mental health nurse education in the United Kingdom: going round in circles or on the straight and narrow? Nurse Education Today 23(5):338–346.

Derrida J 1972 Dissemination. University of Chicago Press, Chicago.

Ben Hannigan & Michael Coffey

The case for maintaining P/MH nurse preparation within higher education

Introduction

In the UK, as in many other countries of the world, the education and training of P/MH nurses is an activity shared between higher education institutions and organisations providing health care. We argue in this chapter that this is an entirely appropriate state of affairs, and that any attempt to deprive the discipline of nursing of a foothold in the university sector would be a harmful and retrograde step. In pursuing this argument we do not suggest that nursing is, or should be, a purely 'academic' discipline. Practitioners of mental health nursing engage in skilled interpersonal and practical activities, with the intention of helping those who are experiencing mental distress. It is appropriate, then, that the educational preparation of those intending to practise in this discipline should be largely vocational. But we argue that this vocational, or practice-oriented, preparation should be delivered from a base in higher education, in which the aim is to develop students' reflective and critical thinking skills to enable the generation of knowledge from practice.

Nursing and higher education

It is now over a century since the first accredited course for mental health nurses, the Certificate in Nursing the Insane, appeared in the UK (Nolan 1993). In the intervening years, P/MH nursing practice and approaches to the preparation of nurses have changed out of all recognition. The psychiatric hospital is no longer the sole location for the delivery of mental health care and treatment: over recent decades, increasing numbers of people with mental health difficulties have received care in their own homes. Specialities within P/MH nursing have appeared and nurses now provide care for people with the widest range of needs, including older people with dementia, adults with long-term and disabling mental illnesses, and children and young people with psychological difficulties.

Courses of preparation have evolved, reflecting the growing complexity and diversity of P/MH nursing practice. Some universities were relatively quick to recognise the benefits to nurses of following degree level education programmes. From the 1950s onwards, academic departments of nursing began to appear in Edinburgh, at the Welsh National School of Medicine (now the University of Wales College of Medicine), in Manchester, in London and elsewhere. Pioneering programmes offered in these university departments were intended to equip newly qualified graduate practitioners with a range of clinical and analytic skills, underpinned by an advanced knowledge base (Roberts & Barriball 1999). For most UK P/MH nurses, however, initial preregistration preparation for practice up until the 1990s meant following 3-year courses delivered in National Health Service (NHS) schools of nursing, leading to the non-university accredited qualification of Registered Mental Nurse.

The late 1980s and early 1990s were important times for nursing education in the UK. Dissatisfaction with the 'apprenticeship' style of preparation, in which nurses largely learned their craft 'on the job', led to searches for a new way of preparing nurses for practice. The outcome of these deliberations, Project 2000, brought forward an approach to preregistration preparation in which qualifying nurses were to be awarded both professional and academic accreditation, typically at undergraduate diploma level (United Kingdom Central Council for Nursing, Midwifery and Health Visiting [UKCC] 1986). The statutory requirement for Project 2000 nurses to complete their studies at Diploma in Higher Education level at least became, in turn, one of the major drivers for the integration of UK NHS-based schools of nursing into the higher education sector; a process formally completed in the mid 1990s (Burke 2003). The process of adjustment on the part of educators and others to working in a higher education environment has, however, taken much longer. Nonetheless, in the UK now, all preregistration P/MH nursing students are enrolled on programmes delivered in higher education departments. All students are required to demonstrate both clinical and academic abilities in order to obtain a licence to practise. Whilst Project 2000 preparation has recently disappeared in favour of a more competency-oriented preparation (UKCC 1999), the role of universities and other higher education institutions in preparing practitioners remains.

Nursing and higher education: some criticisms

A steady flow of criticism, from both within and outside the nursing world, followed the relocation of schools of nursing into higher education establishments, and the corresponding raising of the academic standard required to be met by all newly registered practitioners. Allen (1997) summarised some of these criticisms, noting the claims of some non-nursing commentators (such as Nigella Lawson and Richard Horton, editor of *The Lancet*) that as, in their view, nursing is largely concerned with the non-technical practical provision of care, its practitioners have no particular need for academic accreditation.

Criticisms such as these are based upon complex cultural as well as professional attitudes related to concepts of caring and the traditional role of women within society and the workplace. It is perhaps a well rehearsed argument, and as such the move of nursing into higher education is an easy target for non-nurses to hit. Essentially, the argument suggests that caring is an inherent trait that cannot be taught. Underlying this position, however, is a value judgement that caring is menial work and requires little intellectual effort or educational preparation. From a cultural perspective, the main carers in our society are female, as are the majority of nurses. The expectation of subservience of women in male dominated societies and professions (for example, medicine) has a long history, and the attempt of nurses to gain improved professional or academic status challenges this orthodoxy.

We question the claim that 'nursing' equals 'caring', and that 'caring' is an uncomplicated, practical, and 'natural' activity for which no particular educational preparation is needed. We have already noted a first objection to this position above, in that the criticism of nursing and higher education preparation reveals ingrained yet challengeable cultural assumptions regarding the role of women and the nature of 'women's work'. These cultural assumptions extend to the generation of knowledge and the subsequent use of this knowledge in the education of nurses. Berragan (1998), for example, in discussing epistemology in nursing has suggested that the emphasis on what knowledge is useful to nursing is itself predicated upon value judgements related to gender roles. That is, positivist empirical knowledge has an inherent male bias and is therefore afforded greater value than interpretative and subjective 'female' orientated, qualitative forms of knowledge. P/MH nursing, in particular, has attempted to accommodate broader perspectives on what constitutes useful knowledge for practice. This knowledge may be judged in some quarters to carry less weight than positivist approaches. Perhaps it is judgements about the worthiness of such knowledge that have, in part, prompted questions about the place of nursing in higher education. As we shall see, however, it is this very breadth of knowledge that requires nursing to be placed in higher education where the parallel traditions of knowledge generation and critical thinking can be developed to enhance nursing practice.

In addition, while we accept that providing care is indeed at the centre of nursing, we also question whether caring is a sufficient quality on its own for nurses working in contemporary health services settings. As Allen (1997) points out, evidence of the abuse of children and of older people calls into doubt the idea of 'caring' as a natural, commonly encountered attribute. Allen also observes how the changing nature of health care and health care delivery, and the changing place of nursing in a complex division of health and social care labour, call into question the idea that 'caring is enough'. Arguably, the challenges posed by demographic change, technological developments, the promotion of evidence based practice and shifts in occupational boundaries all point towards nurses needing to be *better* educated. In mental health nursing, for example, there is great interest in practitioners becoming more knowledgeable and skilled in the use of specific psychological and social interventions aimed at helping people with schizophrenia and other severe mental health problems, and their carers (for a discussion, see Gournay & Sandford 1998). UK P/MH nurses may, in the future, also have the opportunity to prescribe medications from a specified formulary (Gournay & Gray 2001), or to play a significant part in making decisions on the use of compulsory powers to oversee the treatment of people with mental health difficulties (Department of Health 2002). Extensions of P/MH nursing activity such as these are hotly debated within the field (and within this book!); our point is, however, that nurses need the kind of educational preparation that enables them to engage with the issues, and, if necessary, modify their practice accordingly. This requires the development of critical analytical skills, something in which higher education has a long tradition. Such skills have enabled other professions to engage in constructive debates about the focus of professional practice. P/MH nursing operates in a contested field of expertise (for example, the very nature of mental illness and the consequent responses to it) and as such requires its practitioners to be capable of critically evaluating the evidence base for practice.

It is tempting to suggest that arguments against nursing having a place in higher education and its practitioners being required to achieve both clinical and academic competencies are the sole preserve of self-appointed social commentators and medical professionals. Tempting, but not wholly convincing, as many similar views are probably held within the nursing profession itself, from, one would think, supposedly better informed nurses. Miers (2002) suggests that one reason for these criticisms is that there is, in essence, an anti-intellectualism in nursing and that this may itself be fostered by nursing academics valuing abstract thinking skills above the practical skills on which nursing depends. Clarke (1999) suggests that the move into higher education was orchestrated without much consultation with the wider discipline and that this essentially represented the interests of the academic elite within nursing. This, therefore, may be one of the reasons for an anti-intellectual stance within much of nursing: a defensive reaction to academic culture.

The concerns about mental health nursing in higher education range wider, however. Ward (1999) notes that a particular concern for some has been the much touted theory–practice gap, with many practitioners expressing the view that newly qualified nurses completing Project 2000 courses have been unable to practise competently. Other concerns include a mismatch between the philosophies of health promotion in educational curricula and the illness focus of clinical practice (Clarke 1999), and the preference for abstract theories over practical P/MH nursing/clinical interventions (Gournay & Sandford 1998).

Why universities?

There are, then, a number of criticisms of the place of nursing in higher education, and of the expectation that newly registered nurses achieve academic as well as clinical qualifications. In this section of our chapter we consider the purpose of higher education institutions, and put forward a number of arguments as to why such places are suitable locations for the preparation of mental health nurses.

The role and purpose of universities is much debated in the UK and beyond. Expansion of the higher education sector has seen not only nursing brought within its ambit, but other 'non-traditional' practitioner and applied disciplines too. The present UK government sees further growth in post-compulsory education as a major policy goal, and has declared a wish to see 50% of 18–30-year-olds participating in higher education. However, debates rumble on with regard to the funding of higher education, and the appropriateness (or not) of delivering what is, now, a remarkably broad range of disciplines through the university sector.

Two key functions of universities are education, and the generation of new knowledge through research. With respect to the first of these functions, we note that nursing is not the first applied discipline to educate its future practitioners in universities – far from it. As Professor Martin Harris, former Chair of the Committee of Vice-Chancellors and Principals of the Universities of the United Kingdom (now known as Universities UK) put it in a speech to the Royal College of Nursing in 1999 (Harris 1999):

'Remember that in coming into universities, schools of nursing were entering not ivory towers, but institutions with a long and distinguished tradition of professional education – starting in the middle ages with medicine, theology, law, and progressively embracing teaching, engineering, accounting and so many more; a tradition which has more recently extended to meeting the training needs of business and industry and society in general in so many ways'.

To suggest that nurses should not be educated in universities when, as Harris points out, practitioners in so many other disciplines are, seems to us to be rather nonsensical. If medical practitioners, occupational therapists, physiotherapists, lawyers, teachers, social workers, engineers, accountants and town planners (and so on) are all prepared in universities, then why not nurses, too?

There are distinct advantages to preparing nurses in institutions where other practitioners are also educated. For example, opportunities for interprofessional learning are that much greater. In the practice setting, P/MH nurses work closely with psychiatrists and other members of the medical profession, and with psychologists, social workers and others; formal and informal shared learning with representatives of these other professional groups is more likely to happen when all are enrolled in higher education institutions. There are advantages, too, for nurses to be able to participate in the overall higher education 'scene', including the informal social and cultural world of university life. We argue that providing education in stand-alone institutions, divorced from other disciplines, runs the risk of encouraging students to develop narrow, blinkered perspectives. Participating in education alongside students following programmes in a wide variety of disciplines is, we suggest, a potentially enriching experience that benefits both the individual and the profession.

One of the purposes of a university education is to help students develop skills in critical thinking. Bradshaw (1999) argues, in a frankly idealised view of a Nightingale-inspired tradition of nursing, that nursing is not an 'intellectual' activity because it is primarily a 'physical' activity. This, she suggests, is one reason why nurse training (nurses should not be 'educated', it seems) should be returned to hospital schools of nursing. We would argue, however, that nursing is both an intellectual activity and a physical one. What P/MH nurses, in particular, think about their work is important, and this thinking requires intellectual effort and development. These critical thinking skills are needed to enable nurses to assimilate complex technical and interpersonal data in their work. They must then sift through these data to decide what is of relevance within a specific context so that they can make clinical judgements that accommodate and reflect the best interests of the person or persons they are working with. Critical thinking is one way in which nurses can avoid practising in ritualistic ways based upon unexamined beliefs and traditions. It is an essential intellectual activity that can be applied to clinical practice with the aim of analysing and understanding it (Boychuk Duchscher 1999).

Brookfield (1987) suggests that there are four elements to critical thinking. These are: the ability to identify and challenge assumptions; recognition of the importance of context in shaping our view of (and our response to) the world; a willingness to explore alternatives to received 'truths'; and a reflective scepticism that acknowledges the limits and uncertainties of current knowledge. Critical thinking is what higher education has been developing in practitioners of other applied professions for years, and P/MH nursing care should benefit from such examination.

It is in the pursuit of knowledge to inform practice that critical thinking skills are of particular importance. As such, critical thinking skills are essential to the development of P/MH nursing practice. P/MH nurses can build knowledge from clinical practice experiences through the application of critical reflective thought. They can also do this by applying these skills to the development of empirically grounded, clinically focused, investigation. What we freely acknowledge in making this case for nurses to be educated as 'critical thinkers' is that, although it is part of the function of universities to enlarge students' critical capacities, the value of this in nursing practice is where this 'critical thinking' is applied to the everyday world of clinical practice.

We reiterate here our view that nursing education should be the product of strong partnership between institutions concerned with the provision of education, and organisations providing mental health care. We recognise the problems posed by a 'theory–practice gap', and acknowledge the importance of P/MH nursing education being rooted in practice. In this respect, we applaud strategies which explicitly bring together higher education and health care providing organisations, such as the appointment of lecturer–practitioners. However, we also recognise that the 'theory–practice' gap has positive, as well as negative, aspects. Education driven solely by the immediate demands of health care providers is likely, in our view, to be limited in its scope, and organised to meet largely short-term needs. The 'critical distance' that university-based schools of nursing have from the everyday world of health care provision allows them the space and independence to take a long-term view, and to place emphasis on the education needs and development of each individual student as well as on the immediate demands of service providers.

There are further difficulties with the idea of the 'theory–practice' gap in mental health nursing. There is, perhaps, a false dichotomy (but one that exists nonetheless) which on the one hand advocates that nurse education should be informed by practice, while on the other that practice should be informed by and follow theory. There is much to be said for both arguments, and a combination of the two should not be so difficult to accomplish. However, although both sides in the debate on mental health nurse education may see value in their positions, both are frankly missing the point. Education and training of P/MH nurses should be informed not by practice exigencies or educational theory alone, but by the expressed needs of those in receipt of services. To argue otherwise would be to ignore the voices of service users and reinforce the paternalistic assumptions that have riddled mental health care for generations.

Alongside the provision of education, a further function of universities is the generation of new knowledge through research. It is remarkable, given the number of nurses working in the UK (and indeed throughout the world), how little is known about the impact of nursing work on the experience of health service users. Over 1% of the UK population are registered nurses (Cowley 1999); however, only a tiny fraction of these are engaged in funded research activity. This is a major cause for concern, as nursing – P/MH nursing included – *needs* a knowledge base generated through research. We recognise, absolutely, the importance of other forms of knowledge for P/MH nursing work, such as the knowledge generated by the experienced practitioner engaging in reflective practice. However, we argue that systematic empirical enquiry into aspects of P/MH nursing activity is a vital prerequisite for the flourishing of the discipline, and for the improvement of service users' experiences of P/MH nursing care.

Having put forward this position, we note, again, how varying degrees of value are often accorded to different forms of knowledge, with knowledge generated from within a positivist paradigm often being received in a more favourable light than knowledge produced from within alternative, interpretative traditions. Our view is that nursing benefits from knowledge generated through a variety of methods; for example, both randomised controlled trials and in-depth qualitative case studies are capable of producing findings of importance for mental health nursing practice. What *is* important is that research, of whatever type, is conducted to a degree of excellence and rigour. In our view, it is the function of universities and of nurses working in them to take the lead in this to ensure that the research which informs and underpins practice is of comparable quality to that practised elsewhere.

Research led by university-based P/MH nurses has the capacity to change practice for the better and to improve the experience of service users. A small number of examples illustrating this will suffice. Brooker et al (1994), using an experimental design, demonstrated how community P/MH nurses using structured family interventions were able to have a positive impact on the health and well-being both of people with schizophrenia and their carers. Brooker and colleagues' findings were important in informing developments in P/MH nurse education and training, including the creation and extension of evidence based programmes such as those constructed under the umbrella of the Thorn initiative. More recently, Barker et al (1999) have used qualitative methods of enquiry to generate knowledge of the 'need for psychiatric nursing'. This body of work has shed new light on the significance of interpersonal relations in nursing, and the importance of P/MH nurses being able to 'relate' at a number of different levels.

There are compelling reasons for locating nursing education in the same institutions as those which are home to individuals and teams responsible for the production of nursing research and for nursing scholarship. Students learning in research-active higher education departments have the opportunity for exposure to research-led teaching, and the opportunity to learn alongside nurses who are personally engaged in the production of 'new knowledge', new concepts and in other forms of scholarship. We suggest that early immersion in a research-led environment is critical in inculcating in nurses an appreciation of the value of research as a driver for practice development, and as an important (but not the only) guide for everyday nursing care.

Just as we have made a case in the context of nursing education for strong partnerships between higher education institutions and health care providers, so too do we make a case for the importance of strong links between university based nurses and practising nurses in the context of undertaking research activity. Many, or most, important nursing research questions are likely to arise from the observations of nurses with a solid grounding in everyday practice. Whilst practising nurses are often best placed to generate research questions, or to identify areas where research knowledge is most needed, it is often the case that nurses with the expertise and resources to initiate actual research projects are based in the university sector. We welcome the appearance of practitioner–researchers (as we do the growth of lecturer–practitioners), as people who are particularly well placed to bring together the worlds of practice and higher education. It seems likely to us that the most fruitful type of research endeavour is that where P/MH nurses with different skills and interests located in different organisations come together in pursuit of shared goals.

Issues for the future

Burke & Harris (2000) have shown that purchasers of nursing education see degree-level education benefiting nursing practice with regard to leadership, assertiveness, and reflective and critical skills. Currently in the UK, it is hotly debated whether *all* newly registering nurses should qualify at undergraduate degree level, or whether the current minimum academic level for qualification should more appropriately remain at undergraduate diploma level. This is an issue which arouses strongly held feelings, and the debate seems likely to rumble on for a considerable time yet. In addition, reconciling the competing demands of maintaining a wide entry gate to nursing education and of producing ever-increasing numbers of graduate level nurses is an issue which universities will be grappling with for the foreseeable future. We have shied away from debating the merits or otherwise of pursuing an all-graduate mental health nursing workforce in this chapter; instead, we have limited ourselves to making an argument for university based nursing preparation irrespective of the level of academic award made to students on completion of their studies. However, we acknowledge the importance of this debate in UK nursing and elsewhere. We also note the confusions which exist over 'academic levels' in nursing, and particularly the notorious difficulties which exist when trying to capture and measure concepts such as 'graduate-level practice'. In our view, clarity over terms and concepts should be an important part of these discussions.

There also remains an important message in Bradshaw's (1999) regressive evocations for nurse education; this is her clear and unambiguous argument for nursing to maintain its focus on caring as the basis for its activity with people. The education of P/MH nurses must not ignore this fundamental emphasis in the preparation of its future practitioners.

A further issue of considerable significance for P/MH nursing education and practice is the relationship between nursing and other disciplines. We note the rise of interest in recent years in interprofessional approaches to both mental health service delivery and the preparation of practitioners. In this context, it is unclear how far P/MH nursing will be able to retain its specific identity in both the clinical practice setting, and in terms of preparation for practice. 'Generalist' nursing, in which practitioners are prepared for practice in, ostensibly, any area of health care, is also on the agenda in the UK (as it has been for many years elsewhere in the world). The blurring of occupational boundaries in the mental health arena, and the possibility of the 'generic' nurse (see debate 3), both have implications for the identity of P/MH nursing, and hence for education. Issues of this sort are, we believe, far more pressing for P/MH nursing than is the issue of whether or not higher education is the best place for the delivery of nursing education.

Conclusions

We have pursued the argument in this chapter that the preparation of P/MH nurses is most appropriately located in the higher education sector. We have suggested that preparation for practice should be a shared activity, in which universities and institutions providing health care work together in a form of partnership. We have reviewed, and roundly rejected, the idea that nursing is an activity for which no particular advanced education is needed. Although caring is indeed a central part of nursing, the complex demands faced by those working in contemporary health care settings make education more, not less, important than ever before. We have particularly made a case for the importance of critical thinking skills, and have suggested that universities have a special role to play in developing these. While acknowledging concerns over the existence of a theory–practice gap in P/MH nursing, we have also sought to demonstrate how benefits can accrue to individuals and to health care organisations, and indeed ultimately to users of mental health services, from preparation for practice which is not solely driven by the immediate demands of the health service.

We have also drawn attention to the role of universities in the creation of knowledge through research. Debates continue in P/MH nursing over the 'right' sort of research for mental health practice (see Debate 9); our view has been that good research, of whatever type, has the potential to inform and improve the delivery of care and the experience of service users. Education and research are closely related activities, and it is appropriate, we have argued, for P/MH nurses to have the opportunity to learn in institutions in which research is being undertaken.

References

Allen D 1997 Nursing, knowledge and practice. Journal of Health Services Research and Policy 2(3):190–193.

Barker P, Jackson S, Stevenson C 1999 The need for psychiatric nursing: towards a multidimensional theory of caring. Nursing Inquiry 6:103–111.

Berragan L 1998 Nursing practice draws upon several different ways of knowing. Journal of Clinical Practice 7:209–217.

Boychuk Duchscher J E 1999 Catching the wave: understanding the concept of critical thinking. Journal of Advanced Nursing 29(3):577–583.

Bradshaw A 1999 The virtue of nursing: the covenant of care. Journal of Medical Ethics 25:477–481.

Brooker C, Falloon I, Butterworth A, Goldberg D, Graham-Hole V, Hillier V 1994 The outcome of training community psychiatric nurses to deliver psychosocial intervention. British Journal of Psychiatry 165:222–230.

Brookfield S D 1987 Developing critical thinkers: challenging adults to explore alternative ways of thinking and acting. Open University Press, Milton Keynes.

Burke L M 2003 Integration into higher education: key implementers' views on why nurse education moved into higher education. Journal of Advanced Nursing 42(4):382–389.

Burke L M, Harris D 2000 Education purchasers' views of nursing as an all graduate profession. Nurse Education Today 20:620–628.

Clarke L 1999 Challenging ideas in psychiatric nursing. Routledge, London.

Cowley S 1999 Nursing in a managerial age. In: Norman I, Cowley S, eds. The changing nature of nursing in a managerial age. Blackwell Science, Oxford, p 3–17.

Department of Health 2002 Draft Mental Health Bill. The Stationery Office, London.

Gournay K, Gray R 2001 Should mental health nurses prescribe? Maudsley Discussion Paper No. 11. Institute of Psychiatry, London.

Gournay K, Sandford T 1998 Training the workforce. In: Brooker C, Repper J, eds. Serious mental health problems in the community: policy, practice and research. Baillière Tindall, London.

Harris M 1999 Nursing education in the learning society. Address delivered to Royal College of Nursing conference, 6 February 1999. Online. Available: http://www.universitiesuk.ac.uk/speeches/show.asp?sp=25 accessed 2004

Miers M 2002 Nurse education in higher education: understanding cultural barriers to progress. Nurse Education Today 22(3):212–219.

Nolan P 1993 A history of mental health nursing. Chapman & Hall, London.

Roberts J, Barriball K L 1999 Education for nursing: preparation for professional practice. In: Norman I, Cowley S, eds. The changing nature of nursing in a managerial age. Blackwell Science, Oxford, p 123–149.

United Kingdom Central Council for Nursing, Midwifery and Health Visiting 1986 Project 2000: a new preparation for practice. UKCC, London.

United Kingdom Central Council for Nursing, Midwifery and Health Visiting 1999 Fitness for practice: the UKCC Commission for Nursing and Midwifery Education (Chair: Sir Leonard Peach). UKCC, London.

Ward M 1999 Mental health nursing: education. Nursing Standard 13(43):61.

CHAPTER

9

Linda Marie Lowe

Theory versus practice – gap or chasm? The preparation of practitioners: academic and practice issues

Background

I qualified as a Registered Nurse in the UK nearly twenty-five years ago. The *modus operandi* for registered nurse preparation during the mid seventies was the traditional 'apprentice' route and at that time I believed this was the only option available to me. Had you asked me about my impression of higher education during that time, I would have stated that obviously it was a requirement for the *professions*, for instance medicine, dentistry and law, but not for nursing. My own training had me placed on a ward and engaging in clinical work within 6 weeks. Six months into my training, I was on night duty and holding drug keys. I was aware that not one of my tutors had obtained a degree, as the minimum requirement for teaching nurses in the UK at that time was a Registered Nurse Tutor diploma. However, their extensive clinical experience had a great impact upon me and the rest of the student body, and they were held in high esteem. After qualifying (and I purposefully do not use the term 'graduating' here), I don't believe I encountered one nurse with a degree in any of the facilities where I was employed.

Moving to Newfoundland, Canada in the early 1980s certainly opened my eyes with regards to the possibility of degree nurses, as they were already well established. Working in a large teaching hospital, where the ratio of diploma to degree nurses was approximately 4 to 1, I soon became aware of the subtle differences in the way nurse teams interacted and operated. Although it was not openly verbalised, if one had a degree nurse on one's team, an extra level of supervision was factored in. It was generally understood that these nurses had not had sufficient clinical time prior to graduation and would need extra overseeing until they developed enough experience and honed their skills.

The essential need for clinical experience was reinforced when, in 1986, at the age of thirty-one, I was admitted to a university-based nursing programme to complete a three-year post RN BScN programme. Our group, each of whom was an older nurse, having worked clinically for an average of ten years, felt strongly that post RN was the route to go. We were of the understanding that we had sufficient clinical time and that this experience was invaluable as a framework upon which to 'hang' the nursing theory. Like my colleagues, I had not had any formal academic preparation for undergraduate life and found the programme quite demanding. It didn't take long before we were of the opinion that there was inadequate clinical preparation available to baccalaureate nursing students and that they were grossly unprepared for the reality of professional clinical nursing.

The 'old chestnut' issue

What has changed since those days? We are now in 2006 and the question needs to be asked: has this chasm between theory and practice narrowed? I believe not. One only has to search the contemporary literature to see that the old tensions remain, and regardless of every well intentioned author who attempts to provide solutions, there they linger, expansive and hungry. To provide context as to the nature of the two philosophical and epistemological approaches for nurse preparation, I will undertake a brief retrospective analysis. It is hoped that this will help envision future possibilities (Cutcliffe 2003). Further, it needs to be acknowledged that the education (preparation) of P/MH nurses has been significantly influenced by the education of other types of nurse (e.g. general nurses).

Accordingly, the purpose of this chapter is to provide a brief overview of the history of general and psychiatric nursing. Following this, I highlight the views of two predominant proponents of nurse education and draw attention to the emergence of increasingly sophisticated nursing education programmes. Then, I discuss the value and importance of clinical experience within nursing programmes, and finally discuss possible future educational directions for the discipline. I argue that if we cannot reconcile the two principal positions that underpin nurse preparation (i.e. practice or theory emphasis), then at least we can provide some possibilities for crafting tentative links.

History: general nursing

Nursing, as a practice orientated discipline has traditionally had its roots in 'hands-on' or front line clinical work. Watkins (2000) purports that the training of nurses within the UK, as introduced by Florence Nightingale in the latter part of the 19th century, was via the 'apprenticeship model'. The model transferred to North America but unfortunately the general public viewed nurses in a dim light. In her insightful history of nursing in Canada, Mansell (2003, p 25) presents the views of a 19th century physician. She states:

'Age and frowziness (meaning – 'messy') seemed to be the chief attributes of the nurse, who was ill-educated and was often made more unattractive by the vinous odor of her breath. Cleanliness was not a feature of the nurse, ward or the patient; the language was frequently painful and free . . . Armies of rats frequently disported themselves about the wards and picked up scraps left by the patients and sometimes attacked the patients themselves.'

This model continued for nearly a century on both sides of the Atlantic. In 1919, the UK moved to formalise nursing training and the clinical experiences within the 'apprenticeship model' were seen to fulfil the registration requirements of general nurses. At the same time, North America moved away from this model with the introduction of the first university based nursing programmes. These programmes contained increased emphasis on theoretical preparation (professional registration then came under the auspices of the University of Alberta) and similar developments were already taking place in the USA, Australia, and New Zealand (Watkins 2000).

The UK was slower off the mark. It was not until the mid 1980s that a report entitled 'Project 2000. A new preparation for practice' (UKCC 1986) concluded that instead of an apprenticeship model, students of nursing should have a higher education focused student experience. Many arguments and explanations have been offered as to why this move occurred, including Elkan & Robinson's (1993) position that the underlying thrust to discard the apprenticeship model was driven by the notion that nurses could acquire additional status through higher education.

History: psychiatric nursing

It can be argued that, throughout history, the treatment of the mentally ill has been heavily influenced by the views of society. Forward thinking luminaries such as Plato (*c.* 400 BC) viewed the *'psyche'* as the struggle between our noble and base desires, not unlike Freud's views of the *id, ego, and superego* (Darton 1999). Plato's recommendations for the treatment of mental infirmities included music and sleep, with very little discernible stigma. Contrast this approach to the beliefs of the 16th and 17th centuries, when society understood that mental disorder was principally caused by demons and the mentally ill were often burned as witches. Fast forward to Darwin's 1859 *Origin of the Species* giving rise to the general assertion that insanity was hereditary; therefore, *Bedlam* or incarceration was the only answer.

Our contemporary understanding of mental health problems can be summarised into two apparently polarised views, and Dr Liam Clarke provides a useful summary of these. According to Clarke (2000), the first group believes they have the answers to most of the big questions in mental health (and health care for that matter). They believe the physical sciences offer up these answers or are on the cusp of solving whatever remains. Similarly, this group sees behavioural/cognitive sciences as having produced a workable range of cognitive and socially focused interventions. The second group, suggests Clarke (2000), believes that the search for the answers in mental health has only just begun. He states (p 75):

'it's not that they see biological discoveries as unworthy; it is simply that they are inappropriate questions for nurses'.

Barker (1999) offered similar remarks, suggesting that, although technology may offer intriguing insights into what appears to be happening on a biological level, it tells us little or nothing about the human experience of mental health problems.

Not surprisingly, these historical and contemporary views of mental health and illness have influenced how P/MH nursing was brought into operation within the UK. Traditionally, individuals with a lack of formal training cared for the mentally ill. It was not until early in the 20th century that the growing dissatisfaction with lack of formal preparation and care of mentally ill clients brought about radical change. Up to that point, male and female attendants were considered to be hard working yet poorly paid; they identified with working class ideology. Entry requirements included physical fitness, ability to play games and mastery of a musical instrument; the range of duties was mainly functional, such as cleaning, feeding, restraint, and organisation of games (Chatterton 2004).

Across the Atlantic in North America things were similar, in that until the early 1880s there were no formally trained psychiatric nurses in the USA. Resistance to women caring for the 'insane' was high. However, this resistance was overcome with the first psychiatric training school for nurses founded in Boston in 1882. In 1913 general nursing training incorporated a formal psychiatric nursing component (Laurence 2002). Masters degrees in Psychiatric Nursing became a possibility after the Mental Health Act of 1946 and the first graduate programme was offered by Hildegarde Peplau in 1954.

A new debate or more of the same?

Historically, the argument about the appropriate emphasis within nursing programmes and the concomitant debate about 'which is best', the actual 'hands on', clinical work or the theoretical preparation, was not an issue. When nurses were awarded their certification, principally for their physical stamina and endurance of long hours, for their ability to endure backbreaking work and receive little in the way of remuneration, the need to be well versed in nursing theory was largely irrelevant. The latter part of the 20th century saw the advent of diverse subspecialities in P/MH nursing, each requiring more advanced academic preparation. In North America, we now have advanced practitioners, clinical specialists, community specialists, and more. However, the overall thrust over the past five decades towards an increasingly formal academic preparation brings with it an uneasy tension between what is an appropriate academic grounding and the need to produce safe practitioners. This has led to important questions including: Have we gone too far one way with our insistence upon such rigorous formal preparation at the expense of valuable clinical experience?

These extant tensions generate laudable arguments for each side of the theory versus practice debate. However, it is worth considering whether having appropriate content material for curricula is at odds with the absolute need to produce an efficient and safe practitioner at the end of the programme (RNABC Standards for Registered Nursing Practice, 2004, p 18). These arguments are not new; one can locate their origins at the time when the apprenticeship model was the nurse preparation model of choice. At that time, there were general disagreements about what could be considered an appropriate amount and quality of classroom time in one form or another. Fast-forward a few decades, and with entry to practice being at baccalaureate level in many places we now see the clear division between prominent nurse educationalists. There are those who argue that current programme emphasis is rightly the focus upon a rigorous academic discipline with a pronounced de-emphasis on clinical practice. Conversely, there are those who argue that practice, clinical practice experience, remains as always the *raison d'être* of nursing and that this must be reflected in nursing programme curricula.

Generally, the luminaries in our discipline are fully supportive of, and dedicated to, raising the bar for the overall standard in nurse education. Although the following two are a hundred years (and a continent) apart, we will see that their insight, forward thinking, and application of rigorous standards paved the way for the natural evolution of our discipline in the truest sense of the word.

The argument for rigorous academic preparation: from Nightingale to Peplau

You may hold a particular view of Florence Nightingale, either as

'a consummate confidence-trickster; an hysteric, a bully, a liar, a manipulator, an ingrate, an intriguer, a bluffer, a betrayer, dogmatically

ignorant, avid for fame, a paranoid deceiver, above all as one who set about deliberately and consistently distorting and perverting the historical record to her own advantage' (Smith 1982, p 2)

or perhaps as someone who

'worked tirelessly to change conditions in hospitals and in places that cared for the wounded and sick in the Crimean War and throughout England and India. She used her interest in mathematics and applied statistics to create the changes she thought were needed' . . . *Her great accomplishments in the fields of nursing, sanitation, and statistics 'reflect the strong conceptual and design skills, supported by exhaustive and accurate research'* (Milton 2002, p 41).

For better or for worse, Nightingale is considered the mother of modern nursing. Granted, she had a privileged, albeit restrained upbringing; however, her adherence to the principles of a formal educational preparation for nurses (something unheard of for women in the early 19th century) arguably laid the foundation for nurse preparation that is grounded upon a sound theoretical basis. Many researchers and nurses have difficulty with Ms Nightingale as she was definitively anti-feminist, vehemently opposed to the concept of female physicians, and against the professionalisation of nursing. This, strangely enough, is diametrically opposed to her renowned indefatigable drive towards excellence in nursing. Also, what can be off-putting is the heavy religious overlay to her words that can obscure the message and meaning. However, if one places that patina of piety aside, one can uncover some kernels of truth. In her writings she determined that knowledge, and the inclusion of this knowledge in the formal preparation of nurses, was an essential element not only for nurses, but for the public at large. She was perhaps the first woman to consider that medical knowledge had a wider realm than just physicians and surgeons. Consider what she says in her 1860 publication 'Notes on Nursing: What it is, and what it is not' (Nightingale 1860, p 3):

'But how much more extraordinary is it that, whereas what we might call the coxcombries [conceitedness] of education – e.g., the elements of astronomy, are now taught to every schoolgirl, neither mothers of families of any class, nor schoolmistresses of any class, nor nurses of children, nor nurses of hospitals, are taught anything about those laws which God has assigned to the relations of our bodies with the world in which He has put them . . . They call it medical or physiological knowledge, fit only for doctors'.

Fast-forward nearly a hundred years, and nurses are obtaining undergraduate degrees in North America and Europe. Hildegarde Peplau, known as the mother of modern P/MH nursing, earned an MA in

Nursing in 1943, then went on to design and offer the first graduate programme for Masters Degrees in Psychiatric Nursing at Rutgers University in 1954. Dr Peplau will be forever associated with her interpersonal theory; a clear workable conceptual framework that could be utilised for either general or P/MH nursing and which, arguably, took nursing to new heights through its clarity and purpose. Her objective of transforming the 'occupation' of nursing to a profession was underpinned by her stringent belief in the value of formal educational preparation. A holder of seven doctoral degrees, a visionary and prolific writer, she was not able to publish her seminal work *Interpersonal Relations in Nursing* until 1952, although it was originally written for publication in 1948, as at that time it was considered too 'avant garde' to publish without a physician as a co-author! Until her death in 1999 she was a vigorous supporter of academic preparation for nurses; Peplau believed that in order to provide considered and deliberate remedial care of clients, rather than the then prevalent 'custodial' care (Sills 1998), a sound educational preparation was necessary. Peplau's experience with graduate education was formative in that her obvious disappointment in her own graduate preparation in nursing may have provided the motivation not only to create new programmes for P/MH nursing, but to set the bar higher for nursing education as a whole.

Indeed, Peplau declared:

'I had graduated from the master's program at Teacher's College which I took in 1946 and '47, and it was really very, very bad. It was a series of lectures by nurses who came in, and some of them talked about their golf games, some of them spent the time berating us because we had been in WWII and had an easy time of it, in Europe or Asia, while they were at home and overworked. Others just sort of filled in the time with whatever came into their heads'
(Sills 1998, p 170)

Whatever the motivation, we look upon this courageous and spirited individual as

'. . . a woman of uncommon intellect, socialized outside the traditional 1940s model of nursing in the United States, who developed a paradigm of professionalism . . . that has permeated every aspect of her long and distinguished career'
(Sills 1998, p 171)

Where are we now?

The consideration of the current nature of education and nurse preparation is prefaced by a number of key contextual points:

- First, there is an abundance of literature and substantiated research that attests to the ill preparedness of new nurses for the demanding and sometimes harsh workplace environment. Yet even the authors of such research and reports would be loathe to suggest that we turn back the clock to the days when nurses received 'training' as opposed to education (Nelson 2002 p 3).
- Something of a schism can be seen to exist within nursing academia. Many proponents of an emphasis on academic preparation for nurses believe that, as with other professional programmes, a professional higher education should be considered *de rigeur*, as only then can a nurse function from a sound educational knowledge base and a position of autonomy (see, for example, Watson 1989). However, it is still widely recognised that even today nurses remain the least educated among professional health care providers (Nelson 2002, p 5).
- With regard to P/MH nursing, there is a common belief that today's generic baccalaureate degrees have had such an effect as to dilute the mental health components of nursing curricula (Chan et al 1998, Cutcliffe & McKenna 2000a, 2000b, Norman 2005).
- The nature of nursing education currently appears to be concerned with the processes of 'learning and personal development', yet teaching *per se* is not necessarily synonymous with learning.
- Educational input does not necessarily equate with a positive learning outcome.

Although not at a literal starting point, we are yet again faced with another round of reports, recommendations, suggestions, projects, studies, etc. The consensus of opinion that things need to change is evident from the plethora of literature, but the direction of change is far more equivocal. Governments and institutes of higher learning, on both sides of the Atlantic, are all for promotion of improved nursing education (theory based); ironically even though the literature suggests that more theory courses are not what is needed. In the UK, an ongoing study, involving 16 pilot projects, is currently underway at institutions wishing to facilitate the development of the new model of education.

The deep sense of irony is not lost on the author that this requirement for a new model of nurse education is occurring only twenty years after the publication of the then 'innovative' Project 2000 document. The numerous publications from 1995 onwards agree that there is a need to tighten the theory–practice interface within nurse education programmes. Interestingly, however, there is no clear consensus as to what the practitioners produced by the new programmes will look like. The Royal College of Nursing, too, shares the vision for a better educated workforce. The precise nature of this education, the equipoise of theory and practice courses within such education and the value of clinical education and experiences are less clear or visible:

'The RCN strongly believes that nursing education is central to enabling skilled expert nursing care in order to improve outcomes for patients and staff. A better-educated nursing workforce, which has equity in terms of opportunities, will lead to higher standards of patient care and improved health outcomes'

(RCN 2002, p 2)

Researchers, authors, academics, and frontline clinical nurses are taking stock of the current aptitudes of the 'new nurse' and asking the question: just *how* able are our new graduates to function in an increasingly complex health care delivery system that has many competing facets? The findings from a variety of studies, such as they are, are equivocal, but tend to indicate that employers have some reservations about the 'work readiness' of many new graduates (Lenburg 2002, p 1).

Mutually exclusive or fruit from the same tree?

Clearly, the debate about having the 'correct' emphasis within P/MH nursing preparation is bound up with not only understanding the value of practice and theory, but at the same time recognising the interplay between the two. Cutcliffe (2003) points out that despite the sometimes entrenched positions of the 'practice advocates' and the 'theory advocates', these phenomena are not mutually exclusive; they are fruit from the same tree; the one does not exist without the other. Even accepting this as axiomatic, the question still remains as to *how much* professional competence finds its origin in either *or* both camps. Accordingly, this begs linked, preliminary questions such as: can one develop *professional competence* from programmes with a theory emphasis? Accepting that some exposure to clinical placements is necessary – how much exposure is required to facilitate the development of *professional competence*? Given the evidence that some employers believe that recent nursing graduates lack 'work-readiness', one might conclude that current programmes have insufficient clinical emphasis to enable the development of adequate *professional competence*. This warrants further consideration.

The necessity of clinical experience

The fundamentally negative aspect of the mechanistic model of nursing preparation prior to Project 2000 was that the hospital system engineered the production of a multitude of nurses trained in *care giving*.

However, it is now widely accepted that these nurses were not encouraged or taught to think critically. Critical thinking is included in most, if not all, Western baccalaureate nursing curricula. Nevertheless, what our colleagues lacked in academic rigour, they certainly made up for by their early and complete immersion in clinical experience, as this was introduced within 2 months of starting their programmes (and incidentally provided the clinical facility with a cheap workforce). Today, the 'flipside of the coin' sees baccalaureate level as the entry point to practice in many places and this immersion in higher education has indeed produced nurses who can *think critically*, but this has not been without cost. First, there is an abundance of evidence indicating how we have lost vital clinical exposure essential for the development of clinical expertise. For example, nursing students in the UK experienced a 40% decline in clinical time over the 3-year period following the introduction of Project 2000 (Elkan & Robinson 1993, Elkan et al 1994). Second, we are facing a global nursing shortage that is expected to balloon when the first of the baby boomers start to retire. This will create a situation where our health services have far fewer practitioners with extensive clinical experience. Third, in British Columbia, Canada, for example, the amalgamation of Community Health Councils and Community Health Service Societies within the province has created the situation where, importantly, acute and community sector mental health placements for nursing students are dwindling alarmingly. Furthermore, this centralisation means there is a lack of available community mental health care professionals to care for those discharged from facilities and, at the same time, provide preceptorship (mentorship) for students. Students are thus gaining their 'mental health' clinical experiences in what might be considered to be insufficient, inappropriate and unsuitable placements and are having inadequate preceptorship and mentorship.

Subsequently pressure on available placements is growing exponentially, with programme coordinators scrambling to place their students. For example, throughout Canada, it is increasingly difficult to place students for their clinical experiences. This situation is exacerbated by dramatically increasing student numbers. As a result, and using a Northern British Columbia university as an example, students are supposed to undertake 1261 clinical exposure hours (which translates into only 5.6 months' clinical experience on a four-year degree programme). However, even this scant amount of time student nurses actually spend in clinical placement is coming under threat due to increased student numbers and decreased numbers of appropriate clinical placement options. This leads to the extremely real danger of universities graduating nurses who are less than clinically competent; this means, unsafe!

The provincial facilities, already aware of this current practice deficit, are attempting to 'plug the dyke' by stretching the resources of their already overworked and stressed nursing workforce. It is current practice to impose a preceptorship model. (Preceptorship is a one-to-one relationship between an experienced nurse [the expert] and a lesser experienced/newly graduated nurse in order to learn the roles and responsibilities of clinical nursing in a particular area of practice.) The preceptor usually oversees the practice (and therefore accepts responsibility) for the novice. The lack of popularity of this approach is evident by the many letters of complaint from harassed colleagues to their professional journals, stating that their workload has effectively doubled in that they now have two primary responsibilities; caring for their own clients and keeping the clients safe, by overseeing the practice of new graduates.

The necessity of education – Part One

At this point, it would be relatively simple to conclude this discussion and state that evidence has shown that substantial clinical practice is considered the most valuable attribute for the modern nurse, particularly when *professional competence* is considered. This appears to be reinforced each time an employer hires a new graduate and assigns him/her to one of the various aspects of the preceptor model in order to develop baseline competencies/safety in the new employee. Ergo, it would be reasonable to state that even the most academically lauded new nurse is virtually unemployable unless this academic preparation is accompanied by professional competencies and skill levels. Herein lies the dilemma. By function, P/MH nursing, just like any other specialty was, is, and will be for the immediate future, grounded in the practice domain (Barker 1999). Thus, there will always be a requirement for P/MH nurses to engage in specific and specialised practice-related activities (which are currently not within the realm of training or practice of either health care assistants or licenced practical nurses). Concomitantly, there is an expectation (from employers, clients, and the public) that, inherent within the implementation of such advanced skills, nurses have grasped the theoretical components, underpinnings, and rationale of the intervention. Ironically, one can argue that this widely held belief fails to consider that with the increased academic demands in contemporary nursing curricula, the opportunity to put into practice what one learns in the classroom has diminished substantially.

The necessity of education – Part Two

After extolling the virtues of a practice-based discipline, one in which the doing perhaps takes precedence over the knowing, how can one possibly present a case for the opposite – for the continuation and development of higher learning in nursing? By way of a response to this question, we need to acknowledge that, in nursing education, the goal is not facilitating the acquisition of knowledge for its own sake, but facilitating the acquisition of knowledge that is then applied in practice. As with all applied or professional programmes, the acquisition of theoretical knowledge is not an end in itself. Furthermore, we should also recognise that the acquisition of knowledge through practice alone had severe and significant limitations as a model for nurse preparation.

Though I recognise its vintage, Bloom's 'Taxonomy of educational objectives' (Bloom 1948, cited in Anderson & Sosniak 1994) still has relevance to this debate (see Fig. 9.1). Interestingly, it should be noted that Bloom positions knowledge as the precursor to application. In other words, acquiring and understanding (theoretical) knowledge is important, but this is superseded by the need to use the knowledge and apply it in a meaningful way. According to Bloom then, if the educational process (and resultant outcome) stops at the acquisition and understanding of knowledge, then the student is less than halfway to achieving the 'ultimate' educational objective.

Equally importantly, if the educational process (and resultant outcome) stops at the application of knowledge stage, then the student still remains only halfway to achieving the 'ultimate' educational objective. If the 'ultimate' educational objective is to be achieved, then in Bloom's view, this requires analysis, synthesis and evaluation:

Fig. 9.1 Bloom's taxonomy of educational objectives.

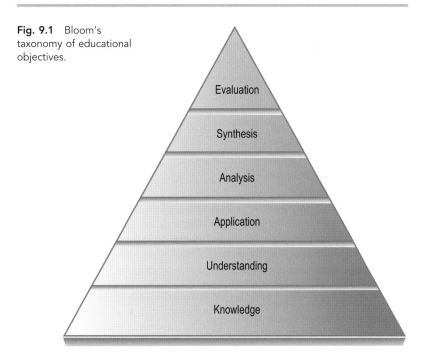

Evaluation

Synthesis

Analysis

Application

Understanding

Knowledge

educational processes that are widely recognised as synonymous with higher education, and are the minimum academic requirements for baccalaureate level education.

So what?

Where does this leave P/MH nurse education today? The author believes the clock cannot be turned back, regardless of the myriad pressures and concerns facing the discipline today. A return to the apprenticeship model would only serve to delay the inevitable, that is, a progressively educated workforce that pushes not only the boundaries of nursing knowledge, but the very nature of nursing practice itself. Our roles as nurses have, by sheer necessity, changed exponentially over the decades. This metamorphosis will and should continue, so it is vital we (continue to?) produce graduates/nurses who are not only knowledgeable and theoretically sound, but who are also professionally competent and above all, safe. This appears to necessitate the willingness and ability to see the vital components and associated educational value of both theory and practice in P/MH nurse education. Furthermore, finding effective methods of synthesis and the integration of theory and practice within curricula remains a pressing concern; of helping students experience the reality of a reciprocal relationship, where theory is applied in practice and practice in turn informs theory. Only then can the 'theory versus practice' argument be laid to rest and relegated to the occasional seminar filled with epistemological musings. Nevertheless, my closing point is that this matter is currently far from resolved and that evidence contained in this chapter indicates how the pendulum has swung too far towards theory rather than practice-driven curricula.

References

Anderson L, Sosniak L 1994 Bloom's taxonomy: a forty year perspective National Society for the Study of Education. University of Chicago Press, Chicago.

Barker P 1999 The philosophy and practice of psychiatric nursing. Churchill Livingstone, Edinburgh.

Chan A, Buchanan J, Forchuck C, Moore S, Wessell F 1998 Essential psychiatric/mental health nursing (PMHN) education for entry-level nursing programs in Canada. Canadian Federation of Mental Health Nurses (Education Committee), Toronto.

Chatterton C 2004 Caught in the middle? Mental health nurse training in England 1919–51. Journal of Psychiatric and Mental Health Nursing 11(1):30–36.

Clarke L 2000 Challenging ideas in psychiatric nursing. Routledge, London.

Cutcliffe J R 2003 A historical overview of psychiatric/mental health nurse education in the United Kingdom: going round in circles or on the straight and narrow? Nurse Education Today 23(5):338–346.

Cutcliffe J R, McKenna H P 2000a Generic health care workers: the nemesis of psychiatric/mental health nursing? Part one. Mental Health Practice 3(9):10–14.

Cutcliffe J R, McKenna H P 2000b Generic health care workers: the nemesis of psychiatric/mental health nursing? Part two. Mental Health Practice 3(10):20–23.

Darton K 1999 The history of mental health. http://www.mdx.ac.uk/www/study/mhhtim.htm accessed 2004.

Elkan R, Robinson J 1993 Project 2000: the gap between theory and practice. Nurse Education Today 13(4):295–298.

Elkan R, Hillman R, Robinson J 1994 Project 2000 and the replacement of the traditional student workforce. International Journal of Nursing Studies 31(5):413–420.

Laurence J 2002 Pure madness: how fear drives the mental health system. The Independent Faculty of Public Health Medicine Annual Scientific Conference, King's Fund Lecture, London.

Lenburg C B 2002 Redesigning expectations for initial and continuing competence for contemporary nursing practice. Online Journal of Issues in Nursing, article published 31 May 2002.

Mansell D J 2003 Forging the future: a history of nursing in Canada. Thomas Press, Chicago, Michigan.

Milton D 2002 Florence Nightingale (book review). Noetic Sciences Review 62:41–42.

Nelson M 2002 Education for professional nursing practice: looking backward into the future. Online Journal of Issues in Nursing 7(3). Available: http://www.nursingworld.org/ojin/topic18/tpc18_3.htm accessed 2005.

Nightingale F 1860 Notes on nursing: what it is, and what it is not. D Appleton, New York.

Norman I J 2005 Models of mental health nursing education: findings from a case study In: Tilley S, ed. Psychiatric and mental health nursing: the field of knowledge. Blackwell, Oxford, p 129–149.

Registered Nursing Association of British Columbia, Standards for Registered Nursing Practice 2004. Online. Available: http://www.rnabc.bc.ca/registrants/nursing_registration/continuing_competence/tutorial/standards-and-cc.html accessed 2005.

Royal College of Nursing 2002 Quality education for quality care: a position statement for nursing education. RCN Press, London.

Sills G M 1998 Peplau and professionalism: the emergence of the paradigm of professionalization. Journal of Psychiatric and Mental Health Nursing 5(4):167–171.

Smith F B 1982 Florence Nightingale: reputation and power. Croom Helm, London.

United Kingdom Central Council 1986 Project 2000. A new preparation for practice. UKCC, London.

Watkins M J 2000 Competency for nursing practice. Journal of Clinical Nursing 9(3):88–95.

Watson J 1989 New paradigm of curriculum development. In: Bevis E O, Watson J, eds. Toward a caring curriculum: a new pedagogy for nursing. National League for Nursing, New York, p 37–49.

Commentary
Maritta Välimäki

Introduction

The psychiatric health care system in many countries has undergone a process of de-institutionalisation, which started in the early 1960s, was continued in the 1990s, and is still ongoing in the 2000s. Especially in the 1990s, the process was enhanced as a result of pressures from an economic recession and ideological issues in North America, Europe and many Asian countries. During this process psychiatric bed rates were decreased or came under pressures to do so, and as a result people with mental health problems are now being treated in various social and health care sectors.

At the same time, the work environment for P/MH nurses has become more hectic. Demands for efficiency and economy, needs for evidence-based practice, and the development of health technology have created new roles for P/MH nurses. Today, health problems are more complicated, and mental health problems are entangled with other problems in society. For example, drug abuse, social exclusion, and burdens at the workplace occur everywhere in society, e.g. it has been shown in Finland that employees in mental health care and the drug abuse sector find their work most mentally demanding compared to other areas (Ministry of Social Affairs and Health 2001).

I am convinced that there is no doubt about the need for personnel who are able to make rational and quick decisions in high pressure situations and who have reflective and critical thinking skills to enable the generation of knowledge from practice. The complexity of health problems and the health care services, and also the many technological innovations require that nurses possess (and apply) multidisciplinary knowledge, an ability to work in multiprofessional and multicultural groups, skills to manage large problems and an ability to work on different levels in health sectors. In order to plan and develop client-centred, need-based health care services for patients, families and consumer groups, the personnel must also be able to identify and analyse problems using research skills. They need the ability to generate new and innovative treatment methods besides those used and tested methods using evidence-based knowledge. At the same time, the personnel need practical knowledge and they should be skilled in working with those persons who are experiencing mental distress and also with their family members. In addition, multicultural aspects of psychiatric nursing have to be taken into account (Khanlou 2003).

As rapid and wide-ranging changes occur in health care systems, the nursing discipline must display a new and comprehensive vision that projects its values, beliefs and relationships; with commitment to patients and co-workers (Moshe-Eilon & Shemy 2003). Therefore, our discipline needs theoretically and practically skilled personnel who are motivated to work in this demanding area. The basic question is still open: where should such personnel be educated and what should be the emphasis of this education?

Higher education seems to be an excellent place to educate P/MH nurses. There are, however, a number of reasons why there are special difficulties answering the following question:

- Should psychiatric nurse education be based in higher education and have a stronger theoretical than practical focus?

This question is not a simple one, and therefore my answer is both yes and no. In this commentary, I shall look at the question from different perspectives and identify some reasons why there is no straightforward answer to the question. I hope that, by so doing, we can open up this important issue for wider discussion, because its effect on the quality of nursing is decisive.

Educational policy perspective

First, we can look at the question from the perspective of educational policy. In so doing we can easily find that the educational system for P/MH nurses varies a great deal between countries, for reasons of history and economy. By arguing that P/MH nurses should be educated within higher education we may then narrow our focus. The fact is that many countries are still struggling with less systematic education for P/MH nurses, not to mention those nurses who have no opportunities to study nursing at the higher academic level. Today there are countries in the European Union (EU) where people with mental health problems are treated by nursing staff with no vocational education in the field of health care. Should we then leave P/MH nurses without any education or do we help them to organise academic education, even though the structure for basic education is unclear?

In these countries, I think, it would be important first to organise short-term vocational education to ensure even a minimum educational level for staff taking care of people experiencing and suffering psychiatric distress. After that it would be more convenient to develop an academic education for P/MH nurses. These countries, however, need support from those academics and countries where nursing education within higher education has long traditions. Even now we can find countries where doctoral students develop their academic education (Master's degree) without a professorial post in nursing science. In order to satisfy the need for an academic higher education system for

P/MH, we need structures and content to develop this in a way that is realistic in principle and possible in practice.

It has also been discussed whether or not a whole P/MH nursing education should be offered at the academic level. This would mean that the number of nursing students would be hundreds of times higher at the universities than it is today. This leads to a range of hitherto unanswered questions: Do we have enough academic teachers? Do we have infrastructure for that? Do we have enough universities for this demanding job? Who will educate teachers of nursing? Do we have enough professorial posts?

We cannot resolve these questions only by changing the name of nursing school to university. The whole idea of science, knowledge and discipline should be fitted into the curriculum of P/MH nursing education. Before that, however, a number of educational policy questions should be resolved.

The health policy perspective

Second, there are some health policy issues which we have to take into account. Although there are similar trends in different countries in health problems and health care services, each country may still have its own unique health problems to be tackled. Suicide rates and length of hospital stays, for example, may vary between countries, as may the rates of diagnosis of schizophrenia or depression. The number of patients with mental health problems and other health problems, such as substance abuse or HIV/AIDS may also vary depending on the country (e.g. South Africa and the Scandinavian countries). Moreover, mental health problems may well be paid different degrees of attention in different countries. And again, the realisation of hospitalised patients' rights may be a very big problem for some countries, while others are struggling with the fact that their patients have difficulties gaining access to psychiatric treatment. Therefore, different national health trends and health policy issues should be taken into account in the curricular development for P/MH nursing.

The labour policy perspective

Third, employers' perspectives need the same approach. All employers want their employees to be as skilled and highly educated as possible – as long as they come cheap. Today, about 65% of health care costs in Finland are due to the costs of health care personnel. Having nurses who have university degrees may increase pressures for higher salaries, which will duly raise health care budgets. Employers already have problems in meeting the wage costs of their nursing personnel now. So, looking at the issue from the employers' perspective leads to another important question: can we afford to educate nurses within higher education?

In addition, in the next ten years we shall face a serious shortage of nurses when the 'baby boom' nurses start to retire. Preparing nurses in universities means a longer timeline before they qualify. This will do nothing to alleviate the labour shortage. Quite the reverse, it will make matters worse, possibly leading to a situation in which it becomes necessary to plug the gaps by employing untrained personnel to care for patients.

The career perspective

Fourth, nurses' opportunities for a career must be taken into account in educational decisions. In Finland, nursing science became an academic discipline twenty-five years ago. Traditionally, nurses did not have so many options to advance in their careers. A master's degree programme at university level has opened up new opportunities for nurses to take academic degrees: first Master in Nursing Science and then Doctor of Health Sciences. The problem is, however, that many of those nurses with a Master's degree who are working as registered nurses may still have the same salary after three to four years of full-time university studies. The situation is very frustrating for well educated nurses. Therefore, many of them have moved to administrative tasks, such as working as ward managers, nursing directors etc. This has caused a situation in which the knowledge which was intended to support clinical nursing has moved to administrative tasks. No doubt this knowledge is important for nursing administrators, but we also need nurses face-to-face with patients and their families who are skilled in their practical work and can develop treatment on the wards, in the outpatient clinics etc. Therefore, if P/MH nursing education is located within higher education, we have to ensure that the basic structures, such as salary, career structures and responsibilities are in the right balance.

Fifth, new trends in nursing education have raised a debate related to the theory–practice gap. The concern is whether we need theory based knowledge at all and whether or not new graduate nurses from higher education are able to manage their work in practice. However, the gap between novice and experts is not a new one. As long as we have had novice practitioners in health care, more experienced persons have doubted the capacities of novices. This can also be seen in collaboration problems between old and new areas, professions, disciplines, and organisations. On the other hand, a novice may have unrealistic goals for their job and become frustrated and even leave their jobs. The more experienced practitioners may impede the participation of the new arrival and so 'support' him or her to go elsewhere. Indeed, competition and power structures persist on different levels in the health care environment.

"Dealing with violence and aggression in psychiatric/ mental health nursing: the cases for 'control and restraint' and 'de-escalation'

CHAPTER 10

Managing violence – a contemporary challenge for psychiatric/mental health nurses: the case for 'control and restraint'

James Noak, Sean Conway & John Carthy

CHAPTER 11

Issues and concerns about 'control and restraint' training: moving the debate forward

Andrew McDonnell & Ian Gallon

Commentary

Malcolm Rae

Editorial

The act of choice, we are told, is what separates us from our animal brothers and sisters. In a more sophisticated vein we are reliably informed that our ability to choose is based upon our knowledge, likes and dislikes, level of freedom, discriminatory abilities and the occasional television commercial. Choosing can be fun, especially if it involves chocolates; it can be more difficult if the options are wider, and it can be almost impossible when there are serious consequences for our actions. But all of these considerations are nothing unless we consider the influence of attitude on our decision-making processes. It seems that without attitude there is no necessity to make a selection, whatever it may be. In the case of this particular debate the issue is whether or not P/MH nurses should use either de-escalation techniques, when confronted by violent and aggressive patient behaviour, or the more physical approach of controlling by some form of human restraining activity. The authors in these next two chapters clearly set out their stalls, both for and against these approaches, and the Commentary critically evaluates their key points and offers an alternative. However, what the reader will soon realise is that whichever approach, or combination of approaches, is used within a clinical situation, the issue of choice and its attendant attitudes will play a great part in what takes place.

An evaluation of the literature on staff attitudes towards aggression in health care carried out by a team in the Netherlands (Jansen et al 2005) found that within the 74 studies of their sample, three-quarters of the attention was placed on cognitions rather than attitudes. Whilst telling us quite a lot about the validity of health care research generally, the information in the review does tend specifically to highlight a very salient point in relation to these chapters. This is that staff attitudes towards definitions of aggression, and therefore its causes, related intervention options and care evaluations, will have a profound influence on whether or not nurses choose to use physical or de-escalating techniques in aggressive circumstances. The review concludes with some interesting data about staff attitudes and characteristics, particularly the work undertaken by Whittington (2002). He concluded that staff with over 15 years of clinical experience were far more tolerant of aggression than staff with less experience. Now, tolerance does not necessarily equate with choice, but it is linked to freedom, and the more of this commodity you have, the wider your selection options become. If your nurse education programme teaches you to function in one way towards a problem, then that is how you will act. As you progress through your career and become more able to make choices based on exposure to different ways of working and attitudes towards people, their behaviour and the nature of your relationship, then things start to become slightly blurred.

Eventually it comes down to choice – the choice of the individual practitioner as to which way he or she is going to handle a given situation. In the case of a violent or aggressive patient much may depend on organisational protocols, but left to personal choice nurses will make the one they feel most comfortable with. Some might argue that this will depend on their relationship with the patient, whether or not they see them as equals, and their understanding of why the person is being threatening in the first place. Logically, however, if the nurse's attitude is that none of the above matters then they are more likely to do something physical (though not necessarily clinically acceptable) than if it is not. Yet this is far too simplistic. The editor is neither stating nor not stating that the above is the case, nor suggesting that relationships with patients, education, organisational procedures or peer pressure could influence a decision about the use or non-use of a physical intervention. What the editor is saying is that careful reflection and a sensitive approach to the choice of intervention in such complex situations may well be what separates not just a nurse from his/her animal relatives but also the skilled from the unskilled. Enjoy the debate and remember, there is never one answer!

References

Jansen G J, Dassen T W N, Jebbink G G 2005 Staff attitudes towards aggression in health care: a review of the literature. Journal of Psychiatric and Mental Health Nursing 12:3–13.

Whittington R 2002 Attitudes towards patient aggression amongst mental health nurses in the 'zero tolerance' era: associations with burnout and length of experience. Journal of Clinical Nursing 11:819–925.

James Noak, Sean Conway & John Carthy

Managing violence – a contemporary challenge for psychiatric/mental health nurses: the case for 'control and restraint'

Introduction

In mental health care the physical management of violence and aggression is an emotive and controversial subject both nationally, in the UK, and internationally. In the UK recent government campaigns such as that of 'zero tolerance' have emphasised the unacceptability of violence against health care staff. Although this is a laudable campaign and should be positively embraced, it is unreasonable to expect that interpersonal violence against staff, or patients' violence to each other will be eradicated by such initiatives from central government.

Unfortunately, violence in health care generally, and specifically in inpatient mental health settings, is not uncommon and is unlikely to go away. Indeed, physical violence has long been recognised as an 'occupational hazard' for staff working in health care (Health Service Advisory Committee 1987, Department of Health 1999a, Wright 2003). It is clear from professional literature and from clinical experience that nurses are the main group of health professional staff who routinely have to deal with violence in their clinical work; this includes nurses as victims of violence and as the members of staff who have to deal with both the perpetrators and other victims of violence. Although this is an unattractive part of nurses' clinical experience, it is an experience that most, if not all, will face during their careers. Given this background it is our view that nurses need to be equipped with sophisticated strategies and tools to address the full range of human emotions, feelings and behaviour in critical situations of interpersonal violence. Just as nurses cannot measure vital signs without the appropriate instruments, techniques and recognised training, they should not be expected to manage interpersonal violence and its associated risks without the appropriate tools and training.

Within the UK, as in many other countries, inpatient mental health care is delivered in a variety of settings, such as open acute and rehabilitation wards, where patients can enter and exit at will, as well as low, medium and high security hospitals, or mental health units situated in prisons. Within this range of services providing treatment for patients with complex clinical characteristics, nurses will often care for individuals who may be violent. Few would challenge the view that patients and staff in inpatient health care settings are entitled to a safe and harm-free environment; where violence is seen as unacceptable rather than as an inevitable and acceptable occupational hazard. It is therefore important to have some professionally acceptable strategy for dealing with violence when it occurs.

It is beyond the scope of this chapter to explore the causes and prevalence of interpersonal violence; this text provides personal views from its authors on the management of physical aggression and the use of control and restraint (C&R) as one method of managing violent patients. We hope to offer the reader a practical perspective on C&R whilst proposing that it is a suitable method, which can provide an effective way of resolving violent incidents in the clinical setting if used appropriately. When speaking of acts of physical violence that require C&R intervention we refer to actual assault that may be unremitting in nature, and where the victim is likely to suffer harm and/or sustain physical injury.

Background to 'control and restraint'

Control and restraint did not come into health care in the UK by accident; it was originally developed in the prison service in the early 1980s to help assist prison service staff to deal with violent prisoners who might harm themselves or others and who may compromise the security of a prison establishment. Prior to the development of C&R in prisons there had been a reliance on numbers of staff to manage a violent situation, which resulted in situations where too many staff were involved, thereby increasing the likelihood of injury to staff and prisoners. It was also felt that having large numbers of staff involved in managing violent situations tended to cause a breakdown in the professional relationships between staff and prisoners. Similarly, the submission of violent patients in mental health services was historically achieved by overwhelming numbers of staff, usually physically large male staff, holding, grabbing and lying on the patient. As in the prison service in the UK, there were no special restraint methods (techniques) available to staff; nurses faced with violence had to use 'brawn over brain' to control the situation. This was, and remains, an unacceptable way of managing violence in a professional context.

The introduction of C&R into the National Health Service (NHS) followed concerns about the adequacy of training for staff in the physical management of violence. Training crossed over from the prison service to the special hospitals in the UK in the mid-1980s, prompted by the death of a patient in a high-security hospital in 1984. (Special hospitals in the UK are high-security mental hospitals that provide care and treatment for patients who present as a grave and immediate danger to the public.) The inquiry following the tragic death of this patient recommended that all nursing staff in the special hospitals should be trained in the use of control and restraint (Ritchie 1985). Prior to this inquiry the special hospitals in England had expressed an interest in the introduction of C&R techniques to manage violent incidents. Following the introduction of the techniques into the special hospitals, C&R training was adopted by conventional mental health services from the mid 1980s, to the extent that a survey of 11 inner-city Trusts in London in 1998 showed that only one Mental Health Trust did not routinely train staff in its use (Gournay et al 1998).

In adapting control and restraint to the health service, national bodies such as the English National Board for Nursing incorporated some elements of the original C&R into postregistration training for nurses in the UK. (Previously responsible for accrediting nurse training courses in the UK, English National Boards have been replaced by the Nursing and Midwifery Council.) This national professional recognition legitimised the use of C&R as a form of clinical intervention that nurses could use to manage violent patients. It meant that C&R was more acceptable to acute and medium-secure services than when it was originally used in high-security hospitals.

What is control and restraint?

There was and continues to be a professional and ethical dilemma surrounding the symbolism of the training title (control and restraint) that may be perceived to prescribe a course of action without regard to the patient's ability to manage their own aggression. The title suggests an inevitable conclusion, which is the submission of the patient to numbers of staff employing restraint techniques to ensure compliance. If, as the authors suggest, C&R is an intervention of last resort, used to prevent imminent violence or further violence, its meaning becomes relevant: to bring safe control to an out-of-control situation by the use of effective physical restraint techniques. Some training organisations have changed the title and some of their training techniques from 'control and restraint' to 'care and responsibility'. This title, also abbreviated as C&R, may not best describe the methodology and techniques, but offers a different perception of the meaning, aim and philosophy of the clinical intervention.

Although there are several systems for physically managing violence, there appear to be four essential elements that either individually or in combination can be used for any restraint system (Ledbetter 1995):

1 The immobilisation of the subject (patient) by weight or strength
2 The restriction of movement of the long bones by some form of hold or lock
3 Maintaining the subject in an off-balance position
4 The use of reasonable force, which may include pain, to encourage compliance.

This chapter deals with the C&R system that was developed from prison service origins. Whatever system is used, it should directly relate to the needs of the client or patient group. More important than the system chosen is the quality of the training provided to the staff who may have to undertake these interventions.

Training should be provided by competent and experienced trainers, and should place an emphasis on theory, ethics, prevention and non-physical interventions for managing interpersonal violence. The physical techniques we discuss in this chapter usually involve a form of wristlock where pressure can be applied to the wrist and where the elbow is simultaneously immobilised, thus offering a very secure 'hold'. The wristlock has the potential to be used (and misused) as a form of pain-controlled compliance. The 'pain element' can be active, i.e. deliberately applied to prompt a response from the patient (e.g. to stop struggling or to move in a certain direction, such as to a safe area) or passive, i.e. excessive movement by the patient whilst in restraint will result in pain. For the authors it is the active use of pain to gain compliance that represents the most difficult dilemma in using C&R.

Rationale for control and restraint

Some may argue that there is never any justification for the use of C&R in any form. C&R might be described as an assault against the person, a negative response to internal distress by a nurse, or a wilful act of hostility toward the patient. However, it is our consideration that those who promote these views are not likely to be habitually faced with actual clinical violence, since they are unlikely to work in direct contact with the acutely disturbed and potentially violent individual. The academic debate over violence and the moral and ethical considerations about how to manage such violence are areas that require continued reflection and further research. Those who facilitate debate and research should be minded that contemporary clinical evidence is as valid as research evidence when formulating their recommendations.

The reality is that staff are at times faced with actual violence or the threat of it. What nursing staff most need is an acceptable, effective and ethical means of managing those situations safely. Actual clinical violence is not a game that can be paused, replayed and switched off: it is critical, imminent, and it's directed at 'you'. Just as C&R is not an appropriate response to the early warning signs of aggression, so counselling and de-escalation techniques are not appropriate responses to actual physical violence. The authors therefore do not claim physical control and restraint is a panacea for managing all risk factors associated with violence; they acknowledge and promote the efficacy of a range of other interventions to deal with non-physical aggression (irritability, shouting and threats, etc.), but they argue against the proposal that a non-physical approach is the clinical 'holy grail' in all instances, especially when violent behaviour is exhibited as a physical assault on the person.

C&R should never be used because of problems or defects in the environment, lack of appropriate resources or because of limited expertise, skills or training. When restraint is being contemplated, a full assessment of the person's problems, taking into account factors such as physical illness, discomfort or pain, side effects of drugs, psychological distress, poor relationships and incompatibility between the person and their carers, other residents or the environment needs to be made.

Staff who are trained in the use of C&R must accept the principle that restraint, if it has to be used, is an intervention of last resort. Prior to the actual use of restraint staff should actively engage alternative interventions and strategies for dealing with the prevention and management of violence. If a physical restraint system is to be used it should be a recognised and effective 'taught' technique: last resort intervention it may be, but left to chance it should never be.

Confidence

Although there is limited empirical evidence for the value of C&R, it is our view that staff who have been trained in physical intervention techniques tend to be more confident in dealing with potentially violent situations, often without needing to intervene physically. The authors can point to their experience of witnessing staff confidently using de-escalation techniques on patients who have been highly aroused and are on the verge of becoming physically violent. Personal reflection by staff involved in such situations has shown that they were able to de-escalate the threat of violence, since ultimately they were confident about managing the situation if it developed into a physical assault. The authors propose, therefore, that staff who have been appropriately trained in the use of C&R techniques are more likely to prevent violence in potentially violent situations than their untrained peers. Trained C&R staff will have confidence in their own skills and the competence of their colleagues, and this confidence appears to override their natural fear of physical conflict, allowing them to engage with a difficult and potentially violent patient.

It is by coincidence that whilst writing this chapter one of the authors was visiting an acute admission ward, when one male patient became aggressive, assaulting another by holding his neck and banging his head against a wall. Staff intervened by using C&R techniques to stop the assault and separate the patients. At the time the assaulting patient was highly aroused and was not responding to verbal instructions to desist. In this scenario it was difficult to appreciate how the situation could have been resolved quickly to prevent further injury without the physical restraint intervention.

Being confronted by violence is a frightening experience for all staff; nurses are usually in the front line dealing with physical hostility and are entitled to have training in specific techniques that provide them with safe and effective ways of both preventing and dealing with aggression and violence.

The authors have observed a variety of approaches to managing physical aggression and the risk of aggression. Comprehensive risk assessment will provide nurses with an understanding of the context within which patients might express violence and of the associated risk factors. Risk factors may accumulate, if unchallenged, to create the context within which violent behaviour is exhibited.

A detailed risk assessment allows the nurse to interpret early warning signs and to manage these before they escalate to the point of violent behaviour. The type and range of risk factors are well documented within the literature (Steadman et al 1994) (see Box 10.1). There is a range of assessment instruments available to assist nurses and clinical teams to identify risk (including the risk of violence). An individual risk management care plan can subsequently be developed that combines empirical and clinical evidence together with a pragmatic, common sense approach to managing the risk of violence. Each patient who presents a risk of violence has a unique risk 'signature'; their journey towards aggressive behaviour and the context within which they express violence is unique to them.

By understanding their individual risk factors the individual's 'violent risk signature' can be interpreted and expressed as a hierarchy of factors ranging from low or early warning signs to imminent risk of violence. If risk factors can be graded in this way, nurses will be able to plan appropriate interventions designed to 'interrupt' the journey towards violence or de-escalate the risk of violence (see Box 10.2).

Evidence base

There has been some evaluation of the evidence base for C&R (Silas & Fenton 2001, Wright 2003). Wright (2003) describes an early study of the effectiveness of C&R training in a mental health setting by Mortimer

BOX 10.1   Risk factors for violent behaviour

Dispositional factors

Demographic
Age, sex, race, social class, marital status

Personality style
Anger, impulsivity, psychopathy

Neuropsychological/physical
IQ, neurological impairment, central nervous system damage, size and strength

Contextual factors
Support (actual and perceived), family support, social networks, career networks, employment networks, activities of daily living
Availability of perceived victims, availability of weapons, availability of drugs/alcohol
Perceived stress

Interests including: sexual, violence, cruelty, social domination, racism

Historical factors
Family history, child-rearing, child abuse, family deviance
Work and education
Psychosexual development
Previous hospitalisation, treatment contacts
Crime/violence including: arrests, prison history, self/other reported violence, previous sexual assaults, violence against self

Clinical factors
Delusions, hallucinations, tension, depression
Paranoid distortion, religiosity, jealousy
Anger, rage, impulse control
Substance misuse
Fantasies including: violent, sadistic and deviant/sexual

Adapted from work by Steadman et al (1994).

(1995), in which Mortimer portrayed the effect of various policy changes, including the expansion of C&R training, on the number of violent incidents in a psychiatric intensive care unit. He observed a reduction in assaultive behaviour following the introduction of C&R trained staff and describes how assault frequency had fallen by 27% and the seriousness of assaults had lessened, with life threatening assaults falling from 5% to 2% and serious assaults falling from 41% to 15%. Mortimer concludes that since the proportion of exceptionally assaultive patients had remained constant, his findings were attributable to the increased number of C&R trained staff. Parkes (1996) also observed a reduction in staff injuries during violent incidents following the introduction of C&R training. However, Silas and Fenton (2001) criticise the lack of available evidence supporting the efficacy of C&R.

BOX 10.2 Care plan

Risk
Mr Butcher has assaulted two male patients with kicks and punches within the last month; there is a history of eight similar assaults during the last 12 months.

Context
Following these incidents Mr Butcher has said that his victims had followed him around for several days with the intention of sexually assaulting him. He was observed to be acutely paranoid at the time of the assaults and described delusions about male patients planning to rape him.

Aim
To manage the risk of violence presented by Mr Butcher by detecting risk factors and intervening to prevent escalation.

Risk factor	Intervention
Mr Butcher is uncommunicative for periods exceeding 6 hours	Proactive engagement for 10 minutes each hour in order to assess mental state, appreciate potential problems and intervene to reduce distress
Mr Butcher is irritable, gesticulating and grimacing when in the vicinity of other male patients	Engage Mr Butcher to provide feedback about his behaviour. Seek perception and explanation. Agree boundaries and an action plan for dealing with further episodes. Assess mental state. Review with MO, consider periodic nursing observations
Mr Butcher is observed to shout derogatory accusations at other male patients	Intervene to de-escalate this situation. Provide debriefing to elicit perception and explanation. As this behaviour indicates a high risk of violence, implement regular nursing observations (e.g. every 15 minutes). Provide feedback and discuss preventative measures with patient each hour
Mr Butcher is threatening to assault other male patients	This behaviour indicates imminent violence. Employ de-escalation techniques; encourage him to move to another area. Provide debriefing, elicit mental state. Implement 1:1 nursing observation. Review management with MO
Mr Butcher is observed physically assaulting another male patient	Summon help and respond immediately to prevent further aggression by giving firm verbal instructions to disengage. If this fails staff will intervene using physical restraint to bring the situation under control

The effectiveness of C&R can and should also be viewed in relation to the quality of the training received by the staff who have to carry out the interventions. Dowson et al (1999) found serious deficiencies in standards of professional practice and training in their evaluation of the management of violence. The study observed an apparent relationship between lack of training and the possibility of staff injury during restraint. This may not surprise the reader. As in any clinical intervention, the quality of the act will be based on the knowledge, skill and attitude of the clinician, and the clinician's skill will be based on the quality of training received and the ability to translate this to practise effectively.

It can be seen that there is little empirical evidence to support the effectiveness of physical restraint in reducing violent incidents and the paucity of current evidence does not yet allow firm conclusions to be drawn. However, none of the above-mentioned studies reported an increase in violent incidents following the introduction of C&R training.

It is important to remember that, although reduced frequency of assaults following C&R training would be desirable, its validity as an outcome measure may not be demonstrable, or at least will be difficult to prove scientifically, as there are likely to be a number of complex variables influencing the possibility of violence. However, we propose that the introduction of good-quality C&R training and practice is a significant factor in positive outcomes.

The introduction of C&R training was not initially aimed at reducing the number of violent incidents, but to provide better and safer management of such incidents when they occur. This is an important point. C&R was brought into the health service as a result of recommendations following the death of a patient. Tragically, there have been patient deaths following restraint; sadly, there have also been fatal assaults on nursing staff by patients: the associated reasons have been and will continue to be examined case by case so that lessons can be learned. Single case studies sometimes offer the best way of examining critical incidents, as in the Ritchie inquiry (1995). Some inquiries have criticised the general management of patients and the use of restraint. Criticism of restraint often focuses on the individual event and how restraint was carried out, rather than the use of restraint per se.

Another criticism surrounds the early or overuse of restraint, without attempting other non-physical interventions (e.g. de-escalation techniques) to prevent and reduce violence. Restraint can be used oppressively, as a threat, rather than (as the authors propose) a safe means of resolving incidents of violence. The authors would argue, therefore, that it is not the principle of restraining a patient that is at issue: rather it is the choice of when and how it is used.

Experiential evidence

Although there is limited (if any) empirical evidence to support the use of C&R, clinical and personal reflection offers a valid means of examining clinical practice. Indeed the National Service Framework for Mental Health in the UK (Department of Health 1999b) suggests that expert opinion (Level V) is one type of evidence that can be used in evidence-based practice. The authors have reflected on a range of personal clinical experiences in their roles as observer and participant during the physical management of violent behaviour. We argue that unless staff are trained appropriately, so that they possess competence and confidence in their ability to manage violence, the success of the physical intervention will at best be less than effective and at worst could have serious or tragic consequences for the patient and/or staff members. Staff groups who are well trained in C&R techniques will often report an increased confidence in their ability to engage and de-escalate the potentially violent patient; they will also point to an increased confidence in their colleagues to act in synergy should the need to intervene physically arise.

Whilst acknowledging that there are approaches other than C&R, the authors would recommend that all staff working in a ward or department should be trained in the same technique(s), as anecdotal evidence suggests that several staff, each possessing different skills, converging on a violent incident with a patient, are likely to achieve little more than a confusing melee, and may indeed make a difficult situation worse. In addition, patient feedback indicates that some have preferred the short term C&R intervention rather than the longer term effects associated with the forcible administration of intramuscular medication to achieve control of violent incidents. When a patient exhibits serious self-harm or becomes violent toward others, we would recommend that staff need a clear method of managing the situation. In the face of interpersonal violence and when all other forms of de-escalation have been tried and failed, it is imperative that the situation is brought under effective control. Staff fear and uncertainty during violent incidents can contribute to dysfunctional responses to aggression from patients. C&R offers one systematic way of managing the physically aggressive individual.

In writing this chapter the authors are cognisant of the criticism and concern expressed within the professional literature and elsewhere about the appropriateness of using C&R in the clinical setting. We are equally aware of the false sense of security that inappropriate approaches to the management of violence can cause. It is unacceptable that either patients or staff are assaulted because of the inadequate or inappropriate training of staff.

Ethics

All people who are in hospital, in care homes, or receiving care in the community retain their full human rights unless these have been restricted by a legal process, and then only to the extent allowed by the law. Self-determination and freedom of choice and movement should be paramount unless there are compelling reasons why not. The ethical principle of justice means that the patient receives that to which he or she is entitled. The authors argue therefore that the quality of C&R interventions must achieve the highest ethical standards. The individual's autonomy constitutes a prima facie ethical principle, though in certain circumstances this may need to be superseded by other principles. We would argue that for an individual to be autonomous they must possess insight into the potential and actual consequences of their actions. The clinical and other factors contributing to an expression of interpersonal violence may therefore interfere with an individual's insight (e.g. 'blind with rage') and it may be appropriate in those circumstances to override his/her autonomy by referring to the principle of non-maleficence (doing no harm) when intervening to resolve the violent behaviour. The aim of a physical intervention (C&R) in these circumstances is to prevent harm to the patient and/or others, to restrict the patient's ability to express further violent behaviour and ultimately to facilitate the restoration of self-control. In our view there is little that is attractive about managing violent conduct, even for staff who have been well trained in safe restraint techniques. The vast majority of potentially violent situations are safely de-escalated and the individual concerned is able to regain self-control without the need for physical intervention; nursing staff will always seek to achieve this outcome. There are circumstances that give rise to impulsive, unpredicted or wilful violence despite efforts to prevent or reduce the threat. In these circumstances a timely, proficient physical response may be the only option that will bring the violent incident under rapid control.

Providing C&R is implemented in a way that reflects its underlying aims and principles, it can be said to be an intervention that is ethically defensible.

Conclusion

Providing that the training staff receive includes components of theory, causative factors, ethical considerations and physical techniques, the C&R intervention can provide a safe and appropriate way to resolve incidents of violence. The application of physical techniques (C&R) designed to reduce the harm caused by actual violence can be viewed as legitimate and therapeutic providing that the principles of non-maleficence and reasonable force are applied. Criticism of the use of C&R is welcomed, and should continue to provide those clinicians who may have to use it with an opportunity to reflect on their practice. However, criticism without proposing realistic alternatives is of limited value. Clinical staff will face challenging situations on a daily basis and need a range of options and skills to deal with those situations safely and effectively. Mental health nurses will inevitably be confronted with violence at times, and it is insufficient to hope these situations will arise rarely or never. It is unacceptable to expect that the quality of the therapeutic relationship alone will neutralise all episodes of potential violence, and it is inappropriate to suggest that all potentially violent situations can be successfully de-escalated. Nurses need a proactive, reliable, effective and ethical response to deal safely with violence in the clinical setting. C&R in its refined and contemporary form can, in our view, meet all of these needs.

The authors suggest that the use of pain compliance as a means of control appears to be the most controversial aspect of dealing with violent individuals. Following the UKCC Study on the Therapeutic Management of Violence (2001), the National Institute for Clinical Excellence (NICE) have developed measured and useful clinical guidelines for the short-term management of disturbed/violent behaviour (National Institute for Clinical Excellence 2005). The authors support the guidelines, which reinforce that any use of force that is applied must be justifiable, appropriate, reasonable and proportionate to a specific situation and should be applied for the shortest possible time).

Every effort should be made to use skills and techniques that do not deliberately apply pain. The application of pain has no therapeutic value and at times can aggravate a situation. NICE suggest that pain should only be used for the immediate rescue of staff, service users or others. C&R is not a first-line approach to manage the potentially violent individual, but the last approach, and it needs to be used once all other options have been considered and/or tried. It is important that nurses and patients have safe environments in which to practise and be treated. Despite the best intentions of clinicians, politicians and researchers, it is unlikely that physical violence will be fully eradicated from the clinical setting. Without the use of some form of recognised physical intervention the management of actual physical violence will again rely on brawn over brain.

References

Department of Health 1999a Survey of sickness, absence, accidents and violence in the NHS. HMSO, London.

Department of Health 1999b National Service Framework for Mental Health. Department of Health, London.

Dowson J H, Butler J, Williams O 1999 Management of psychiatric inpatient violence in the Anglia region. Psychiatric Bulletin 23:486–489.

Gournay K, Ward M, Thornicroft G, Wright S 1999 Crisis in the capital. Inpatient care in inner London. Mental Health Practice 1(5):10–18.

Health Service Advisory Committee 1987 Violence to staff in the health service. London, HMSO.

Ledbetter D 1995 Technical aspects of physical restraint. In: Lindsay M, ed. Physical restraint practice: legal, medical and technical consideration. Glasgow Centre for Residential Childcare, University of Strathclyde, Glasgow.

Mortimer A 1995 Reducing violence in a secure ward. Psychiatric Bulletin 19:605–608.

National Institute for Clinical Excellence 2005 The short–term management of disturbed/violent behaviour in in-patient settings and emergency departments. London, NICE.

Parkes J 1996 Control and restraint training: a study of its effectiveness in a medium secure psychiatric unit. Journal of Forensic Psychiatry 7:525–534.

Ritchie S 1985 Report to secretary of state for social services concerning the death of Mr Michael Martin. Special Hospitals Service Authority, London.

Silas E, Fenton N 2001 Seclusion and restraint for people with serious mental illnesses (Cochrane Review). In: The Cochrane Library, Issue 1. Update Software, Oxford.

Steadman H, Monahan J, Applebaum P 1994 Designing a new generation of risk assessment research. In: Monahan J, Steadman H J, eds. Violence and mental disorder. Chicago University Press, Chicago, p 207–218.

United Kingdom Central Council 2001 The therapeutic management of violence. UKCC, London.

Wright S 2003 Control and restraint techniques in the management of violence in inpatient psychiatry: a critical review. Medicine, Science and Law 43(1):31–38.

Andrew McDonnell & Ian Gallon

Issues and concerns about 'control and restraint' training: moving the debate forward

Introduction

Many nurses are exposed to violent behaviour in their day to day work (Health Services Advisory Committee [HSAC] 1987) and there is some limited evidence that such behaviours are increasing in frequency. In the UK there exists a wide range of training that includes the physical management of aggressive behaviours (Wright et al 2002), with 'control and restraint' (C&R) being the most common training system employed in UK psychiatric services. Training typically contains skills to defuse a situation, physical management strategies such as breakaway skills, and physical restraint. However, a significant proportion of other training courses contain only physical interventions, whose concentration on physical skills is of particular concern as the rationale for teaching such skills appears to be relatively unclear. This chapter will focus on a number of issues and concerns about C&R training.

Problems of definition

C&R training comprises a collection of physical techniques apparently derived from the 'martial arts' of Aikido in 1979 (Gilbert 1988). The training was developed primarily in the prison service and Special Hospitals, and the original training system was never intended for general consumption in caring environments (A Healy, personal communication 2002). At present there are at least three different training systems that use the abbreviation 'C&R'. These include approaches used in the prison services, so-called 'care and responsibility' training used in one of the special hospitals, and control and restraint (general services), which has been described as a modified version of 'control and restraint' for health and social services in the UK.

In attempting to define control and restraint a number of ambiguities arise. First, different schools of practice use the same acronym. Second, it is our experience that many front line nursing staff appear to be unable to define the term, tending to associate the expression 'control and restraint' with physical techniques such as wrist-locks and physical restraint holds. It is quite rare for staff to associate this term with defusing skills. A recent violence survey of psychiatric nurses conducted for the United Kingdom Central Council of Nursing (now known as the Nursing and Midwifery Council) found that fewer than 21% of training courses formally taught defusing skills. Third, the term is often used as a collective noun to cover any training in management of violence. In England and Wales the Mental Health Act code of practice appears to use the term in this generic manner. Lastly, the authors have found it extremely difficult to get practitioners to talk openly about, describe or debate specific physical interventions. (Later in this chapter we hope to break this veil of secrecy.) So, what is in a name? The ambiguity created by the expression has led to difficulties both for clinicians and researchers. One of the authors experienced this at first hand when a member of staff in a secure facility stated that 'I used control and restraint to calm the patient down'. Such a response begs the questions, which type? Which school of practice? Which physical interventions were used?

A new definition?

It is the view of the authors that the expression 'control and restraint' is tired, outdated and horribly ambiguous. One definition that may be useful to consider is the use of the terms *progressive* and *traditional* control and restraint. *Traditional* control and restraint is typified by training in physical management that is broad based and tends to use a 'kitchen sink' philosophy (teaching for as many situations as possible) typified by a 'one size fits all' emphasis and a lack of hierarchical structure to physical interventions. There is also little practical emphasis on teaching skills for defusing situations. Finally, many traditional systems avoid openly restricting and banning certain physical interventions. *Progressive* control and restraint would be regarded as systems that avoid 'high risk' (to the patient) physical management techniques and specify a clear hierarchy of physical interventions, clearly emphasising the teaching of strategies to defuse trouble, and not just 'rhetoric'. In our opinion more progressive schools of control and restraint should be judged by techniques that they are prepared to 'ban'. It is our contention that the practice of many training schools literally gets caught 'between these two stools'.

The marketplace

A number of systems would appear to lack historical background, with some systems developing from control and restraint training and others having more ambiguous beginnings. Training systems have been reported in the literature that have been developed outside the 'control and restraint' systems. These include the SCIP (Strategies for Crisis Intervention and Prevention) approach (Baker & Bissmire 2001) and the Studio3 System (McDonnell 1997). There is also a lack of accurate information on the numbers of training systems that provide services to staff in the UK. A recent survey of participants (n = 115) in a series of national workshops in England on physical interventions in the learning disability field identified a number of training systems that were in use in their services. These included: control and restraint (45%), care and responsibility (16%), strategies for crisis intervention and prevention (SCIP) (37%), Studio III (6%), non-aversive psychological and physical interventions (NAPPI) (11%), protection of rights in care environments (PRICE) (5%), preventing and responding to aggressive behaviour (known as the Welsh centre method) (5%), natural therapeutic holding (5%), Timian training (3%) and crisis aggression and limitation and management (CALM) (1%), other methods (17%) and none (19%). The authors have found no similar marketplace evidence in the psychiatric field and suggest a similar survey is urgently required for psychiatric services in the UK.

Staff training outcome research

According to Wright et al (2002) 84.5% of psychiatric nurses do receive some form of training in the management of aggression in their nursing careers and there is no doubt that a substantial service industry has been developed in this area. This presents academic researchers with an additional problem, namely, that researchers often evaluate their own preferred system. Indeed, some researchers do not always mention to their readers their own affiliations to a training organisation or system, so it is not surprising that genuinely independent research is almost absent in this field. In this section we will review the current research knowledge on staff training.

Some researchers appear to be very positive about the benefits of Control and Restraint training. Wright et al (2002, p 26) stated that 'research into C&R has suggested that training in the methods is beneficial'. It is difficult to justify such a statement when the research in this area could at best be construed as 'poor'. Wright et al (2002), in their own review of research conducted for the UKCC, cited only four studies as positive examples. One of these (Judd 1996) described an internal service audit, whilst two others (Mortimer 1995, Parkes 1996) were cited as providing positive evidence. In a rather poorly controlled study Mortimer (1995) did report reductions in patient to staff violence after training in C&R; however, patient to patient assaults actually increased after training! Parkes (1996) reported reductions in the use of break-away skills, but did also report increases in staff injuries after training. A general problem with evaluating training research is that the majority of published studies occur in both psychiatric and learning disabilities fields and in our view this research needs to be reviewed as a whole. The evidence of staff training from the learning disability field leads to only a few conclusive findings. First, carer confidence does appear to increase after training in physical interventions (McDonnell 1997). There are some reports of reductions in the use of physical restraint (Allen et al 1997). Similar studies have been reported in mental health literature in the USA (Infantino & Musingo 1985), with one study even reporting an increase in physical interventions after training (Baker & Bissmire 2001). Second, we can find no studies that formally and independently assess the retention of physical intervention skills after staff have completed their training. Lastly, usage of physical skills, particularly breakaway skills, appears to be relatively low.

Overall, the outcome research that is cited specifically for C&R training would appear to be extremely poor methodologically. The more general research involving other systems is similarly crude. A recent report on the management of violence in psychiatric nursing in the UK provided a relatively thorough review of C&R training (Wright et al 2002). This report found that only 54% had received training in breakaway techniques and 40.3% had received training in physical restraint since commencing work with their current employers; few staff received refresher training. Paradoxically, the report also admitted that many of the respondents to their survey did not use 'breakaway skills' in the workplace. The authors rightly pointed out the great variability of training delivery in terms of content, and one of their major recommendations was the adoption of a standardised syllabus for C&R training to contain the teaching of defusing skills, breakaway and restraint skills. There were a large number of physical interventions included in this speculative syllabus, ranging from being punched and defending against kicks, to '5'-person restraint teams and 'awareness of weapons'. The evidence base for this syllabus would appear to be the survey responses of psychiatric staff, with no hard evidence of direct usage of such skills in the workplace. More importantly, the views of consumers were not a focus of this report.

Defusing skills

Staff who are assaulted by patients rarely suffer physical harm (HSAC 1987). Despite media hyperbole, which tends to focus on fatalities or serious incidents, it is more common for psychiatric staff to experience verbal aggression (Adams & Whittington 1995). Defusing a violent situation would appear to be a much more desirable outcome than having to provide emergency medication or physically restrain an individual.

The likelihood that psychiatric staff will experience verbal aggression is not always reflected in the training syllabus. The speculative syllabus for the UKCC acknowledged the importance of defusing skills; however, the recommendations for a training syllabus focused primarily on physical restraint and breakaway skills. More worryingly, in their national survey verbal de-escalation was only briefly mentioned or not mentioned at all in 22% of courses (Wright et al 2002). It is possible that there is a serious lack of knowledge about the constituents of such skills, though anecdotal evidence indicates that the assault cycle is quite commonly taught on training courses. This normally suggests that there are five phases, ranging from a triggering phase to a recovery phase and post-incident depression (Kaplan & Wheeler 1983). Whilst this model would appear to have considerable 'face validity', it is debatable how much evidence exists for the use of such a universal model for such heterogeneous subjects as violence and aggression.

One of the authors of this chapter, McDonnell (1997), proposed a four-element low arousal approach as a staff-based model for defusing incidents. The elements were: (1) the reduction of staff demands and requests at 'high risk' times; (2) the adoption of strategies that avoid verbal triggers to assault; (3) the avoidance of threatening non-verbal cues; and (4) the need to challenge the negative attributive beliefs of staff.

There is some limited evidence that training in defusing skills may reduce the risk of assaults on staff. Whittington & Wykes (1996a) evaluated the impact of a one-day training course for psychiatric staff that emphasised the verbal and non-verbal behaviour of staff, and found that after training staff reported a 31% reduction in assaults. There are several obvious methodological problems with this study, including the lack of a control group and the crudity of the incident measure. However, these data suggest that training may have an impact on staff behaviour. As there is some compelling evidence to suggest that violent assaults on staff and patients are often preceded by aversive interactions with nursing staff (Whittington & Wykes 1996b), it is possible to conclude from the above that it is the staff who sometimes need to change their verbal and non-verbal behaviours.

More research is needed on the direct effects of staff training in defusing skills. The assumption that physical interventions should be taught as a standard component of training for dealing with violence and aggressive behaviours requires more scrutiny, for it is our belief that core training in defusing skills should be increased on all training courses. There has been some acknowledgement that more emphasis needs to be placed on training nurses in non-aversive means of setting limits (Wright et al 2002) and that challenging the negative belief systems of psychiatric staff is a key component of a low arousal approach (McDonnell 1997). A radical suggestion for training providers would be to change the balance of training to reflect the fact that verbal aggression is more commonplace. It would be possible to design training courses in which at least 50% of the skills taught were for defusing situations, with the remainder emphasising physical interventions.

Do we need to teach breakaway skills?

The expression 'breakaway' skills is often used by researchers with little attempt at a formal definition. Breakaway skills consist of a menu of physical techniques that will help a member of staff to break free from an assailant, but the term is in such common usage that it has become reified. The expression 'breakaway' is used in a manner that suggests that there is an agreed set of skills taught using this name. Are we literally just teaching nurses to break away from a violent situation or is this a misnomer? Presumably the blocking of punches and kicks is different from staff releasing themselves from holds, while, in contrast, some systems still teach the use of strikes and blows to care staff for so-called 'exceptional circumstances'.

Real confusion exists about the content of breakaway skills. On a number of occasions the authors have listened to different nursing staff state that 'they had been taught' breakaway skills, which creates the impression that they have been taught the same physical interventions. It is difficult to guarantee that the skills taught to staff on different training courses (and sometimes within the same training system) are identical, as the methods of teaching delivery may vary quite dramatically.

What is the rationale for teaching staff breakaway skills? Many C&R trainers appear to believe that teaching these skills may help nursing staff protect themselves from injury. The current limited evidence strongly indicates that few staff appear to use breakaway skills on a regular basis (Gallon & McDonnell 2002), whilst the evidence for reduced injuries in the workplace is almost nonexistent. The clearest rationale for teaching these physical skills would appear to be that they may increase carer confidence. In the UK 'breakaway skills' appear to be taught, literally, to 'get out' of situations. This has led to many training courses teaching a large number of physical skills based on the *what if* scenario. Staff will pose hypothetical or real life situations and request that C&R trainers show them a breakaway skill. These 'what ifs' can become extremely divorced from the realities of training and can be compared to the teaching of physical techniques for rare situations. Many training courses teach 'wrist releases' in which nursing staff are given a variety of 'grabs' and are then given a breakaway solution. The first author of this chapter was once taught seven techniques on one short training course. It is concerning that such situations occur very rarely in the workplace, and in addition, the more physical interventions taught on training courses the more difficult skill retention becomes. In the experience of the authors many psychiatric nurses often have difficulties remembering 'breakaway skills', whilst sometimes the physical techniques recommended by trainers can involve inflicting a considerable degree of harm to an individual. There are a number of 'high risk' techniques that are still recommended by some trainers in situations where a nurse may need to escape from a 'bear-hug'. Staff are taught that they could smash the back of their cranium into a patient's face to break such a hold, yet it is possible that teaching such a 'vicious' response could potentially place the member of staff at even greater risk of physical harm. Do we really believe that a disturbed individual would 'calm down' after having a nurse's cranium 'smashed' into their face? We believe that teaching highly aversive techniques for rare situations is a poor training rationale.

The context of training is also important. There is a difference in training staff in controlled, almost sterile, training environments and translating this into real life situations. If individuals are taught to release themselves from a choke hold, is there evidence as to how successful this would be in a 'real life' situation? It appears that many C&R training courses offer a menu of physical techniques, which presumably course participants are supposed to remember, yet there are so few published data about skill retention and the use of physical interventions. It is more likely that breakaway skills are simply being taught to improve the confidence of staff (McDonnell 1997). In this instance, it is hoped that nurses who perceive themselves as capable of managing a crisis situation physically will be more likely to attempt defusing strategies. Unfortunately, the opposite may also be true, though there is little hard evidence to support this. Staff who are overconfident about managing a situation physically may be more likely to confront an individual.

Do we need to teach breakaway skills at all? The evidence base would suggest that for many staff such skills are completely irrelevant. We can conceive of 'high risk' staff teams requiring such training, but as a general rule it is probably better to teach a small number of environmentally relevant breakaway skills that people are likely to remember and use. In our own study (Gallon & McDonnell 2002) we found the most common physical assault on psychiatric nursing staff was being punched in the face, and would advocate concentrating on an area such as this, rather than teaching people numerous 'what ifs'.

Is C&R a form of self-defence training?

There are similarities between self-defence training and a broad range of training courses used in the Health Service, and C&R systems could be viewed in this manner. There appears to be a syllabus of 'set moves', a formal assessment and pass/fail grading system, regular 'refresher' training, and a hierarchy of competencies for instructors. There are, of course, concerns with such a similarity. First, self-defence training is concerned primarily with the safety of the person who is being attacked. The expression 'mind over matter' has been applied to these situations: 'I don't mind what I do to the other person because they do not matter'. In caring environments the relationship with the service user should be of paramount concern, therefore protection of the service user and of the nurses are both of equal concern to service providers. Anecdotal evidence suggests that a significant proportion of senior instructors in C&R have some form of martial arts qualification. The authors do not make a case for the pros and cons of such qualifications; however, it is hard to believe that the respective martial arts knowledge of these instructors has not influenced the culture of C&R systems.

Is training in C&R 'high risk'?

Staff training in physical interventions can lead to increases in staff injury rates after training (Parkes 1996) as well as to reductions (Allen et al 1997). An area that has been relatively overlooked by researchers is the potential for injury on training courses. A survey in secure facilities conducted in the UK produced a startling pattern of injury on training courses, where 27% of nursing staff reported that they received injuries whilst *participating* on training courses in the management of aggression (Lee et al 2001), with 7% requiring medical attention. The UKCC national survey reported injury statistics of 18.8%, with an incredible one in six requiring medical attention (Wright et al 2002). Although the national evidence would indicate that many of these injuries may be minor in nature, more serious injuries do appear to occur on training courses and it would be useful to separate tissue damage from non-tissue damage in any future research. Given these reservations, it is concerning that staff may actually be more at risk of injury on a training course than in the workplace. Perhaps the most important question to be investigated involves what is causing these injuries. Are there specific physical techniques that account for many of these injuries? Is it a question of the competence of trainers? One intriguing line of research involves the use of 'matted' areas on training courses (cushioned mats used to protect participants whilst falling). Most psychiatric wards do not have such areas. It is our belief that 'matted' areas may create an 'illusion of safety' on training courses, which may encourage participants to practise movements vigorously, leading to injuries, as well as increasing the risk of harm when applied in 'real world' settings.

Physical restraint: some relevant background information

Physical restraint has been defined as:

'actions or procedures which are designed to limit or suppress movement or mobility'   (Harris 1996, p 100)

The physical restraint of people who present a danger to themselves or others may well be socially undesirable, but at times a necessity (McDonnell 1997). Discussion about restraint techniques is not a recent event as there are descriptions of 'floor restraint' methods taught to psychiatric nurses in North America that appear to pre-date the development of C&R systems in the UK. It is the anecdotal experience of the authors that physical restraint is often defined by carers as the use of specific physical restraint techniques. If a person is prevented from leaving an acute admission ward by a staff member physically holding them, this clearly is a form of physical restraint and this has implications for nurses, who are expected to record incidents of restraint. It is acknowledged that there is some under-reporting of violent incidents (HSAC 1987) but it is concerning that nursing staff may be recording 'hold downs and take downs' and under-reporting other forms of physical restraint.

The vast majority of training systems in the UK appear to use variations of so-called 'floor restraint' methods. The aetiology of these methods is difficult to trace, although there are methods described in the literature that date to the early 1970s. Recent concern in the USA about 'positional asphyxia', where an individual may have their respiration interrupted, leading to hypoxia and cardiac difficulties, has led to fears that specific postures can contribute to sudden death (Reay et al 1992). In the UK the recent report into the death of a black psychiatric patient in a medium secure facility concluded that he was held in a prone position for approximately 25 minutes. The report recommended that physical restraint in the prone position should last no more than 3 minutes (Sallah et al 2004). Face down postures would appear to be associated with the risk of respiratory problems. Anecdotal evidence suggests that rapid tranquilisation often occurs with an individual in a prone posture. Prone (face down) restraint postures have been linked to a number of sudden deaths in the USA, though the reasons for these deaths may be quite complex and (as Sallah et al indicate) prone position interventions may be permissible in certain circumstances.

However, this typifies an approach that is based on a 'worst case scenario'. Typically, advice suggests avoiding procedures rather than banning them, because of the possibility that in extreme circumstances such methods may have to be used. There are several difficulties with this argument. First, it is debatable whether basic C&R training can provide solutions to extreme situations. The recent tragic death in the

UK of a local councillor who was attacked with a samurai sword, illustrates the pitfalls of this approach. Would we really consider teaching public officials how to disarm such lethal weapons as an option? Indeed, how much training would be required to train people to an adequate and safe standard? Second, in secure environments there is a tendency for staff to be expected to deal with extreme violence without involving external agencies, the involvement of the police being relatively rare on UK psychiatric wards. It is our belief that overconfident staff may attempt to control a situation that may be better dealt with by the police.

Recently, some authors have tried to argue that non-aversive restraint methods can be developed for staff who work within the learning disability field (McDonnell 1997). Stirling & McHugh (1997) described a floor restraint method as 'natural therapeutic holding', as an alternative to C&R but, as in the case of previous papers, the description of the restraint method was vague, and uncontrolled descriptive statistics of therapeutic outcomes were reported. This reliance on anecdotal and poorly controlled studies is concerning, especially as there have been a growing number of fatalities at the hands of practitioners attempting to use physical restraint. Supine positions have been advocated as safer than prone postures. Allen et al (1997) reported teaching an alternative method that also involved the use of the floor. In both studies the methods used were poorly described, making clear comparisons difficult; however, it would appear that restraint holds invariably involve the use of a bed or floor in their practice.

Is pain compliance valid?

There are serious issues about the infliction of pain on individuals. The Royal College of Psychiatrists (1995, p 6) has been particularly scathing about such procedures:

'There is no evidence in the literature that the use of Control and Restraint has been examined to determine its relevance. Its role becomes particularly problematic and hazardous where the patient's perception of pain is altered (as might occur with learning disability, autism or various psychiatric states).'

There is always the risk that the infliction of pain may exacerbate an already inflamed situation. Guidance implying that physical techniques that inflict pain should only be employed if other pain free techniques have been tried allows too much leeway for bad practice, since there are a number of problems with teaching pain compliance physical interventions. First, pain is an aversive event to the vast majority of people; second, condoning the use of physical techniques that employ pain is potentially exposing nurses to allegations of physical abuse;

third, despite the subjectivity of individuals' experiences of pain, we have to rely on what patients are telling us; and, lastly, how can staff develop a positive therapeutic relationship with a patient whom sometimes they have to hurt?

Avoid teaching locking procedures

The abnormal rotation of joints and other forms of hyperflexion are often referred to as arm or wrist locks. Literally, a person may be unable to move without having quite severe pain inflicted on them. A common argument of C&R trainers is that 'a lock only hurts if the person moves'. Whilst this may initially sound quite plausible, the argument unravels relatively easily. It is difficult to hold a person who is struggling violently using such methods without a psychiatric nurse inadvertently inflicting pain on the person. These locks and holds are designed to use pain in a controlled manner and it is also possible that the infliction of pain may actually exacerbate a situation and make an individual more aggressive.

Are physical techniques socially valid?

The social validity of behavioural interventions was first highlighted by researchers in the learning disabilities field who were exploring the views of consumers and of society on interventions. Such studies are required in the field of psychiatric nursing. The views of service survivors (and front line staff) require examination. Indeed, it would be interesting to evaluate many of the so-called *breakaway methods* by asking service users, staff and members of the public to rate their acceptability. Social validity is a useful tool for discriminating amongst methods of physical restraint, and in the absence of clear outcome data on safety and effectiveness, the social validity of such methods will be of increasing importance. Limited attention has been given to the role of consumers in the literature (Baker 2002) and in both UK and USA studies some consumers reported both positive and negative experiences about their own restraint, although there is also evidence suggesting that patients see this as punishment. In sum, the role of service users in giving feedback on the use of procedures and even assisting in training may be of importance in the future.

Issues and concerns

The authors hope that this chapter will encourage debate even though it is difficult to criticise a training system that appears to be well established in many services in the UK. However, the fact that training is relatively popular does not mean that it is effective. This chapter has raised a number of important issues and concerns about C&R training:

- There are problems defining the subject area. The term *control and restraint* has almost become meaningless.
- The overall outcome data on the effects of staff training are relatively poor in general.
- The outcome data for control and restraint training are extremely limited and methodologically crude.
- There would appear to be little compelling evidence for teaching a large number of breakaway skills on training courses. It may be better to teach a small number of skills more intensively to increase staff confidence.
- It is extremely concerning that staff and patient injury data, both on training courses and in the workplace, have received little attention. People are being injured on training courses. They are also being injured in the workplace. The authors are amazed at the lack of national concern about injury data.
- Traditional C&R 'kitchen sink' training in physical interventions would still appear to be popular in the UK and is both inefficient and ineffective.
- There is little compelling evidence for the retention of physical interventions among nursing staff.
- There are clearly some physical techniques such as wristlocks that rely on pain to be effective.
- The social validity of physical methods is poorly understood. It is the contention of the authors that the views of service users represent a key area of evaluation.
- Finally, prone restraint holds have been implicated in restraint-related deaths in the UK and the USA. Where do we draw the line? The prima facie evidence would appear to indicate that such methods should be limited in their use or even banned.

Disclaimer

The views of the authors reflect their personal opinions and not those of any official national body or professional organisations.

References

Adams J, Whittington R 1995 Verbal aggression to psychiatric staff: traumatic stressor or part of the job? Psychiatric Care 2:171–174.

Allen D, McDonald L, Dunn C, Doyle T 1997 Changing care staff approaches to the preventions and management of aggressive behaviour in a residential treatment unit for persons with mental retardation and challenging behaviour. Research in Developmental Disabilities 18:101–112.

Baker P 2002 Best interest? Seeking the views of service users. In: Allen D, ed. Responding to challenging behaviour in people with intellectual disabilities. British Institute of Learning Disabilities, Kidderminster.

Baker P, Bissmire D 2001 A pilot study of the use of physical intervention in the crisis management of people with intellectual disabilities who present challenging behaviour. Journal of Applied Research in Intellectual Disabilities 13:38–45.

Gallon I, McDonnell A A 2002 Developing non aversive behaviour management training in psychiatric services. Online. Available: http://www.studio3.org accessed 2004.

Gilbert P 1988 Exercising some restraint. Social Work Today 30:16–18.

Harris J 1996 Physical restraint procedures for managing challenging behaviours presented by mentally retarded adults and children. Research in Developmental Disabilities 17(2):99–134.

Health Services Advisory Committee 1987 Violence to staff in the health services. HMSO, London.

Infantino J A, Musingo S 1985 Assaults and Injuries among staff with and without training in aggression control techniques. Hospital and Community Psychiatry 36:1312–1314.

Judd M 1996 Mental health service control and restraint training: retrospective survey of nurses. Clinical Audit Department, Camden and Islington Community NHS Trust, London.

Kaplan S G, Wheeler E G 1983 Survival skills for working with potentially violent clients. Social Casework 64:339–345.

Lee S, Wright S, Sayer J, Parr A M, Gray R, Gournay K 2001 Physical restraint training in English and Welsh psychiatric intensive care and regional secure units. Journal of Mental Health 10:151–162.

McDonnell A, Sturmey P 1993b The acceptability of physical restraint procedures for people with a learning difficulty. Behavioural and Cognitive Psychotherapy 21:225–264.

Mortimer A 1995 Reducing violence on a secure ward. Psychiatric Bulletin 19:605–608.

Parkes J 1996 Control and restraint training: a study of its effectiveness in a medium secure psychiatric unit. Journal of Forensic Psychiatry 7:525–534.

Reay D T, Fligner C L, Stilwell A D, Arnold J 1992 Positional asphyxia during law enforcement transport. American Journal of Forensic Medicine and Pathology 13:90–97.

Royal College of Psychiatrists 1995 Strategies for the management of disturbed and violent patients in psychiatric units. Council Report CR41. Royal College of Psychiatrists, London.

Sallah D, Sashidharan S, Stone R, Struthers J, Blofeld J 2004 Independent inquiry into the death of David Bennett. Norfolk, Suffolk and Cambridgeshire Strategic Health Authority, Cambridge.

Stirling C, McHugh A 1997 Natural therapeutic holding: a non aversive alternative to the use of control and restraint in the management of violence for people with learning disabilities. Journal of Advanced Nursing 26:304–311.

Whittington R, Wykes T 1996a An evaluation of staff training in psychological techniques for the management of patient aggression. Journal of Clinical Nursing 5:257–261.

Whittington R, Wykes T 1996b Aversive stimulation by staff and violence by psychiatric patients. British Journal of Clinical Psychology 35:11–20.

Wright S, Gray R, Parkes J, Gournay K 2002 The recognition, prevention and therapeutic management of violence in acute in-patient psychiatry: a literature review and evidence based recommendations for good practice. United Kingdom Central Council for Nursing, Midwifery and Health Visiting, London.

Commentary

Malcolm Rae

Introduction

The prevention and effective management of violence is one of the most important challenges facing modern Mental Health Services. Never before have we had such a heightened focus, scrutiny, pressures for change or the political will to make improvements and develop new methods, manoeuvres and holds. The recommendations from the inquiry into the death of David Bennett, a service user at the Norvic Clinic in Norwich (UK), and other deaths in local authority care, police custody and other services, have all provided a wake up call to mental health services. In addition, various professional reports have also raised the profile and level of concern and have frequently highlighted inconsistencies in practice, the language used, a general lack of understanding of the causes of violence, unclear definitions of techniques and the absence of accreditation and regulation for those delivering training. Reports have also highlighted a lack of focus on prevention of violence initiatives, poor physical care in the event of a physical collapse, and inadequate reporting systems. Further concerns are the increasing use of illicit drugs and weapons, an apparent increase in police involvement in supporting staff in some acute units, and an increased media interest.

Undermining effective prevention and management of violence is the paucity of evidence available. Currently, there is a massive mixed bag of responses, care and support being provided to people who are aggressive and violent, and to staff who are expected to manage violent and threatening behaviour. Some individuals get a 'top class' service and support, while others are badly served. Arguably, by now, there should be no major problems in describing what good care should look like, as there is a collective intelligence and widespread agreement amongst the leaders in the speciality of management of violence of what is unacceptable, and a consensus forming on some of the more contentious issues. Most contributors to the debate point out the need for a greater attention to be given to prevention and minimisation of aggressive behaviours rather than the physical responses to controlling the situation. There is a major challenge in ensuring that, where training and practice is working well, it is made known to other areas where there is poor performance. This can be a feature within and across organisations. Effective practice in one service should be replicated and embraced by others, of course, taking account of the specific needs of users in each service. There is still a need for benchmarks and identification of contemporary standards of positive practice and a transfer of shared learning.

Analysis of the two sets of authors

Both sets of authors share a number of valid concerns and agree on a range of issues that one can endorse. They accept the prevalence of violence in mental health services and that nursing staff are the main staff group subjected to violence and aggression. They both, rightly in my view, argue that the environment should be as safe as possible and violence should be regarded as unacceptable, not inevitable or accepted, as many do, as an occupational hazard. They both agree that there is a need for ethically based training and sophisticated strategies to give staff the skills and confidence to deal with interpersonal violence in order to protect both service users and staff from harm. They agree that curricula should enable tailored responses for specific client groups, including women, and age differentials. They accept that, in some instances, the use of restraint is necessary, as doing nothing or withdrawing may be more dangerous, and they appreciate that it is the choice of method and how it is used that is the frequent source of problems.

Both sets of authors fear the development of well meaning academic or ethically and legally driven approaches that may inadequately equip front line staff; staff who regularly face real life intimidation, threats and actual violence, and have to manage incidences of disturbed behaviour in a safe way. They both express their dismay at the absence of reliable quality research that takes account of different client groups and settings, and they observe that where research has been undertaken it has often had mixed outcomes and paradoxical findings. There is very little evidence of the effectiveness of techniques.

They both believe that where there is effective training it usually raises the confidence of the individual to attempt de-escalation techniques, with a service user who is aroused and expressing intimidating language. It is also acknowledged that appropriate training is likely to lead to other members of the clinical team having confidence in the individual and the viability of the team, to manage the disturbed behaviour episode together. They both appear to acknowledge the current variations in training and procedures and a need for unambiguous terminologies and consistent approaches to avoid different interpretations and uncertainty amongst trainers, front-line staff, managers and service users.

However, they bring different perspectives on how to move forward in the future, and they are at variance in their favoured methods of approach and the acceptability of pain as a method of containment and control. The protagonists for C&R do accept the ethical dilemmas, but, in contrast, argue the overall value and benefits of effectively preventing harm to others by its use. The second set of authors assert that there is too much emphasis on physical intervention and ineffective breakaway or disengaging techniques, (the current preferred language), and that insufficient balance is given to the importance of defusing techniques. They suggest more emphasis should be given to the verbal skills and non-verbal behaviours of clinical staff. One can assume that this means the giving of respect, courtesy, warmth and preventing the person losing their dignity and privacy; of valuing relationships rather than reacting in a hostile manner, as some staff sometimes seem to, being overzealous and petty in applying rules and regulations, which service users claim results in them not being spoken to appropriately. The second set of authors also argue that there should be a limited range of techniques taught, as they consider that focusing too much on 'what if' situations overwhelms practitioners, is often irrelevant, and leads to poor retention of skills or confused application. They contend that much of current training is divorced from reality. They also assert that there are too many injuries sustained by staff in the current process of training in many areas.

Although both sets of authors enthusiastically articulate their cause with conviction, it seems that they have fallen into the common trap of viewing training as a panacea for the ills associated with the management of violence. This narrow approach, overemphasising the importance of training and not considering the 'whole systems' approach reflects the state of affairs in most organisations throughout the UK. Both sets of authors mention the importance of risk assessments and understanding the causes of violence, and hint at an appreciation of the importance of the environment and resources, together with service user feedback and involvement, but they do not go far enough. They have not given these factors the priority they deserve or articulated how they would include them in their respective training programmes.

There now appears to be a growing awareness amongst enlightened contemporary thinkers and practice leaders in the field that training is just one dimension, albeit a critically important one. Other authoritative writers and exponents of innovative practice, who advocate more modern and progressive approaches, point out the mistake of seeking simple solutions to complex organisational problems and complicated individual presentations of violence and aggression. They argue that the structures, systems and leadership of an organisation also need to be vigorously and imaginatively addressed.

The best and most progressively oriented individuals and organisations in the future will be those that constantly seek to review, evaluate and learn lessons from local, national and international experiences, and then regularly fine tune their systems and means of support for staff. I have no preferred method. My experience to date has exposed me to many different approaches. My respective experience as Trust board director, researcher and policy-maker has insulated me from bias and has given me a sense of objectivity. I wish to espouse a wider alternative view, which emphasises a strategic whole systems approach, and highlights the importance of those who occupy senior management positions taking more seriously their leadership roles and having the management of violence more clearly focused on their radar screens.

The way forward

The challenge for managers is to take a radical new look at the magnitude of the challenges confronting clinical staff. Managers must make sure that they themselves are involved in the debates and new developments, and in their various roles and responsibilities promote safe systems and adopt the whole systems structured approach. However, all too often in many services there appears to be a fragmented organisational approach, with individuals sometimes competing against each other or unnecessarily duplicating effort. Managers should ensure that policy, practice and training are enmeshed with local clinical governance arrangements.

For a start, managers should examine the current position, perhaps by methods of audit, and identify:

- The number of injuries sustained as a result of assault
- An analysis of incidents by type, location and time
- How much absence and lost time is due to injury and associated stress
- The impact of violence on staff leaving and recruitment to their service
- How much time is spent on the investigation of complaints, grievances, or the attendant bureaucracy
- How many injuries are sustained in the process of training
- How to appraise staff morale and measure the impact on performance associated with violence in their workplace
- How safety might be enhanced, whilst ensuring an appropriate balance between therapy and security
- How to measure the impact of violence on service users/carers.

Without access to detailed data, it is difficult to understand how they can plan services, identify an appropriate skill mix or fulfil their clinical governance or health and safety responsibilities? For nurse managers, there is an extra obligation to meet their code of conduct and leadership responsibilities.

Essential action for managers

For ease of access these issues have been itemised:

- Ensure the integration of communications standards, environmental factors, policies, protocols, training programmes and care pathways and the clarity of clinical organisational structures.
- Ensure that acute care forums agree that clear admission policies are in place with clear criteria of which, and when and how, individuals should be admitted.
- Ensure effective risk assessment procedures are in place that reduce risk to the lowest practical level and that they are reviewed on a regular basis.
- Ensure that patient-centred and therapeutic values and principles underpin the ward clinical philosophies, culture and polices.
- Be sure that recording and reporting systems, to help with legal requirements, to inform practice, and to identify themes and trends, are in place.
- Ensure an effective skill mix and staffing levels are in place in order for clinical teams to have the capacity to deal safely with the challenges they face.
- Identify replacement costs for staff to receive necessary training and updates.
- Ensure the environment and therapeutic milieu and the necessary resources are available to meet the needs of clients whose behaviour is challenging.
- Ensure that clinical and line management supervision is available to focus on challenging behaviour.
- Ensure a regular scrutiny of workload and assess the amount of time spent on non-patient focused activities and in making sure the administrative burden is not unreasonable.
- Review costs and ensure that revenue is being used in the most effective way.
- Prioritise standards and regularly assess progress and put in place measures to seek improvement (link to essence of care framework).
- Have in place a vigorous performance management system(s) so that people know what is expected of them.
- Ensure that strong clinical leadership is present and effective support is given to staff and service users who are victims of violence.
- Ensure active service user and carer involvement in service incident reviews and evaluations, and where appropriate, that they receive education, including positive motivation, etc.
- Have in place systems for monitoring complaints and incidents, and by paying meticulous attention to the contributing factors ensure that lessons are learned, and that important factors to identify patterns and problem areas are noted and acted upon.

- Develop root cause analysis and avoid blame cultures, and where performance does not meet the required standards, ensure this is dealt with fairly and sensitively.
- Ensure that lessons are learned from clinical review, and that they in turn inform changes in clinical practice, procedures, the training curriculum or skill mix and promote the concept of reconciliation.
- Seek feedback from course attendees in respect of the appropriateness and calibre of the training and its usefulness and facilitate follow-up support from trainers to enmesh teaching with practice and realistic settings.
- Obtain feedback from courses, including reports from the instructors on the performance of those taking part, both strengths and any areas of concern, gaps in knowledge or skills, or a need for improvement in any particular area. (You cannot assess work competence just by attendance at a course. Managers are responsible for their staff and must be actively involved in appraising the application of skills taught, the demonstration of appropriate attitudes and relationships, performing as a team player and how an individual responds to stress and difficult situations.)

The future essential actions for trainers/instructors

Instructors should extend their roles, widen their clinical repertoire and increase their influence, by going outside their traditional training areas, and in some instances changing their base. They should actively support front line staff, through mentorship and coaching, to develop their skills, esteem and confidence levels. This would also permit a positive acknowledgement of front line staff's current capabilities. Working in partnership with clinical and managerial staff, they should help to devise organisational and clinical strategies to reduce risk, and assist in matching solutions to local circumstances, problems and need. They should seek to present role models for positive engagement and defusing skills. A further innovative extension of the role for trainers would be to undertake sessional work with individuals or groups of service users, carers, or their advocates, to identify what social, emotional or stress factors or motivations cause them to become distressed and disturbed. This approach could be of value in teaching methods of stress reduction and enable the service user to have a better understanding of the reasons underpinning their behaviours. It will reinforce the point that the 'one size fits all' approach does not work.

Working in partnership, with clinical staff engaging with service users, could also lead to a better understanding of what systems and personalised interventions and behaviours from staff are likely to be effective in preventing or managing disturbed episodes and supporting individuals in dealing with their frustration, anger or anguish, suspicions, insecurity, inappropriate communications, shame or previous traumatic life experiences or whatever else motivates their aggressive behaviours. It could result in negotiated care plans in the form of advanced directives. Other potential benefits from this approach include gaining insights and ideas from the experiences of service users, to assist in designing or changing services and environments and shaping the care they receive. While there are many difficulties to overcome and resistance to change to break down, through these proposals, nevertheless, services providers should consider the many potential benefits to the quality of services available to vulnerable service users. In addition, the real benefits of crucial improvements in the confidence and optimism of hard-pressed clinical staff should be taken into account. It is also suggested that deepening and expanding the role of instructors as described would achieve an increase in their competence, respect (both of self and from others), credibility and job satisfaction. Surely, it makes sense that instructors cannot exercise the same level of influence by being based entirely in training centres or classrooms. They need to seek, in a proactive way, to extend their influence, share their talents, and in so doing build the capacity and capability of services.

Conclusion

Services must avoid drifting or spinning out the 'status quo' wheel, or taking easy options. Instead they must constantly be searching for excellence and seeking out new ways and solutions to deliver safe and effective support to service users and staff. Those involved should look everywhere possible, learn from other sources and buy into a collective intelligence. In addition, services must increasingly respond to the choice agenda and other service user-centred initiatives and interpret them in a way that will enhance safe care, using them for leverage for additional resources for further training, organisational and personal development. Services must tackle the emerging ethical and practical dilemmas of new technologies such as alarm systems and CCTV, while also considering the controversial option of mechanical restraints in their duty of care responsibilities. Organisations must also consider the safety aspects of supporting people in, or being transferred from, community locations. To date, much of the emphasis has been on inpatient care settings.

Significant benefits can be produced from an enhanced and expanded role for trainers and an astute management focus on organisational issues, together with combining improved know how of those most at risk, that is, improving knowledge of high-risk individuals and areas that have the highest risk. Despite the complexities, mental health services are heading in the right direction. An increased focus on values and ethical principles, and the development of modern techniques and approaches in delivering safe care must be the goal of all professionals. This too, is what the public both expects and wants from us. We need to convince them that we are up for it and can match their expectations.

"

Expansion or diminution of our character, essence and core: the matter of nurse prescribing in psychiatric/mental health nursing

CHAPTER 12

Gently applying the brakes to the beguiling allure of P/MH nurse prescribing

Tom Keen

CHAPTER 13

Psychiatric/mental health nurses as non-medical prescribers: validating their role in the prescribing process

Katharine P Bailey & Steve Hemingway

Commentary

Dawn Freshwater

"

Editorial

There appears to be wide-scale consensus within the psychiatric/mental health (P/MH) nurse community that there is room within our current scope of practice for expansion, evolution and development. The precise direction of this expansion, however, and the nature of this development are more contested matters. One such 'hotly debated' area of development is that of nurse prescribing within P/MH nursing. Whether one sees this as a challenge to the very essence of our discipline, or as a problematic amalgamation of reductionalistic and holistic philosophies (arguably the different philosophical underpinnings of psychiatric medicine and P/MH nursing – see Cutcliffe & Campbell 2002), or as a unique opportunity to expand our scope of practice, it is fair to say that this is one of the most far-reaching issues facing contemporary P/MH nurses. Interestingly, as with each of the debates covered in this book, once the substantive issue begins to be scrutinised and considered, the associated matters arising out of the discussions are both broad and, yet, central.

Tom Keen offers a compelling argument when he asserts: 'Rather than seek to impersonate medical practice, it might be preferable for nurses to focus their attention on those areas of people's functioning that exist despite their diagnosis . . .'. Similarly, it would be imprudent for P/MH nurses to ignore the emerging evidence cited by Katherine Bailey & Steve Hemingway when they highlight how some service users have benefited from their experience of P/MH nurse prescribing. A further, hitherto largely absent, element to this debate is introduced in Dawn Freshwater's thought-provoking commentary when she reminds us of the evidence relating to nurses' poor arithmetic skills and how this might influence their 'ability' to prescribe. Given the documented body of evidence developed over the past five years, which suggests that some nurses lack numeracy and cognitive skills, and that the minimal level of mathematics required to enter nurse training was failing, it seems something of a 'long reach' to expect the same nurses to be able to engage safely and competently in prescribing.

However, even though the issue of nurse prescribing is a relatively new phenomenon in most countries, it is far from being restricted to having meaning for contemporary P/MH nurses – to borrow a term from Tolkien's parlance, this issue has *'applicability'*. Without wishing to impose our own interpretation on this issue, and thus compromise the freedom given to readers that applicability provides, it strikes the Editors that this issue may be symbolic of many historical and perhaps future 'developments' in P/MH nursing. With this in mind, the searching and insightful questions that are raised in this debate could similarly be applied to other historical developments (e.g. nurses' holding power). Moreover, similar questions might be asked of any future, proposed 'developments'.

It is rarely spelled out in our literature that our discipline, as a self-governing body, has an inherent duty to monitor and question the direction(s) in which we develop; that each of us, as registered P/MH nurses, needs at times to act as 'watchdog' of our own discipline. Accordingly, to follow blindly and without question any proposed development, especially those developments that have an external genesis, would be to renege on one's own duty as P/MH nurses in one of the most damaging ways possible.

CHAPTER

12

Tom Keen

Gently applying the brakes to the beguiling allure of P/MH nurse prescribing

Introduction

It would be naive to argue against P/MH nurses being able to prescribe anything at all in any circumstances. Throughout my career, it has always seemed absurd that in everyday clinical situations nurses lack the prescribing power granted to ordinary citizens as parents or carers. First, having to ask a doctor whether or not a client could have a headache pill is just one of many humiliating bureaucratic nonsenses to which nurses have long been subjected. Second, most nurses of anything but absolute inexperience know how often many medical colleagues (particularly the inexperienced ones) rely on their advice, or deferentially disguised suggestions, about which drug to prescribe, and in what dose. Third, it rapidly becomes obvious to any half-way decent nurse when a prescription needs varying because of the occurrence of unpleasant or crippling side-effects which can threaten the therapeutic benefit, concordance with the medication regimen, or even the person's life. Similarly, intervening happenstances, such as infections, often call for commonsense prescriptive variation.

There is some evidence, albeit somewhat ambivalent (Cutcliffe 2002), that people feel more comfortable (and are therefore more likely to 'comply') with medication regimens that can be flexibly fiddled with (or 'titrated', if you prefer less friendly jargon) from moment to moment by on-the-spot staff. Such on-the-spot staff are more likely to be nurses than their much rarer and more detached medical colleagues. Although protagonists of nurse prescription usually limit their case to *advanced*, not basic, practice (Daniels & Williams 2003), and there are various complex definitions of diverse prescriptive protocols under consideration by the UK's Department of Health, nurse prescribing in whatever form initially adopted into P/MH nursing practice will have profound ramifications for our clinical and educational mores (McCann & Hemingway 2003).

Just as nurses in the UK have historically been handicapped by petty rules, regulations and the historically tacit resolution of professional demarcation disputes, so, in contradiction, they have in other national jurisdictions (e.g. USA) long been enabled to prescribe psychoactive medication. Arguing against something that is already the case would be futile. Nevertheless, I contend that to develop nurse prescribing further in the UK, beyond sweeping away certain stubbornly stupid policies, would be to misplace our professional priorities, when there has been, and remains, so much educational and clinical neglect of other areas of unquestioned nursing need – for example, the neglected areas of psychosocial care, practical problem-solving, psychotherapeutic conversation and solution-focused support.

My argument is about common sense and priority – on one hand, the common sense to realise that defensive practice, bureaucratic hog-ties, economic expediency and struggles for status are no basis for quality care; on the other hand, the common sense to recognise that nurses cannot sensibly be trained and educated to perform all caring, healing and helping tasks expertly, and that, therefore, some degree of prioritisation of need must govern what they are expected to do. It may or may not be desirable for nurses to develop greater freedom to practise medically, to diagnose illness and prescribe appropriately. My argument boils down to this: however desirable it is for nurses to become more like doctors (some of whom, of course, already combine aspects of psychotherapeutic practice with the licence to prescribe medicaments), it is nothing like as desirable as that we should become better at what we are already expected to do, yet so often fail to achieve in any high degree or quality.

The argument is about pragmatism versus idealism; on both sides of this dispute: what we can be, or perhaps what we are allowed or coerced to be, as against what we ought to be. The underlying questions are: Who or what determines that moral imperative? Who or what decides what we ought to be – government policies, professional aspirations, users' needs, choices and expectations, economic imperatives, clinical expediency, historical roles, or diversity of specialism, and best fit of professional help to personal need?

Clearly, policy-makers find nurse prescribing economically and politically expedient. There would be a larger and cheaper prescribing workforce, which would also conveniently weaken any potential political weight-pulling by the turbulent medical priesthood of psychiatry. In addition, some nurses would like to be able to prescribe, not simply to remove the bureaucratic anomalies that make the everyday work of nursing and its relationship to medicine sometimes seem so archaically cumbersome, but to satisfy their frustrated personal professional aspirations and achieve what they regard as higher-status job descriptions. But the key questions remain: What do people needing help from mental health professionals want from their nurses? What is it that needs doing for them, that otherwise may not get done so well? What was it that brought nurses into existence? And do these needs persist, or is our grasp of human biology so complete, and our certainty that pharmacological equanimity is the proper state of humankind so absolute, that basic human needs are now best met by a medical prescription? And, if so, where is the evidence that enabling nurses to issue that prescription is as safe or safer, and as efficacious as, or more so than the current situation?

Nurse prescribing: what are the issues?

What is it to nurse? What is it to prescribe? Although my contribution to this debate will address both of these questions, especially the first, I have shunned a detailed examination of all the various formal aspects, definitions, subcategories and policy proposals (for example, the distinctions between substantive and complementary prescriptive authority, supplementary prescribing, etc.) of the UK nurse prescribing project in order to ponder some of the more basic underlying philosophical and professional issues.

The arguments put forward in favour of nurse prescribing condense down to these:

- Nurses need to expand their role
- Users would like nurses to prescribe, or would be more compliant if they did so
- Nurses need to embrace the expansion of biological knowledge about mental illness, and medication management has always been at the heart of nursing
- So-called 'holistic practice', which in this case means an increased emphasis upon, and application in nursing care of, the biological nature of human life
- Government policy already favours the development of nurse prescribing in some form or other.

Nurses need to expand their role . . . but what is it?

The traditional way of presenting the argument about nurses' proper role is that of a polarisation of 'care' and 'cure' (see Hemingway 2003b). *Either* people are ill and need treatment designed to eliminate their disease, and thereby cure them, or at least palliate the effects of their regrettable malady, *or* they are ill, and therefore need to be cared for while they recover or regain sufficient strength, willpower, etc. to cope

less dependently. One of the problems with this supposedly dichoto-
mous thinking is that the problem is always to a large degree located
inside the person, or within his or her immediate personal space. The
person's very real life problems, aspirations and abilities disappear or
fade into secondary consideration, as that other thing – the supposed
illness, disease or disability that has afflicted him or her – becomes the
object of professional preoccupation. People's sensibilities, lives, wishes
and solutions are then potentially ignored or subordinated, either in
the heroic efforts that doctors and their allies make to beat, treat and
eliminate their affliction, or in the valiant pains taken by dedicated,
devoted nurses to perform their caring endeavours consistently.

I have elsewhere suggested that this dichotomy of professional identity in the ranks of P/MH nursing is reflected in the complex noun
customarily employed to describe the job (*psychiatric* nursing seeks to
treat or *cure*, whereas *mental health* nursing emphasises *care* – see Debate
One), and moreover that the split-mindedness, if not operational practices, may well be irreconcilable (Keen 2003). Others propose that the
dichotomy is an artificial one, arising from faulty logic or unrealistic
analyses of human nature and nursing activities (Burnard 2002). So
what is P/MH nursing? What, after all, is its primary purpose? Perhaps
it is *treatment*, administering medicines and other interventions derived
from professional formulations of problems and traditionally prescribed by other professionals. If so, then the move towards prescriptive
authority is only natural and to be expected as the job evolves.

Maybe it is *caring*, although this has become such a debased term
that the concepts underlying it are either, unclear, ill defined and vague,
or quasi-religious certainties held as articles of faith, and therefore
potent causes of conflict. Caring is often identified as an important
component of therapeutic change, if characterised, for instance as
'perceived empathy', whereby clients feel that the worker understands
them – or is trying to – and likes or values them as a person (Burns &
Auerbach 1996). Although arguments persist about what significant
differences there may be between caring *for*, caring *about* or caring
with people, a more important issue, in my opinion, is what may be
called 'benevolent inaction' or 'beneficent intent'. This is demonstrated
in practice when professionals feel deeply about someone's plight or
behaviour, but actually do nothing or little effectively to *help* them cope
better with life.

What service users seem to want and need is quite simply to be
helped. Perhaps they don't accept that conventional medical formulations fit their situation or experience; they aren't ill, although they may
well qualify for a psychiatric diagnosis; they've been messed about by
life or the man-next-door; or temporarily or chronically overwhelmed
by real-life economic or practical difficulties. Equally, they may not
necessarily benefit just because a nurse is able to demonstrate some
degree of warmth, encouragement or understanding, although, as David
Smail (1993) has claimed, it may be that being supported, encouraged

and having help to clarify one's situation are essential components of a helping relationship. Treatment without care is unethical and likely to be ineffective; care without *helping* is righteous, but ultimately ego-centric and self-indulgent.

I believe that what people want from nurses is practical help. Psychiatrists, with their long, biologically based, medical education are ideally placed to provide pharmacological assistance, when acceptable and effective chemical remedies exist. I believe that nurses should provide something else, first, because otherwise there is no point in the two different professions/disciplines or crafts continuing to exist separately, and second, because there is ample evidence that people can be helped by collaborative, person-centred, solution-focused, narrative-based, pragmatic and systemically aware methods – methods that ultimately do not threaten to disempower the person by being based upon diagnosis, dwelling on illness, and focusing on treatment and taking away risk, but emphasise instead the certainty of recovery. So, do nurses need to expand their role, or do they perhaps need to fulfil the one they have historically developed, that professional codes repeatedly stress, and for which there is a sad accumulation of evidence of non-achievement? Protagonists of nurse prescribing may believe that the oft-reported failure by nurses to achieve caring help is partly because of the medical restrictions and limitations placed upon the nursing role. Rather than seek to impersonate medical practice, it might be preferable for nurses to focus their attention on those areas of people's functioning that exist despite their diagnosis, and that, if supported and strengthened by careful nursing action, may help them not only to deal more positively with their supposed illness, and endure less uncomfortably the discomforts of psychiatric treatment, but also become more capable and more contented human beings.

Nurses can usefully prescribe . . . but what?

It is not simply a medical task to prescribe, but one derived from ordinary human activities. In the sense that 'prescribe' means to recommend, many people, including trainers, teachers, coaches, guides and parents, prescribe activities, substances or courses of action to their charges. Only medical practice presumes, although I'd hesitate to use the word 'arrogantly', to substitute for the idea of 'recommend' the much stronger notion 'command', so that people speak of being under 'doctor's orders'. As one contributor to a recent discussion on a web-based discussion list wrote:

'The direction we nurses should be taking is an essentially humanistic one. We need to be more collaborative, embracing respect for others' opinions; and genuinely 'not knowing' their reality until we have proper discussions

with them, and meet them where they are. This is impossible if we begin from the medical position that we 'know' what's best for them – a position demonstrated in the practice of prescribing. Medication may be useful, but then we already have people trained and licensed to prescribe – they're called doctors. Our role may be more useful if, rather than trying to become like doctors, we adopt a collaborative and explorative stance which allows genuine advocacy. If nurses want to prescribe let them go and be doctors.'

(Psychiatric-Nursing Archives 2003)

If prescribing is an essential component of the medical–nursing–patient relationship, is it so important for nurses to be able to prescribe *medicine* as distinct from an unfamiliar way of thinking, a fresh way of relating to people, or a change of recreational habit? If the co-joint power axis of psychiatry and drug companies didn't command a monopoly on most forms of expensive research, if other forms of help were to be regarded as equally significant, and commonly perceived as potentially efficacious, then research programmes could be established that might well demonstrate their equal or greater efficacy than pharmaceutical medicines, and thus establish an evidence base that would gratify service users while at the same time achieve the happy side-effect of helping those nurses who feel lower class to achieve the status and importance they desire.

Once upon a time, a colleague and I observed that, in so-called controlled trials, drugs in development were only ever compared with either placebo, 'conventional treatment' or other drugs. We suggested that if the effectiveness and efficacy of medicaments were to be researched really thoroughly, then medical treatments could usefully be compared with other similarly expensive interventions, gifts, activities, or rewarding or challenging experiences, such as a course of scuba diving, parachute jumping, Antarctic exploration, an ordinary holiday, household repairs, or paying off a debt. Although this notion was developed slightly sardonically, and without having stumbled upon the writings of David Smail, who suggests that most people's so-called psychiatric problems are actually rooted in, or are expressions of real-life social, economic or cultural difficulties, we were making a similar point. Let doctors prescribe medicine, we argued, and let P/MH nurses prescribe gardening instead, or motor maintenance classes, a monastic retreat, a climbing visit to the Pyrenees, dry stone walling lessons, ditch clearing, etc. In the après postmodern unironic 21st century, this pointed joke has recently been given legitimacy under the banner of 'social prescribing' (Cassandra 2003), as well as being accepted practice in more enlightened 'assertive outreach' services. If the nurse prescribing agenda is to be pursued further, perhaps the definition of prescription could sensibly be widened to include such social prescription; services could be funded to include such interventions in their repertoire, and nurses empowered to work with people (and occupational therapists) to identify the most appropriate prescription.

What do users want, expect or need from nurses?

As one might expect, when referring to such a complex heterogeneous sociodemographic group as mental health service 'users', there is conflicting evidence and opinion as to what 'they' require, or desire, from P/MH nurses and about medication prescribing. Some P/MH nurses certainly welcome the task (Gournay & Grey 2001, Hemingway 2003a), whereas others definitely do not (Clarke 2000, Gournay & Barker 2002, Cutcliffe & Campbell 2002). Jordan (2002) suggests that a carefully phased, client-centred introduction of nurse prescribing could allay the suspicions of both users and professionals. Users' views are probably just as conflicted, but less easy to establish or interpret. In the Mental Health Foundation's report 'Strategies for living', Alison Faulkner (2000) quotes an earlier MHF survey on users' requirements:

'At times of distress only 6% of people wanted medication, but 66% needed support and someone to talk to'.

Proponents of a primarily psychiatrically led model of mental health services might, of course, argue that the verbs (*want* and *need*) and the disparate percentages in that sentence are mutually misplaced.

One survey of what mental health service users want from nurses led to subtle and complex conclusions about various aspects of relationship – control, time spent together, depth of understanding – but prescribing medication wasn't mentioned (Barker et al 1999). Different people in different plights at different times would most probably want different things from nurses, but I suspect that if the requirements could be clearly established they would include such qualities as composure, honesty, kindness, firmness and expertise in the abilities that have traditionally been nursing roles, and that members of the public have come to expect from nurses. This includes the provision of physical care and security, as well as psychotherapeutic support and therapeutic activities. At times, some users would perhaps also like nurses to sort out their drug habit, their money, neighbours, partner, parents, children or domestic mess, and strong arguments have been advanced that nurses should, and indeed do, work to these ends. As I have already argued, nurses should *help* – not necessarily simply 'care' or help to 'cure'. And perhaps, although medication compliance is a significant psychiatric goal, there is an admittedly more radical (protagonists of nurse prescribing might disparagingly claim 'more irresponsible') argument that nurses have an important part to play as supporters or advocates of patients' cussed resistance to enforced, coerced or manipulated compliance to medical treatment, which is usually struggled against simply because it feels wrong for them.

A recent UK Department of Health report (Workforce Action Team 2001) concluded that mental health service users experienced a lack of some essential help: patients felt a deficiency of caring *support*; professionals spent insufficient *time* with them; and treatment failed to focus on their *recovery*. With interesting logic, the report concluded that these gaps should be plugged by inventing a new workforce of *support, time and recovery workers*. It is my contention that nurses are the very people who should be focused on the expert provision of these intrinsically therapeutic necessities instead of choosing to, or being forced to, migrate so far from the needs of their so-called 'clients'. Critics might suggest that therapeutic conditions such as empathy, warmth and congruence are simple interactive commodities that can be provided easily and cheaply by anybody, and maintained indefinitely by the magic power of job descriptions. Two decades of providing personal and clinical supervision for workers, singly and in teams, convinces me otherwise. When staff–patient conflict arises or therapeutic progress stumbles, it isn't usually because the nurses lack pathophysiological knowledge or prescriptive authority, but because of the frequent difficulty that even people with deep clinical experience, knowledge and original purity of intention have in maintaining their clear perception, intelligent reasoning, clinical courage, compassion, emotional sensitivity, personal insight or spiritual grace. None of these things is naturally abundant or inexhaustible resources, and it may be that, paradoxically, as workers grow in seniority, the more they need personal and professional replenishment to maintain their complex expertise and preparedness to devote themselves to the needs and hopes of users: support, time and recovery.

How central is biological knowledge?

Proponents of nurse prescribing state authoritatively that medication management, and therefore biochemical knowledge, have always been at the heart of nursing (Gournay & Grey 2001, Hemingway 2003a). I believe, and remember, differently, as do many others (see, for example, Clarke 2000). Knowledge of medication and human biology is a useful requirement of some variants of P/MH nursing, and as such has always featured in its curricula. More central to many other P/MH nursing epistemologies and philosophies, however, has been knowledge of human nature, interactive understanding, psychotherapeutic skills, emotional depth, breadth and resilience, and cultural and integrative awareness (see Cutcliffe 2002). Psychiatric medical practice is an important part of a comprehensive mental health service – and that's what it should be: a part. Unfortunately, the cultural dominance and central, leading role of psychiatry in mental health services has for far too long been uncritically assumed by many nursing and political leaders. Both cause and consequence of this odd thinking has been the increasing dominance of biological formulations and treatments in both nurse education and clinical nursing management. Despite dramatic evidence of the acceptability and effectiveness of psychosocial approaches to 'mental illnesses' and many users' preference for other forms of help, the wider sociopolitical hegemony of science over the humanities seems to have ensured that services continue to be dominated by biomedical formulations – hence the above unquestioned observation by nurse-prescribing enthusiasts. Psychiatry, and therefore those who see their primary professional allegiance as medically based, would be better left to evolve as a subsidiary, albeit significant, mental health profession. Given the complexity of the nature and causes of mental health problems (not really adequately contained in the homely simplicity of so-called 'psychiatric illnesses'), doctors are not logically best placed as the primary helping agents; and medical theory is by no means sufficient to explain, conceptualise or organise the totality of a national service's responses to human psychosocial problems.

Are P/MH nurses well placed to become prescribers anyway, given that their basic training is so brief, compared with medical education? If it takes so long to prepare a psychiatrist, how come nurses can take on the job with apparently an extra module or two of post-qualification preparation? While nurse prescribing in the general nursing arena has been restricted almost exclusively to a limited formulary of largely adjunctive medication, it seems assumed that if the role is to be extended to P/MH nurses then full-on psychiatric treatment, or at least far greater scope to adjust psychiatric prescriptions, will fall within their legitimate prescribing purlieu. Realistically, nurse education managers and curriculum designers would be unable to guarantee sufficient curriculum time to inculcate adequate biochemical, physiological and pathophysiological knowledge, and familiarity with the effects – beneficial and otherwise – of specific medications (including newly emergent ones) at a sufficient depth to enable critical decision-making. Clinical and education managers could do little else but recommend that nurses heed the dubiously motivated remonstrations of pharmaceutical companies and their representatives, a position fraught with difficulties and contentious issues (Ashmore & Carver 2001, Hemingway 2003b). There is already overwhelming pressure from many sources – sociologists, general nursing and compulsive risk avoiders – on P/MH nursing curricula at all levels. Increasingly less time is devoted to inculcating and enhancing those very skills and aptitudes that are said by many P/MH nurses to characterise their job, and that users so often lament the absence of in their professional carers. If nurse education is to continue to swerve towards a more formally biomedical preparation, then it isn't difficult to envisage even less educational time and attention being devoted to interpersonal skills and psychosocial understanding (see Keen 1999).

Political expediency, economics, government policy, etc.

If I were of a more cynical turn of mind, I might suggest as others have (McCarthy et al 1999) that the need for P/MH nurses and other professionals to prescribe psychiatric medication, and thereby swell the numbers of medical substitutes or medical assistants, may be driven by several forces that, while expedient, may also seem unworthy:

- Economic pressures on the government to train and maintain an effective workforce as inexpensively as possible
- Public and media pressure to be seen to respond to the perceived threat of mental illness (Cutcliffe & Hannigan 2001)
- The search for professional identity, meaning and worth by significant numbers of aspirationally challenged P/MH nurses
- Covert government policy to challenge or subvert the power of the psychiatric medical establishment.

Many years ago, as a satirical conference irritant, a clinical psychologist and I devised a therapeutic system called 'money therapy'. In this therapy, instead of prescribing expensive psychiatric drugs or sending someone to hospital for an even more expensive period of waiting-and-observation treatment, we proposed totting up the total cost to the National Health Service (NHS) of whatever course of treatment would conventionally be followed, and offering a marginally reduced sum to the luckless person on a 't.d.s.' or 'b.i.d.' basis, seven days a week – with a special visit to hand over the cash and converse in as ordinary a fashion as possible, rather than monitoring medication administration and the inevitable side-effects. The actual sum allocated could be adjusted to ensure a projected budgetary reduction, thereby saving the NHS money and subsidising the treatment itself (H Proctor, personal communication 1988). We would love to have piloted a scheme, and researched the outcomes, but professional and experimental ethics obviously forbade that. However, one thing I think governments should have learned about reforms to mental health services by now is that – while they (governments) may be cynically accused of having concealed motives to save money and curry public favour by closing down mental hospitals, locking up so-called psychopaths, recruiting cheaper-than-nurses workers to replace cheaper-than-doctors nurse prescribers, and whatever gambits and gambles emerge in the future – quality mental health services are not and never will be achievable on the cheap. The question of adequate pay for prescriptive authority has been fiercely debated by nurses, who increasingly question the disparity between remuneration for advanced, specialist roles both within nursing itself and between their jobs and those of other health care professionals (Psychiatric-Nursing Archives 2003).

Rather than seek to be of economic assistance to governments desperate to reduce the cost of treatments, while simultaneously needing to demonstrate increasing effectiveness (at least in matters of social control and public behaviour), nurses should be concerned with what people want from P/MH nurses, and with why the craft has deviated so markedly from the forging and maintaining of therapeutic alliances, which is one way of summarising that which people seem to find desirable and helpful. If P/MH nurses prescribe medication, then what is left of P/MH nursing practice that distinguishes medical from nursing approaches? Does it matter if nurses function as cheaper, less extensively (and less expensively) trained dispensing agents? After all, other professions are just as well if not better suited to add this particular function to their job descriptions, for instance pharmacists and clinical psychologists. The diversity inherent in a service that provides individually trained experts in each of several different areas of human nature, affairs and malfunction is arguably one of that service's strengths. To dissolve it away by a slow process of unplanned and casually envisioned homogenisation is to risk devaluing the skills and expertise of each specific professional craft, and thereby to short-change the legitimate expectations of their shared clientele.

Conclusion

Are the reasons discussed above sufficient to risk undermining the rich history and value of professional diversity and specific expertise in our mental health services, while countermanding or ignoring the repeatedly expressed preferences of the service's customers? One challenge to the enshrinement of specific professional expertise can be couched in the language of *holism*. If nurses are to practise holistically, some have argued, they must be able to respond authoritatively to all their clients' needs. Maybe, but, if so, why are we not also actively campaigning for a licence to use the legal tools of social workers, the treatment rights of psychologists and the physical jerks of physiotherapists? What does it say about the therapeutic allegiance of nurses to their 'clients' that they seek to treat problems medically (and thereby falsify the trendy nomenclature, and continue to construe them as 'patients', however politically incorrect that appellation) rather than genuinely strive to relate to them as problem-solving people, or as social agents?

As I've already said, it's pointless to argue that nurses should be utterly forbidden to prescribe ordinary medicaments, or modify prescriptions; that may by now be an economically and expediently done deal. In addition, the nurse-prescribing dispute may, sadly, be anachronistically irrelevant to many nurses already practising their hi-tech craft in some states of the USA and other countries (although the quote below perhaps offers an alternative view). This is rather an argument that nurse prescribing is not the best direction in which P/MH nursing in the UK should attempt its onward march, nor the most appropriate aspiration upon which to focus its collective energies, and at the same time an argument that urges a moment of pause and reflection for those countries that appear already to have embraced P/MH nurse prescribing. It is an argument against placing too high a priority on the issue of being able to prescribe psychiatric medication, while there is ample and mounting evidence of a breakdown of relationships and trust between people needing help and the professionals, especially nurses and doctors, expected to provide it.

In short, this is an argument for applying gentle brakes to the pursuit of becoming more and more biochemically medical. An argument for putting up cussed opposition to those who campaign for compliant accommodation to political expediency and the burgeoning might of the pharmaceutical industry. An argument for attempting a rapprochement with ordinary people, so as to not endanger any further the fragile bonds of vestigial trust that leads some users still to extol their experience of the helpful nature of mental health services, at least as embodied in the person of their narrative-clarifying, solution-focused, problem-solving, social-prescribing, time-spending, supportive, encouraging, empathic and listening nurse.

Finally, for those who believe that the USA has embraced prescriptive authority without overmuch difficulty for P/MH nurses, here's a heartfelt, unscientific comment posted 'off-list' by a highly qualified and experienced 'advanced practitioner' during the aforementioned web-based discussion on nurse prescribing:

'Do you want to know what it's like to be the new breed of professional on the neighborhood block; the only one that has the ability to provide full medication management and psychotherapy? Yet is not accepted by all third party payers as 'adequate' enough for reimbursement? Do you want to know how hostile the work environment becomes where territories of practice are traditionally not so blurred? "Psychologists and social workers provide psychotherapy, and medics only do medicine . . . what makes you think you can and will do both?" Do you want to know about the resentments from psych and "regular" nurses who think that because you prescribe, you're a traitor, disloyal to the profession, like having special privileges, or feel that you feel that you're entitled to specialness? Do you want to know about how the union that represents you won't fight for a salary differential for using the prescriptive privilege, because "a nurse is a nurse is a nurse"? Do you want to know about the misconceptions in regards to the glamour of having full responsibility for hundreds of people at any given moment? . . . If your inquiry ever leads down the path of what

it really is like (for a nurse) to prescribe for a living, then I am the person you want to ask. Just don't get too close, I may end up crying on your shoulders.'

References

Ashmore R, Carver N 2001 The pharmaceutical industry and mental health nursing. British Journal of Nursing 10(21):984–990.

Barker P, Jackson S, Stevenson C 1999 What are psychiatric nurses needed for? Journal of Psychiatric and Mental Health Nursing 6(3):273–282.

Burnard P 2002 Not waving but drowning. Journal of Psychiatric and Mental Health Nursing 9(2):229–232.

Burns D, Auerbach A 1996 Therapeutic empathy in cognitive-behavioural therapy: does it really make a difference? In: Salkovskis P M, ed. Frontiers of cognitive therapy. Guilford Press, New York, p 162–186.

Cassandra (pseudonym) 2003 Anyone for tennis on prescription? Mental Health Today July/August, p 37.

Clarke L 2000 Challenging ideas in psychiatric nursing. Routledge, London.

Cutcliffe J 2002 The beguiling effects of nurse-prescribing in mental health nursing: re-examining the debate. Journal of Psychiatric and Mental Health Nursing 9(3):369–375.

Cutcliffe J R, Campbell P 2002 Nurse prescribing: a step in the right direction or undermining the nature of mental health nursing? Mental Health Practice 5(5):14–17.

Cutcliffe J R, Hannigan B 2001 Mass media, monsters and mental health: a need for increased lobbying. Journal of Psychiatric and Mental Health Nursing 8(4):315–322.

Daniels N M, Williams G B 2003 Medication in nursing practice: the nurse and prescribing authority. In: Barker P, ed. Psychiatric and mental health nursing: the craft of caring. Arnold, London, p 488–496.

Faulkner A 2000 Strategies for living. Mental Health Foundation, London.

Gournay K, Barker P 2002 Prescribing: the great debate. Nursing Standard 17(9):22–23.

Gournay K, Grey R 2001 Should mental health nurses prescribe? Maudsley Discussion Paper 11, Institute of Psychiatry, King's College, London.

Hemingway S 2003a Nurse prescribing for mental health nurses: scripting the issues. Journal of Psychiatric and Mental Health Nursing 10(2):239–245.

Hemingway S 2003b Mental health nursing and the pharmaceutical industry. Mental Health Practice 7(2):22–23.

Jordan S 2002 Managing adverse drug-reactions: an orphan task. Journal of Advanced Nursing 38(5):437–448.

Keen T 1999 Nurse-education yesterday? Journal of Psychiatric and Mental Health Nursing 6(3):233–240.

Keen T 2003 Post-psychiatry: paradigm-shift or wishful thinking? Journal of Psychiatric and Mental Health Nursing 10(1):29–38.

McCann T, Hemingway S 2003 Models of prescriptive authority for mental health nurse practitioners. Journal of Psychiatric and Mental Health Nursing 10(6):743–749.

McCarthy W, Tyrer S, Brazier M, Prayle D 1999 Nurse-prescribing: radicalism or tokenism? Journal of Advanced Nursing 29:348–354.

Psychiatric-Nursing Archives 2003 Online. Available: http://www.jiscmail. ac.uk/cgi-bin/wa.exe?A1=ind0311&L=psychiatric-nursing accessed 2003.

Smail D 1993 The origins of unhappiness: a new understanding of personal distress. Harper/Collins, London.

Workforce Action Team 2001 Workforce planning, education and training: underpinning programme: adult mental health services. Department of Health, London.

Katharine P Bailey & Steve Hemingway

Psychiatric/mental health nurses as non-medical prescribers: validating their role in the prescribing process

Introduction

Nurse prescribing may be a relatively recent development in UK psychiatric/mental health (P/MH) nursing, but in the USA P/MH nurses have held prescriptive authority for over twenty years. If we are to examine evidence of the efficacy of prescribing by P/MH nurses then a comprehensive review of its impact on the patient who receives the new provision, the nurse prescriber and the service as a whole needs to be sought. Accordingly, by drawing upon the experience from the USA and discussing the present development of non-medical prescribing in the UK, a picture can be gained that suggests this development is a positive way forward and an exciting new development for P/MH nurses. We present the argument that this is a step forward for mental health care. Further, although concentrating on UK and US perspectives, we believe this debate will have implications for other countries considering implementing this new development.

It should be noted that, currently, all 50 of the United States have existing legislation that allows some form of prescriptive authority for advanced practice nurses. Some of these states allow fully independent practice; others place various restrictions on the scope of practice through limited formularies, required protocols, designated geographic areas (e.g. rural areas) or designated health care sites (e.g. nursing homes), and/or required physician supervision or collaboration. In the USA, the role of nurse prescriber has always been an advanced practice role. That is, in order to be eligible to prescribe, a nurse must have a Master's degree in his/her speciality, pass a speciality certification examination authorised by the American Nurses Association and, in some states, obtain an additional licence in the state in which he/she practises.

For the purposes of clarity, P/MH nurse prescribers from the US will be referred to as 'psychiatric nurse practitioners' (PNPs), and readers can assume that they have the credentials described above. The authors of this chapter define 'Prescriptive authority' as:

'the legal authorization to exercise independent clinical judgment to choose a pharmacologic agent, order it and dispense it to a patient for the treatment of a disease state. It includes full responsibility for the monitoring of the medication and the management of the patient.'

Nurse as prescribers: a UK history

Historically, nurses have assumed a great deal of unofficial critical patient management, including drug related decisions, without formal or legal recognition (Ramcharan et al 2001). This historical situation has changed in places where the former in situ rigid demarcations – with the doctor prescribing, the pharmacist dispensing and the nurse administering medication – has moved to the era of non-medical pre-scribing. The domination of the prescribing process by the medical profession is now being challenged (McCartney et al, 1999, National Prescribing Centre [NPC] 2005), and nurse prescribing in the UK has been supported and developed by the UK Government (Department of Health [DoH] 1999, 2000) and latterly in mental health care to meet the new complexities of health care demand (NPC 2005). (Please also read end note.)

In the late 1980s, a view developed in primary care that some limited prescribing could be adopted by community health nurses and, thus, would save time and money. The time it took for nurses to contact the general practitioner to obtain basic dressings, for example, wasted valu-able time and money. The Crown I Report (DoH 1989) broadened the debate and suggested, in addition to other nurses and allied health care professions, that community mental health nurses could come under pressure to prescribe. It was another ten years before the Crown II Report (DoH 1999), which formally recognised and suggested how prescribing should be developed for nurses. Subsequently, prescription of a limited formulary by generic community nurses (no prescriptive authority was at that point given to community psychiatric nurses) was piloted in several UK sites. Although the medications prescribed by these nurses were only 'over the counter medicines' (e.g. mild analge-sics), topical treatments and a small number of prescription-only medi-cines, the pilot showed that extension of their role to that of non-medical prescribers (NMPs) could improve cost efficiency of nursing care (Luker et al 1997). Once users of the service acclimatised and adjusted to a nurse prescribing, they valued the service, felt nurses could prescribe competently and, importantly, were able to discuss non-medical issues surrounding their care (Luker et al 1997).

The 'Review of prescribing, supply and administration of medicines' (DoH 1999) and 'The National Health Service Plan' (DoH 2000) signalled that the new Labour government administration saw nurse prescribing as a way forward – a way to modernise the health service (DoH 1999). Their reasons for this view were summarised as:

- To increase the range of professionals authorised to prescribe
- To improve the quality and accuracy of the prescribing service
- To make a better use of professional staff and therefore make a significant contribution to the modernisation of the NHS
- To increase the choice and flexibility of prescribing intervention for the service user.

Limited formulary prescribing rights were also granted in the Health and Social Care Act 2001. Nurses, by law, could now prescribe (including community psychiatric/mental health nurses). With the advent of supplementary prescribing (NPC 2005) and the shift in emphasis for P/MH nurses to work with people with long-term and enduring conditions, such P/MH nurses could prescribe medication once a doctor (the Supervisor) had assessed, diagnosed and, in agreement with the service user, completed the clinical management plan. What this meant was that, potentially, the P/MH nurse could prescribe any drug from the British National Formulary, although, in reality, the P/MH nurse, once trained and appropriately supervised, would prescribe medicine within their own scope of practice (Davis & Hemingway 2003).

Psychiatric/mental health nurses' perceptions of nurse prescribing

The history of P/MH nursing indicates that the P/MH nursing role developed alongside the psychiatrist's prescribing decisions about care for the mentally unwell. We argue that medical interventions have also always been a part of P/MH nurses' interventions. With the developments of the antidepressants, antipsychotic, anxiolytic and anti-manic pharmacological agents in the 1950s, and the expansion of 'community care' in the 1990s, the nursing role expanded towards encompassing social, psychological and biological interventions. P/MH nurses, particularly those working in the community, showed they could autonomously embrace different interventions to meet the needs of the person they were working with.

The debate about P/MH nurses prescribing medication has gained increasing prominence in recent years. Central to the debate is whether prescribing will medicalise the P/MH nurse role, diminish the caring aspects (Clarke 2000, Cutcliffe & Campbell 2002) or improve the service delivery given to the service user and validate the P/MH nursing role (Hemingway 2003, NPC 2005). There exists some evidence indicating that some P/MH nurses feel the potential of nurse prescribing is positive; recent studies have shown positive response (Ramcharan et al 2001, Hemingway 2004). These studies, although they can be criticised for having limited or even biased samples (e.g. people attending a conference about prescribing), show that a significant number of the nurses sampled believe that if the adoption of prescriptive authority is appropriately planned and resourced, and if nurses receive adequate training and the service user is central to its inception, nurse prescribing could be effective. It is also important to note there are detractors to the seemingly positive responses.

In the above studies, approximately 30% P/MH nurses were unsure or against P/MH nurses prescribing. In two of the studies, people against felt that prescribing should purely be the doctor's responsibility, and that nurses should attend to the 'psychosocial interventions' rather than the medical interventions. These results echo the concerns expressed by Clarke (2000) and Cutcliffe & Campbell (2002) regarding the potential medicalisation that prescribing could cause.

Opinion originating in the USA further informs this position. An argument for nurse prescribing is that, through their training, P/MH nurses bring a different perspective to patients and to patient care that is additive and complementary to the traditional medical perspective. This perspective includes:

- Commitment and concern for the quality of patients' lives beyond their physical and mental well being
- Attention to total care as the foundation of high quality of care
- Perception of themselves as patient advocates
- Commitment to educate and empower patients regarding their physical and emotional health and their treatment
- Focus on health and health potential
- And, more specifically related to the role of pharmacotherapist, a tendency to use the process of interacting with patients around their medication issues as an opportunity to promote health and growth in other areas of their lives as well.

From the beginning of basic nursing education, nursing practice is defined in terms of the total needs of the patient. Patients with mental illnesses often need medication, which targets the neurobiological aspects of their illness. In order to be fully effective in meeting this particular need, nurses must be able to make independent decisions and interventions regarding psychopharmacotherapy. In other words, we argue that nurse prescribing is a skill and a service that reflects the most fundamental philosophical beliefs of our profession.

Psychiatric/mental health nurses and medication: a positive alliance?

Psychosocial approaches have been described as an essential part of the P/MH nurse role, but we argue here that involvement in pharmacotherapy is what distinguishes the service they provide from that of other mental health professionals in the UK such as social workers, psychologists and occupational therapists (Hemingway 2003). Service users have certain rights and expectations regarding their treatment and medication; further, it has been suggested that P/MH nurses potentially have a part to play in making the prescribing process more inclusive (Harrison 2003, NPC 2005). Interventions in mental health care need to emphasise the person and respect his or her rights; in this case, needs of the person should be included in decisions about pharmacological intervention and treatment (NPC 2005). A concordant approach implies that the service user is the central to the prescribing process (Ramcharan et al 2001). It has been argued that, if the people receiving treatment are given appropriate information to manage their medication, treatment is more likely to be accepted and might reduce non-compliance and relapse rates. The role of the P/MH nurse is key here, and it has been suggested that if the controlling or coercive nature of treatment is to be eliminated then adopting prescriptive authority, using evidence-based interventions, as well as involving the service user fully, can facilitate this process (Harrison 2003, NPC 2005). The National Service Framework for mental health puts an emphasis on using the appropriate psychopharmacological intervention (DoH 1999). P/MH nurses can provide service users with the treatment most pertinent to their needs, with an emphasis on partnership between the nurse as prescriber and the service user as recipient of care (NPC 2005).

Issues pertaining to adequate education and training

Perhaps the most salient argument in support of nurse prescribing is that PNPs have the skills and education to prescribe effectively. Master's programmes in P/MH nursing across the USA prepare PNPs for multiple roles. PNP students take courses that emphasise psychobiological and psychiatric theories of the human behaviour of individuals, groups and families. They are taught several modalities of psychotherapy for individuals, groups and families. Courses in neuroscience, the neurobiological basis of mental disorders and psychopharmacology are also included. Additionally, they study clinical diagnosis and treatment of psychiatric illness, community mental health, the consultation process, programme planning and evaluation, research methods, ethical–legal issues, and management and organisational development. They are prepared to take on the roles of clinician, educator, manager, consultant and researcher.

The speciality curriculum is a combination of theoretical content and supervised practicum experiences. To meet certification requirements, students are placed in a variety of clinical settings where they carry a caseload of patients over time and participate in agency-sponsored learning activities and clinical supervision. In order to obtain the legalisation of prescriptive authority for their profession, advanced practice nurses across specialities have had to challenge the widely held assumption that only physicians have adequate education and training and, therefore, the sole, pre-eminent authority to prescribe. However, in the USA before 1900, consumers could obtain any available drug through their pharmacists without a prescription. Consulting a physician's advice about drugs, although sometimes done, was neither mandatory nor frequently practised. It wasn't until the middle of the 20th century that federal regulations took control from the consumer and embedded the prescription of medications more firmly into the existing medical hierarchy, increasing consumer dependence on the physician.

In the UK the extended/supplementary prescribing training course assumes that students attending the course will have experiential competence, that they will have gained expertise by working in an area for some time, and will have been actively involved in pharmacological as well as other psychosocial interventions in supporting the service user with mental illness (Davis & Hemingway 2003). Evidence is available that nurses have been deeply involved in prescribing decisions that affect the care of the individual service user, and at times de facto prescribe, strongly suggesting or advising the doctor on the appropriate medication for a particular problem (Ramcharan et al 2001, NPC 2005). However, the difference between competence gained through experience and the transition toward making a diagnostic decision and then prescribing psychotropic medication means the educational provision needed to facilitate safe and expert prescribing interventions by the P/MH nurse is paramount.

Interestingly, the content of the available prescribing courses is, on the whole, generic rather than specialism oriented, although some universities have provided a more focused mental health-related content (NPC 2005). The course structure in the UK is a 26-day theory content concentrating on the following:

- Pharmacology (pharmacokinetics, pharmacodynamics, side-effects, adverse reactions)
- Management of the consultation
- Legal and ethical considerations
- Psychological and other issues (transference of the patient, and countertransference of the nurse, influence of the pharmaceutical industry)
- Concordance issues.

The P/MH nurse attending the course is then expected to transfer this knowledge to the clinical area by having 12 days of supervised practice with a doctor who assesses the competence of the nurse-prescribing student. Further, the student needs to maintain a portfolio that shows evidence of reflection on their prescribing activity, and is then observed under examination conditions. The academic level of the course is a baccalaureate degree, this being different from the Master's-level preparation that is required in the USA (Bailey 2004). Two issues emerge here. First, it should be asked: does attending a course that has a generic content truly and adequately prepare the P/MH nurse for prescribing psychotropic medication or should it have a 'stand alone' content? Second, given that, in the USA prescribing is regarded as an advanced nursing role with educational preparation at the Master's level, will this mean that the nurses in the UK are inadequately prepared to practise safely as prescribers? It is unlikely that the resourcing of the UK prescribing course will change in the immediate future, so it will continue to be generic in content; similarly, the emphasis is on the nurse to relate any learning to his or her own clinical area. Accordingly, the use of medical supervision and continued education relative to prescribing will be needed (Hemingway 2004). Postregistration training in the UK differs from that in the USA (where all preregistration courses are at first-degree level). We argue that a considerable number of senior nurses who did not undertake an academic preregistration education in nursing (these nurses trained under the 'certificate system') are in a position where they can draw on their experience of care, and thus not be disadvantaged by the lack of an academic preregistration education. They have developed expertise in the specialism in which they practise, and service users would benefit from these P/MH nurses developing as non-medical prescribers. The differences in preparation for nurse prescribing create an interesting contrast, with the key question being: Can a degree-level trained nurse competently prescribe rather than the Master's-prepared student nurse (Bailey 2004)?

Will service users accept P/MH nurses prescribing?

We argue that this question can be answered only as prescribing by P/MH nurses develops; nevertheless, there have been some encouraging signs. Studies involving people who were visited at home and received prescribing services from district nurses reported competent practice, gains in terms of time spent discussing their health needs (especially non-medical) and favourable attitudes towards nurses prescribing (Luker et al 1997). However, it has been emphasised that P/MH nurses need to have the knowledge and competence to advise about and administer psychotropic medication. Harrison (2003) asked service users what they felt about the possibility of P/MH nurses prescribing, and found them mostly in favour, but they also had questions about the competence of nurses prescribing. This is an important issue, and one that repeatedly arises. The issue of how we can ensure that the P/MH nurse prescriber has the knowledge base and skills to prescribe competently has been recognised by commentators as an area that needs addressing (Ramcharan et al 2001, Hemingway, 2004). Respondents in Harrison's (2003) study also appreciated the possible extended time and the relationship that could be developed with the P/MH nurse versus the limited time the doctor can give. The respondents felt that this, potentially, could equalise care.

Efficacy of nurses as prescribers of medication

Twenty years or so of prescriptive practice, and several outcome studies regarding prescriptive practice by nurse practitioners across specialities, have suggested that four years of medical school and four more years of postgraduate and speciality medical education and training may not be necessary for safe and efficacious prescriptive practice, as many argue. The existing research regarding advanced practice nurses' prescriptive practice has focused primarily on primary care nurse practitioners (NPs). Most of the relevant studies were conducted nearly two decades ago when health services research was in its infancy, and many have methodological flaws. However, taken as a whole, they strongly suggest that the legalisation of prescriptive authority for NPs has increased access to care and allowed nurses to practise to the full extent of their education and training.

A summary report from the US federal Office of Technology Assessment (OTA) in 1986 found that, of 24 studies identified, 22 reported the quality of care provided by NPs and patient satisfaction with NP services to be equal to or to surpass care provided by physicians. The study also reinforced the cost-effectiveness of NP care. Crosby et al (1987) compiled an information synthesis of 248 documents on NP effectiveness that reported findings consistent with those of the OTA study. Another meta-analysis of 53 studies to assess the effectiveness of NP care compared with physician care found that NPs provided more health promotion activities and scored higher on quality-of-care measures (e.g. diagnostic accuracy, completeness of the care process) than did the physicians (Brown & Grimes 1993). Patients of the NPs demonstrated equivalent or greater satisfaction with their health care provider, compliance with health promotion and treatment, and knowledge of their health status than patients of physicians. More recently, two methodologically sound studies clearly indicated equal effectiveness of NPs compared with medical doctors on a range of measures (Mundinger 2000, Horrocks et al 2002).

In summary, the findings from these and other studies indicate that:

- Patients are satisfied
- The interpersonal skills of NPs are better than those of physicians
- The technical quality of their services, including prescriptive practice, is equivalent to that delivered by physicians
- Patient outcomes are equivalent or superior
- NPs facilitate continuity of patient care, as well as improved access to care in rural and other settings and to underserved populations.

Unfortunately, there is a paucity of systematic outcome studies regarding the prescriptive practices of PNPs. What data exist come from questionnaires distributed to random national samples of PNPs (Campbell et al 1998), to a convenience sample from a group of Western states (Talley & Richens 2001), or to the total population of PNPs in an individual state, Massachusetts (Glod & Manchester 2000). Response rates to these surveys ranged from 55% to 81%. Results were similar across surveys and showed that the majority of PNPs were full- or part-time salaried employees in both public and private hospital-based and outpatient settings whose predominant work activity was direct patient care. The majority of PNPs were treating patients who had the full spectrum of psychiatric disorders, with major depression and anxiety disorders the most frequently treated. The most frequently prescribed medications were those from the four main classes of psychotropic agent: antidepressants, anxiolytics, mood stabilisers (including anticonvulsants) and antipsychotics. Interestingly, only between 16.5% and 61% of PNPs who had prescriptive authority were actively prescribing. One study (Talley & Richens 2001) made some comparisons to the practice patterns of psychiatrists, which were very similar in terms of types of patient seen, practice settings and medications prescribed. This general profile suggests that clinical outcomes and patients' acceptance of and satisfaction with PNPs would be comparable to those in the randomised controlled outcome trials for other NPs cited above.

Non-medical prescribing by P/MH nurses is now a reality in certain places and is receiving increasing emphasis (NPC 2005). It has been highlighted as one of the clinical interventions to be reviewed in the forthcoming review of mental health nursing. If we are to evaluate the relative benefits of extending the role of P/MH nurses to include prescribing, consideration of the evidence available from mental health nurse colleagues in the USA practising with prescriptive authority will provide a valuable insight for the UK perspective.

Issues pertaining to comprehensiveness of care

Over the last 20 years, expanding knowledge in the neurosciences and genetics, improved clinical assessment strategies and empirically supported treatments, both pharmacological and psychosocial, have emerged and are being applied more broadly in clinical practice. Despite these advances, according to the World Health Organisation (WHO), of the ten leading causes of disability worldwide in 1990, five were psychiatric conditions: major depression, bipolar illness, schizophrenia, obsessive-compulsive disorder and alcohol abuse. Major depression was second only to ischaemic heart disease as the world's major cause of disease burden. Furthermore, suicide is among the top ten causes of death worldwide. Some evidence exists to suggest that the disability induced by depression or anxiety may negatively impact on the prognosis and mortality of some co-morbid medical illnesses, and that depression may actually predispose individuals to some medical illnesses. Substance abuse is also a pervasive problem that is taking an increasing toll on society and is associated with many of the most serious problems in the USA, among them violence, injury and HIV infection. The use of alcohol and drugs accounts for more deaths, illnesses and disabilities than does any other preventable health condition.

The global population is growing older; for example, in the USA the population over 65 will comprise nearly one in five Americans in the first quarter of the 21st century. Rates of dementia increase substantially with age and represent an enormous public health burden. As many as 30% of older patients with dementia suffer from major depression, and many also experience symptoms of agitation, wandering, paranoia and other psychotic symptoms or sleep disturbance. Each of these can be effectively treated, in part, by pharmacotherapy, even though the basic cognitive deficit may not be altered.

An increasing number of psychotropic agents to treat psychiatric disorders have been developed in the past two decades. However, although newer medications offer comparable efficacy with fewer side-effects and a markedly reduced risk of serious adverse effects, many patients do not adhere to treatment recommendations. The high rates of recurrence and relapse after antidepressant discontinuation highlight the need to address the factors that lead patients to discontinue medications prematurely.

The increasing prevalence, persistence and severity of mental illness and the shockingly inadequate patient access to mental health services around the globe clearly argue for an increase in the number of well trained mental health providers, especially clinicians who can prescribe, manage and monitor medications. The challenges in our profession speak to a need and opportunity for P/MH nurses to improve outcomes, not only within traditional psychiatric settings, but also within general health care, correctional, residential and school-based settings. It is argued, and accepted by some, that most, if not all, major mental illnesses have an underlying neurobiological/genetic diathesis. Further, protagonists of this point of view argue that these are best addressed by pharmacological intervention. In fact, pharmacological intervention plays a primary role in treatment in psychiatry. We believe that, in order for PNPs to be effective practitioners who can deliver comprehensive mental health care, they must have the authority to prescribe medications.

In the USA, historically and currently, funding by private insurance and managed care companies and by local and federal government agencies for psychiatric services, supportive social services, and for education and training of psychiatric professionals has been inadequate. This has resulted in increased limitations on psychiatric patients' access to appropriate and comprehensive services. We believe that these dynamics point towards the utilisation of PNPs as prescribers because they increase the number of clinicians who provide psychopharmacology services, thereby increasing patient access to care, and they deliver these services more cost effectively – given the salary differential between psychiatrists and PNPs.

Personal and professional growth in the service of the patient

In 2003, Brown and Draye conducted a descriptive study that used individual interviews and focus groups to gather data from pioneer NPs about their early experiences in establishing the NP role and their experiences in maintaining and building the role. The findings from this study eloquently demonstrate some NPs' perceptions of the personal and professional rewards that resulted from expanding the scope of their practice. Many of the NPs had become frustrated by the circumstances of traditional nursing jobs, or they were simply 'chomping at the bit' to use their full expertise. Dissatisfaction with previous registered nurse (RN) roles arose from the constant need to obtain physicians' orders before implementing their own interventions. The NPs emphasised that their struggle was not for autonomy for its own sake, but *to make a difference in the quality of patient care*. They derived tremendous satisfaction from increased role autonomy, and felt a great deal of pride in having made important differences in patients' lives. While attitudes towards prescriptive practice were not addressed specifically in the focus groups, prescribing was part of their scope of practice and was one of the skills that increased their autonomy.

Nurse prescribing – the way forward?

The issues, set out in this chapter, need to be overcome if the service user is to receive the full benefit of the knowledgeable, accessible and competent P/MH nurse prescriber. Supplementary prescribing training has already allowed a number of P/MH nurses to be able to prescribe medication within their own speciality. An estimate of between 350 to

400 having undertaken the relevant course to date, these numbers will continue to grow. Supplementary prescribing allows nurses to prescribe once the doctor has agreed, with the user of the service and the nurse, what can be prescribed in the clinical management plan (NPC 2005). Bailey (1999) advises that the novice prescriber starts by knowing one drug from each class (e.g. antidepressant, anxiolytic, antipsychotic, mood stabiliser) well and slowly expanding to other agents as a sensible way to develop expertise in prescribing. Supplementary prescribing provides the opportunity for P/MH nurses to develop their expertise in prescribing within their own speciality in a limited first stage, as described by Bailey, and thus, once proven as a safe and efficacious practitioner, the opportunity to develop as truly independent prescribers could be established.

The organisational and resource implications of P/MH nurses training and then working within a team context must be addressed adequately (NPC 2005). Service provider organisations need to plan for how nurse prescribing can target areas that are suitable, for example where there is an inadequate service provision and lack of medical care, so that the service provision would improve as a result of a P/MH nurse assuming prescriptive authority (Davis & Hemingway 2003). The present prescribing training gives the generic principles of prescribing only, and this clearly is not enough to ensure the knowledge required to understand and assess the service user's needs based on the pharmacokinetics and pharmacodynamics of drugs used in mental health care (Hemingway 2004). Educational initiatives such as the 'medication management programme' show that, with sufficient and comprehensive training, the P/MH nurse can make a positive difference to service users' experience of taking psychotropic medication (NPC 2005). These steps forward in the role of the P/MH nurse help the service user to manage their medication appropriately; these programmes need to be further developed and included by educational providers to supplement the supplementary prescribing training (Hemingway 2004).

Conclusion

This chapter has provided what the authors feel is a realistic, but positive, appraisal of the case for the adoption of prescriptive authority for P/MH nurses in the UK, as well as lessons derived from the experience of colleagues in the USA. The challenge for the novice prescriber is to utilise the appropriate networks of support and regulatory frameworks, keep the service user as the central focus of the care process, and assume the role and responsibility of prescribing practitioner competently in an area where they had only 'de facto' authority with medication. The key to developing into this role successfully is motivation, feeling comfortable with medication as part of a holistic framework of care, and utilising this new-found expertise within their practice. Notwithstanding some methodological problems, the authors believe the evidence originating in the USA regarding the efficacy and cost-effectiveness of NPs as prescribers is strong, and is supported by their patients' satisfaction with their care. Given an unfortunate lack of data for PNPs, we can only assume that PNP outcomes would be similar to those of NPs, and that there would be obvious benefits for the patient, nurses, service provision and mental health care as a whole.

Many nurses who do not prescribe, including those who have the legal authority to do so as well as those who don't, argue that prescriptive practice will rob them of the most satisfying aspect of their work, attending to the comprehensive needs of their patients, and force them to be mere 'physician extenders'. However, some testimony from experienced NPs belies this concern. For example, the pioneer NPs in Brown & Draye's (2003) study described how an established identity as a nurse was crucial, and blending components of nursing and medicine was a satisfying intellectual challenge. In addition, if nurses really want to attend to the comprehensive needs of patients with mental illness, they will need to integrate what we believe is this primary modality of treatment – pharmacological intervention – into their scope of practice.

Many nurses also argue that their nursing programmes do not contain content that adequately trains them for the role of nurse prescriber, and that, therefore, they do not have adequate knowledge and skills for the role (Jordan et al 1999). This may be generally true of nursing education at the pre-Master's level. However, many nurses without prescriptive authority but with significant clinical experience assess patients and make recommendations regarding choice of appropriate medication to physicians, who often solicit their recommendations, before writing a prescription. The UK National Health Service's recent initiation and gradual implementation of prescriptive practice for nurses not trained at the Master's level is a great experiment for the nursing profession. What remains to be determined is how much and what kind of additional education and training they will need, how will it be funded, and what will be the quality of their pharmacological interventions and the resulting clinical outcomes. If they are successful, we believe they will do a great service to their patients by significantly expanding their access to pharmacological intervention and improving the quality of their lives.

END NOTE: Since this chapter was written two major developments have occurred in 2005. Nurses (including P/MH nurses) were 'allowed' to prescribe controlled drugs (Bridge et al 2005). Secondly the Department of Health (2005) arrounced that as of 2006 nurses would be able to prescribe any drug independently.

References

Bailey K P 1999 Framework for prescriptive practice. In: Shea C A, Pelletier L R, Poster E C, Stuart G W, Verhey M P, eds. Advanced practice nursing in psychiatric and mental health care. Mosby, St Louis, p 297–313.

Bailey K P 2004 Should nurses prescribe: reviewing the issues from the US and UK perspectives. Journal of Psychosocial Nursing 42(12):15–19.

Bridge J, Hemmingway S, Murphy K 2005 Implications of non-medical prescribing of controlled drugs. Nursing Times 101(44):32–33.

Brown M A, Draye M A 2003 Experiences of pioneer nurse practitioners in establishing advanced practice roles. Journal of Nursing Scholarship 35(4):391–397.

Brown S A, Grimes D E 1993 A meta-analysis of process of care, clinical outcomes, and cost effectiveness of nurses in primary care roles: nurse practitioners and nurse midwives (summary). American Nurse 25(2):3.

Campbell C D, Musil C M, Zauszniewski J A 1998 Practice patterns of advanced practice psychiatric nurses. Journal of the American Psychiatric Nurses Association 4:111–120.

Clarke L 2000 Challenging scientific advances in mental health. Nursing Standard 15(8):19–22.

Crosby F, Ventura M R, Feldman M J 1987 Future research recommendations for establishing NP effectiveness. Nurse Practitioner 12:75–79.

Cutcliffe J, Campbell P 2002 Nurse prescribing could lead nurses away from core concepts that underpin nursing. Mental Health Practice 5(5):14–17.

Davis J, Hemingway S 2003 Supplementary prescribing in mental health nursing. Nursing Times 99(2):28–30.

Department of Health 1989 Review of the advisory group on nurse prescribing. Department of Health, London.

Department of Health 1999 Review of prescribing, supply and administration of medicines. The Stationery Office, London.

Department of Health 2000 The National Health Service Plan. The Stationery Office, London.

Department of Health 2005 Nurse and pharmacist prescribing powers extended. www.doh.gov.uk accessed 24/02/06.

Glod C A, Manchester A 2000 Prescribing patterns of advanced practice nurses: contrasting psychiatric mental health CNS and NP practice. Clinical Excellence for Nurse Practitioners 4(1):1–8.

Harrison A 2003 Mental health service users' view of nurse prescribing. Nurse Prescriber 1(2):73–75.

Hemingway S 2003 Nurse prescribing for mental health nurses: scripting the issues. Journal of Psychiatric and Mental Health Nurses 10(2):239–245.

Hemingway S 2004 The mental health nurse's perspective of nurse prescribing. Nurse Prescriber 2(1):37–44.

Horrocks S, Anderson E, Salisbury C 2002 Systematic review of whether nurse practitioners working in primary care can provide equivalent care to doctors. British Medical Journal 324:819–823.

Jordan S, Hardy B, Coleman M 1999 Medication management: an exploratory study into the role of community mental health nurses. Journal of Advanced Nursing 29(5):1068–1081.

Luker K, Austin L, Hogg C, Wilcock J 1997 Evaluation of nurse prescribing: final report. The University of Liverpool, The University of York.

McCartney W, Tyrer S, Brazier M, Prayle D 1999 Nurse prescribing: radicalism or tokenism. Journal of Advanced Nursing 29(2):348–354.

Mundinger M O 2000 Primary care outcomes in patients treated by nurse practitioners: a randomized trial. Journal of the American Medical Association 283(1):59–68.

National Prescribing Centre 2005 Good practice guide on the prescribing, administration of medicines by mental health nurses. National Prescribing Centre, National Institute for Mental Health, Department of Health. Online. Available: http://www.npc.co.uk accessed 2004.

Office of Technology Assessment, US Congress 1986 Nurse practitioners, physicians' assistants and certified nurse-midwives: a policy analysis. HCS37. US Government Printing Office, Washington, DC.

Parker S 1991 A participant observation study of power relations between nurses and doctors in general hospital. Journal of Advanced Nursing 16(16):728–735.

Ramcharan P, Hemingway S, Flowers K 2001 A client centered case for nurse prescribing. Mental Health Nursing 21(5):6–11.

Stein L 1978 The doctor nurse game. In Dingwall R, McIntosh J (eds) Reading in the Sociology of Nursing Ch. 7. Churchill Livingstone, Edinburgh.

Talley S, Richens S 2001 Prescribing practices of advanced practice psychiatric nurses: Part I – demographic, educational, and practice characteristics. Archives of Psychiatric Nursing XV(5):205–213.

Commentary

Dawn Freshwater

Drugs are used as the universal remedy for many of life's ills. Taken when one is sick (for therapeutic and diagnostic purposes) and when one is healthy (for prophylaxis, social and recreational reasons), drugs are also a major cause of iatrogenic harm. The focus of the two preceding chapters, that of nurse prescribing in P/MH nursing, is an interesting one when viewed in the context of its potential for increasing or reducing iatrogenic harm. What is clear from reading both chapters is that nurse prescribing (across all specialisms, not just mental health) blurs the boundary between nurses and doctors. However, I argue that it is not only nurse prescribing that is blurring those boundaries, which, in any case, have been contested and debated for many years. The *context* within which nurse prescribing is being implemented, in my view, is absolutely central to the debate, and both chapters make some attempt at grappling with sociopolitical and economic factors. The rapid and fundamental changes that P/MH nurses face within their own everyday practices, and the changes of late in nursing per se, means that it is ever more important for us to reflect upon both the consequences of nurse prescribing and nurse prescribing as a consequence in itself. So, what are the consequences of nurse prescribing for P/MH nurses, and what are the events that have led to the advent of nurse prescribing? These and other questions form the basis of the arguments set forth in Chapter 13 (case for) and Chapter 12 (case against).

Nurse prescribing has, in the main, been embraced by general nursing, and a significant number of nurses are already engaged in the process of writing out prescriptions, legitimising existing nursing practices. It is almost three decades since Stein (1978) described how nurses learned to give advice while simultaneously appearing to bow to the doctor's authority, enabling both parties to avoid conflict and confrontation. Hence, not only were doctors able to evade acknowledging their fallibility, but also nurses did not have to own their own power and knowledge. More recently Porter (1991) argued that, in this way, nurses have participated in *'informal covert decision making'*, what was referred to in Chapter 13 (case for) as *'unofficial critical patient management'*, cooperating with the view of nursing as subservient. Down (2002) notes that, despite many changes over the last thirty years, there is still an inequity between the two leading health professions. Nurse prescribing, of course, has to be seen in the context of this and other ongoing and emerging issues, such as policy and political agendas and current developments in mental health care (for example, the introduction of new mental health workers; Barker & Buchanan-Barker 2004). As was observed in Chapter 12 (case against), one aspect of the debate is the extent to which nurse prescribing has become a political playing field across which the doctor–nurse game continues to be (perhaps unwittingly) thrashed out. I believe that the authors of Chapter 13 vastly undersell P/MH nursing when they write that

'involvement in pharmacotherapy is what distinguishes the service they provide from that of other mental health professionals in the UK such as social workers . . .'

There are many aspects of P/MH nursing that distinguish it from other mental health work, but, as many authors have been at pains to point out, P/MH nurses are not good at making known that which makes P/MH nursing unique (see, for example, Cutcliffe & McKenna 2000, Barker & Buchanan-Barker 2005).

With regard to P/MH nursing, it seems that the question is not really whether we should or should not support this initiative – in this sense I agree with Tom Keen in his 'case against' chapter, when he suggests that arguing against something that already exists is futile. Rather, a more illuminating question might be: How can we work with what is already in existence in a way that empowers P/MH nurses and adds value to the nursing discipline, and simultaneously improves care for the user/carer involved? This again is an interesting and key question to raise: Who benefits from the advent of nurse prescribing? Chapters 12 and 13 concur on the view that nurse prescribing should not take nurses a step closer towards the medical model, diverting, as it appears to, attention away from the core elements of caring. However, if nurse prescribing adds value to the patient's experience and enables the practitioner to practise in a more holistic manner, then can this be described *as* caring?

As I stated earlier, drugs of all types are a major cause of iatrogenic harm, and the arrival of nurse prescribing is anticipated to increase the preventive role of nurses in reducing drug-induced iatrogenic harm (Kelly 2003). Indeed, long-term sustained evaluation of nurse prescribing has already demonstrated some evidence to support this anticipated outcome. However, individuals experiencing mental illness and their carers are often managing complex situations in regard to their medication, for example polypharmacy, issues of compliance/concordance such as forgetting to take medication, not having prescriptions filled and taking incorrect doses. It is not only users that create concerns around non-compliance: some mental health patients are reliant on nurses to administer their medications, and nurses, who after all are only human, are also susceptible to making drug errors and facilitating over- or under-usage. Indeed, many nurses have strong views and opinions regarding both the type and administration of medication to mental health patients, and, while I would not want to suggest that this leads to drug errors, it is well documented (specifically in the USA) that drug-related abuse is one of the main forms of patient abuse by nurses, particularly in the elderly mentally ill.

Kelly (2003), for example, questions, not the notion of nurse prescribing per se, but the ability of nursing to prescribe. This is not surprising given the body of evidence developed over the past five years which suggests that some nurses lack numeracy and cognitive skills, and that the minimal level of mathematics required to enter nurse training is failing to prepare nurses for drug calculations (see, for example, Coombes 2000, Duffin 2000). For P/MH nurses to be appropriately prepared to undertake the role of prescribing confidently and safely, preregistration and postregistration training needs to be reviewed to include relevant and pertinent support in the form of education and development. Chapter 12 (case against) comes at this issue from a slightly different perspective when the authors ask: How central is biological knowledge? Well, given the lack of attention to physical assessment in mental health care, as evidenced in the literature, it could be argued that a certain degree of biological knowledge is of course important, but is it central? The same could be asked of pharmacological knowledge, I suppose.

When scanning the international horizon it soon becomes apparent that there are more differences than similarities with regard to the education and expectations of nurse prescribers. Indeed, Bailey & Hemingway's chapter provides a good example of this difference, not only in education, but also in regard to the health care system. The context within which nurses prescribe in the USA differs enormously, even within and across the states themselves, let alone outside of America. That said, there are undoubtedly lessons to be learnt; I find it especially interesting to note that a good proportion of the nurses who were trained and licensed to prescribe in the USA were not doing so. The training provided and expected in the UK for nurse prescribers is very modest in comparison with that in the USA and, as such, I am not convinced that a universal standard can be created for such interventions; for me, the comparative argument does not hold up, although of course it adds an important and interesting dimension.

Although the increase in mental illness is of concern globally, as is the need for improved outcomes, I am not sure that this is a good base from which to develop the case for nurse prescribing in P/MH nursing. Both chapters agree that the polarisation of caring versus curing is not the way forward, which is interesting because any debate presents dichotomised viewpoints in themselves. Nevertheless, as with this debate, ideas are presented as a place to begin to shape our opinions and develop a better understanding of the values, beliefs and assumptions that underpin our practice.

Turning to the question of what P/MH nurses should be licensed to prescribe, I feel, like the author of Chapter 12 (case against), that limiting prescriptions to medication somehow undermines all the subtleties of the discipline; that would be rather like saying that therapists prescribe insight without paying any attention to the nuances of the therapeutic alliance. Recently medics themselves have moved away from the traditional notion of prescribing medication, to include some more varied approaches to managing the health of the population, including, for example, prescribing exercise. P/MH nurses are adept at sourcing a vast number of resources and alternatives for the patients in their caseload; much of this is subtle, and thus invisible in the larger scheme of things. Perhaps if we had to write prescriptions for those interventions that we take for granted, nurses might focus more on making the nursing in nursing visible.

This brings me to my final point, and one that is well made in Chapter 12 where Tom Keen contends that nurses should become 'better at what we are already expected to do'. Accordingly, we should ask: Nurse prescribing, is this what P/MH nurses are expected to do? Is it what they want to do? And, importantly, is it what the patients want from, what is in many cases in mental health at least, a significant other?

References

Barker P, Buchanan-Barker P 2004 Experts without a voice. Nursing Standard 18(50):22–23.

Barker P, Buchanan-Barker P 2005 What is nursing worth? Oneline. Available: http://www.rcn.org.uk 11 Feb 2005

Coombes R 2000 Nurses need a dose of maths. Nursing Times 96:118–123.

Cutcliffe J R, McKenna H P 2000 Generic health care workers: the nemesis of psychiatric/mental health nursing? Part One. Mental Health Practice 3(9):10–14.

Down J 2002 Therapeutic nursing and technology: clinical supervision and reflective practice in a critical care setting. In: Freshwater D, ed. Therapeutic nursing. Sage, London, Ch 2 p 39–57.

Duffin C 2000 Poor standards of maths put patients' lives at risk. Nursing Standard 14(39):5.

Kelly J 2003 Expanding nurse prescribing and the hidden harm within modern drug therapy. In: Milligan F, Robinson K, eds. Limiting harm in health care: a nursing perspective. Blackwell Science, Oxford, p 79–100.

"

Caring for the suicidal person – the modus operandi: engagement or observation?

CHAPTER 14

Considering the care of the suicidal client and the case for 'engagement and inspiring hope' or 'observations'

John R Cutcliffe &
Phil Barker

CHAPTER 15

Close observations: the scapegoat of mental health care?

Martin F Ward &
Julia Jones

Commentary

Peter Campbell

"

Editorial

Suicide touches the lives of so many people. It has been (under)estimated that each individual completed suicide will impact, in one way or another, on approximately 150 people. Further, the likelihood is that any psychaitric/mental health (P/MH) nurse will have already cared for, or will find themselves caring, for a suicidal person during their career. It is well documented that a completed suicide exacts a devastating toll on individuals, families and society (Maris et al 2000). Indeed, caring for suicidal people is among the most complex challenges that P/MH nurses face. Despite the magnitude of the 'problem of suicide', the P/MH nursing literature has remained mostly 'silent' on this matter. Still less evident, until recently, is any substantive empirical work undertaken by P/MH nurses in the domain of suicidology. Encouragingly, more recently, two distinct, though linked, positions have emerged; they form the cadre of this debate, and they are both worthy of consideration.

In the first of these, John Cutcliffe and Phil Barker construct a compelling case for replacing close observations with an approach termed 'engagement–hope inspiration', an approach that emphasises attempting to help the person deal with the genesis of his or her suicidality as opposed to focusing only on keeping the person physically safe. Interestingly, in addition to highlighting the value of hope inspiration and engaging with the suicidal person, they also provide startling evidence that shows how, often, close observations do not achieve their principal aim, namely, keeping the person physically safe. Martin Ward and Julia Jones, on the other hand, argue that it is not the practice of observations per se that is the problem; it is more the larger system that observations operate in that needs severe amendment. In his perspicacious commentary, Peter Campbell makes some remarks that are difficult to ignore. He states:

'Improving guidelines and training around procedures such as close observation and seclusion can bring appreciable benefits, but positive change may not be sustained until underlying attitudes are addressed and consideration is given to what P/MH nurses think they should best be doing and are capable of doing.'

He continues:

'Denying the ability (to take one's own life) without addressing the desire must be a major reason why service users find close observations unhelpful. Observation without interaction is a cold comfort.'

In the limited debate on this issue that has so far occurred, a further interesting debating 'technique' has been utilised, and this causes the editors a moment of pause. We refer to this as 'catastrophic thinking/ arguing' to make a point, and we wonder whether such a technique actually discourages debate rather than encouraging it. This type of debating attempts to scare people, warning them that if they adopt the alternative position then the outcome will be catastrophic. Almost inevitably, though, no such empirical evidence exists to substantiate the claims of pending catastrophe. Examples of this can be seen within the limited extant literature whereby any replacing of observations is warned against because of the catastrophic rise in suicide rates that would 'be bound to follow'. It can be seen that catastrophic debating then appeals to the emotions at the expense of the intellect, increases the sense of fear, and shuts down meaningful discussions (see also Crichton 2004 for an excellent discussion on this technique). This is not to suggest that emotion has no place in debate (we have already advocated within this book for more impassioned debate, which, it would seem, would be difficult to achieve without involving one's emotion), but it is widely recognised that affect can influence judicious judgement. When considering such an emotionally charged matter as suicide and care of the suicidal person, the editors believe that the last thing the associated debate needs is further unnecessary emotion, particularly when this is 'stirred up' purposefully as a possible ploy to decrease discussion and debate, to prevent serious and thoughtful consideration of the substantive points of an argument or position. Given the documented failure of psychiatric services to offer effective, humane and safe care to suicidal people, it is perhaps even more the case that emotionally charged issues such as this, are *more in need* of debate than other, less emotionally charged, issues. Accordingly, in place of catastrophic arguing, what is required is extensive, thorough and meaningful debate. Maris et al (2000) capture the need for debate in these 'uncomfortable' areas when they argue that it is only in being willing to explore these issues that our understanding grows and, perhaps, our discomfort diminishes. They conclude that, wherever and whatever the truth is, we need to be prepared to go where it takes us.

References

Crichton M 2004 A state of fear. Avon Books, New York.
Maris R W, Berman A L, Silverman M 2000 Comprehensive textbook of suicidology. Guilford Press, New York.

John R Cutcliffe & Phil Barker

Considering the care of the suicidal client and the case for 'engagement and inspiring hope' or 'observations'

Introduction

Psychiatric/mental health (P/MH) nursing has rightly been described as a 'broad church', one that contains many contested matters and areas of differing opinions. One such contested matter is that of the appropriate care for the person who is at risk of suicide. Recent, albeit limited, debate has taken place at mental health care conferences, within some consultation groups and, to a small extent, within the relevant literature (see Barker & Cutcliffe 1999, Standing Nursing and Midwifery Advisory Committee 1999, Dodds & Bowles 2001). Such as it is, the literature indicates two principal (though linked) positions which can be summarised as:

1 The 'engagement and hope inspiration' position
2 The 'observations' position.

Given the P/MH nurse's unique position in providing 24-hour day-to-day care to some suicidal clients, the intensive care provided to some clients in the community, often when such people are at high risk of suicide, and the growing problem of suicide in people who suffer from mental health problems (Department of Health [DoH] 2001), it is both necessary, and perhaps timely, to consider this debate in more detail. Accordingly, in this chapter we focus on the debate regarding appropriate care for the suicidal mental health care client. We begin by examining the 'observations' approach and draw on recent empirical evidence in order to have a better informed 'evidence-based' debate. Following this, we focus on the 'engagement–inspiring hope' approach and point out the key processes of engagement. We then consider the limited and emerging empirical evidence regarding the inspiration of hope. The chapter then describes the range of criticisms that have been levelled at the engagement–inspiring hope approach and considers these criticisms in more detail. As a result of this detailed examination, the chapter concludes with appropriate recommendations.

Principal approaches: 'observation' and 'engagement'

Suicide is a complex, multifaceted phenomenon that requires sophisticated and integrated approaches to care. The complexity of caring for people at risk of suicide or self-harm is axiomatic. Such people need highly specific, and sophisticated, forms of care. There is a growing recognition that the nursing care of people who are at risk of suicide or self-harm needs to refocus on a more manifest form of care and support, rather than upon tightening up the policing strategy of observation (see, for example, the emerging literature from the suicide 'survivor' movement, perhaps most prominent in the USA). Despite this trend, and the epistemological and methodological association that all suicides can be linked to mental health problems, many texts appear to emphasise the need to 'treat' the underlying affective mood disorder. Rawlins (1993, p 281), for example, suggests that a suicidal client needs to be:

'given anti-depressant medication to elevate his mood and make him more **amenable** *to treatment. Electroconvulsive treatment (ECT) is an additional treatment that has proved effective'* [emphasis added].

Similarly, authors such as Pritchard (1998) offer some generic suggestions for the care of the suicidal client, such as input from a variety of clinicians, improved socioeconomic conditions, and social skills training. These broad, and perhaps long-term, interventions (lithium therapy, antidepressant therapy and ECT) have been shown to be effective in the management of depression. However, crucially, Gunnell & Frankel (1994) point out that several retrospective reviews of the treatments received by psychiatric patients have provided no consistent evidence that these therapies reduce the likelihood of suicide (see also Maris et al 2000). Furthermore, ignoring the questionable efficacy of these therapies with respect to 'treating' the suicidal client, it is fair to say that they do not appear to say much about the more acute problems facing P/MH nurses when they attempt to engage with suicidal clients on an hour-by-hour, day-by-day basis.

Some texts appear to advocate an even more 'masculine' approach to caring for suicidal clients. Rawlins (1993), for example, suggests further 'interventions' including the removal of harmful items (such as belts, socks) and placing the client on 24 hours a day observations on a one to one basis. Rawlins is by no means the only author to suggest 'close' or 'special' or 'one to one' observations as the primary intervention for care of the suicidal client. As a result, for people who are deemed to be 'at risk' of self-harm (suicide), harm to others or self-neglect, 'observation' has increasingly become the prime focus of 'care'. Furthermore, these levels of observation are most often 'set' by psychiatrists, perhaps with little regard to the demands this might make on nursing staff, emotionally and logistically (Duffy 1995).

Observation: safe and effective?

Although P/MH nurses' use of observation and 'specialing' has been in evidence for almost 25 years, the therapeutic value of such approaches to care has long been questioned. The practice of observation was developed as a means to inform medical staff of the status of the patient (Barker & Cutcliffe 1999). It served the function of assuring the 'absent' doctor of the physical safety of the patient. Yet, as illustrated by statistics for suicide in inpatient settings (DoH 2001) and the first author's own research experience of attending more than 90 suicide or open-verdict inquests, observation as a caring practice is a woefully weak intervention. Between 20% and 33% of inpatient suicides were committed while the clients were 'under' levels of observation (DoH 2001). Where observation policies exist, there is a great deal of inconsistency in the interpretation of the policies (DoH 2001), and yet further problems with actioning or carrying out these observations.

Key evidence resides, as ever, in service users' experiences of close observation; the limited body of evidence in this substantive area is fairly consistent. Evidence from Newcastle and York (Barker & Walker 1999) indicates that while 'under observation' users felt neither safe nor supported. One user summed up the experience succinctly when he stated (p 36):

'Some do close [observation] *nicely. They talk to the patient like a friend and still carry on with their other duties. But others are like robots; when the patient moves they follow like zombies.'*

Whereas a service user in Fletcher's (1999, p 11) study indicated:

'They didn't actually ask me if I was feeling suicidal. Just went everywhere with me.'

A member of staff stated (p 12):

'I would be happy to say to somebody "Don't try anything because I am going to be with you all the time and I don't want that responsibility on me."'

More recent evidence from Oxford (Jones et al 2000) and Bradford (Dodds & Bowles 2001) further supports this position. Jones et al (2000) found that most of the research subjects in their study did not like the experience of being observed, found it intrusive, and that some nurses did not talk to the users at all during the observation period. This was found to be a particularly negative experience. Similarly, in Dodds & Bowles' (2001) attempt to dismantle observation and move towards a more 'care'-oriented system, the following findings were established. Incidents of deliberate self-harm reduced by two-thirds, violence and aggression reduced by over a third, staff sickness had fallen by two-thirds, absconding had declined by half, and there was no increase of suicides during the corresponding period (18 months). Importantly, they state:

'The effect on patient care has been striking: patients are more engaged with their named nurses, better informed and more involved with their care.'
(Dodds & Bowles 2001, p 178)

As a result, it perhaps comes as no surprise that the therapeutic value of close observations as an approach to 'care' for suicidal clients is being questioned.

The 'who' question

Inextricably linked to the alleged value (or otherwise) of observations is the matter of who carries them out. Extensive shortages of P/MH nurses across the UK and other parts of the world have led to a reliance on 'bank', 'casual' or 'agency' staff. Gournay et al's (1998) study found that bank nurses provided between 23.6% and 36.3% of the staff complement, and the authors quite rightly went on to condemn this practice as unacceptable. (Agency, or 'bank', nursing is analogous to the 'casual' nurse in North America – the nurse who does not have a permanent contract and is asked to 'fill' vacant shifts.) Compounding this situation, in many parts of the UK, observation is carried out in the main by support staff, bank/agency staff and students. These workforce patterns are by no means exclusive to the UK. For example, Cutcliffe (2003) recently pointed out that, in one Canadian hospital, security guards rather than P/MH nurses carry out the 'observations' of the suicidal person. Consequently, observation is invariably regarded as a low-skill activity, often carried out by support staff (rather than registered nurses), or by bank or agency nurses who, by their transient nature, have only limited knowledge of the person. Such a position is, according to Dodds & Bowles (2001), counterproductive and contributes little in the way of assessment and treatment within acute wards, or to the development of new approaches to acute inpatient care. Indeed, this situation leaves nurses in reactionary, custodial roles and, despite the rhetoric of 'supportive observation', the nurse is often construed as a custodian, if not a 'doorman'.

Summary of the 'observations' approach

Thus, to summarise this part of the chapter, observation as a means of intervention for people who are suicidal:

- Is a system that was designed originally to inform medics and now, at least in part, is concerned with meeting the needs of the organisation
- Fails between 20% and 33% of the people it is supposed to protect (and these numbers are even more alarming when one considers the number of people who go on to harm themselves once the 'observation' restrictions have been lifted and the person is discharged)
- Is a crude, 'custodial' oriented form of intervention to meet the highly complex, convoluted and sophisticated care needs of this client group
- Despite the recognised complexity, is operationalised in the main by transient (bank/agency) staff or support workers with minimal training
- Does little (if anything) to address the route or genesis of the user's problems which led him or her to feel suicidal in the first place
- Is highly stressful for the nurses who participate
- Fails to inform P/MH nurses about how to provide care with suicidal people hour by hour, minute by minute, moment by moment.

'Engagement': inspiring hope in suicidal people

Given the complex and sophisticated nature of the problem of suicide, it is perhaps of no surprise that there is no 'singular' treatment or intervention that appears to address the problem. However, there is a growing body of evidence that indicates that there are two linked, basic interpersonal processes that appear to be key in providing care for the suicidal client: engagement and inspiring hope.

Without wishing to offer a concise definition, engagement appears to comprise several processes: forming a relationship (a human–human connection), conveying acceptance and tolerance, and hearing and understanding. Engaging with suicidal clients is clearly concerned with forming a relationship – a human–human connection between the client and the nurse. Any other interpersonal intervention provided to clients to help address their suicidal thoughts, feelings or behaviours will need to be grounded in such a relationship. This relationship not only serves as the grounding for other interventions, but is a powerful intervention in itself. The relationship conveys the message that the nurse 'cares about' the client, that his or her life has value. Providing

P/MH nursing care for the suicidal client then appears to be more focused on 'ways of being' as opposed to 'doing'. The value and importance of this most fundamental of interpersonal processes is described by and alluded to throughout the limited research into care of the suicidal client. Talseth et al (1997) reported the value of compassion and emotional identification when caring for the suicidal client, in addition to the trust that is built through regular contact between client and nurse. Davidhizar & Vance (1993) similarly stress the need for nurses to consider their own attitudes towards suicide in order that they can ensure they do not distance themselves from the client. Duffy's (1995) research alludes to the importance of relating to suicidal clients. Additionally, Talseth et al (1999) purport the value of nurses initiating contact with suicidal clients and attending to clients' basic needs (including the value of physical contact with suicidal clients).

The most recent research on this issue, emanating out of the first study of its kind in the UK (Cutcliffe et al 2006), further supports the value and importance of the relationship between the client and the nurse. In an attempt to answer the question, how do P/MH nurses help move the suicidal client from a 'death oriented' position to a 'life oriented' position, the core variable of 'reconnecting the person with humanity' was induced. One of the key processes of facilitating this reconnection with humanity is, in the first instance, by connecting with the nurse. This reconnection with humanity is brought about by feeling cared about and cared for, experiencing this sense and process of 'co-presencing'. Through demonstrating caring, compassion and concern, the nurse becomes the first 'point' of reconnection with humanity. The client connects with the nurse and thus begins to reconnect with humanity. In essence, this process shows how the nurse becomes a 'representative' or 'emissary' for humanity. When the participant experiences being cared for by the nurse, the nurse is communicating that humanity still cares about the participant. Engaging with the nurse in this way allows the participant to begin to internalise that they can still engage with humanity. The nurse's attitudes, demeanour and behaviour provide an 'inroad' – an opportunity to reconnect.

Engagement in the form of caring practice for the suicidal client is concerned with demonstrating an unconditional acceptance and tolerance, removing any sense of coercion or psychological pressure. Importantly, the presence alone of these qualities in the nurse would not be enough: the qualities also have to be conveyed or demonstrated, and need to be genuine. All too frequently, unfortunately, clients who have attempted to take their own life are met with disapproving attitudes from some formal care staff (see Duffy 1995, Talseth et al 1997, 1999) – attitudes ranging from contempt and believing that the client is taking up valuable space and time that could be used for someone who has 'a real problem', to an attitude stemming from a complete lack of understanding as to why anyone would wish to take their own life. Therefore, the potential therapeutic value of a P/MH nurse who conveys a sense of complete acceptance and tolerance becomes clear. Further condemnation or contempt can serve only to exacerbate the client's feelings of worthlessness and hopelessness that led to their suicidal behaviour in the first instance.

The value and importance of this most fundamental of interpersonal processes is described by and alluded to throughout the limited research into care of the suicidal client. Talseth et al (1997) describe how nurses caring for suicidal clients confirmed, rather than criticised, their emotions and feelings. Davidhizar & Vance (1993) emphasise the importance of communicating acceptance, given that suicidal clients are highly vulnerable to responses from caregivers. Long et al (1998) assert the value and necessity for the nurse to offer unconditional positive regard and empathy to suicidal clients. In addition, according to Talseth et al (1999), nurses must accept suicidal clients' feelings, be open to these people and have time for them.

Similarly, the findings of Cutcliffe et al's (2006) study indicate that suicidal people often need to have their basic needs met, including (if not especially) their fundamental need to feel connected to or engaged with other people. These basic needs are met by the nurse possessing (or adopting) and communicating the following: a sense of warmth for the participant, care for the person, compassion for the participant's situation and experience, a sense of hope and hopefulness for the participant's future, unconditional acceptance and tolerance, empathy, understanding and positive regard. Further, in order to feel connected or reconnected with humanity, the participants need to feel they can trust 'humanity'. Through gaining trust in the nurse, the participant is then reconnecting with a person, taking the first tentative steps towards reconnecting with the wider 'community' of humanity.

The third apparent component of engagement is concerned with listening, hearing and understanding. As with the previous two components of engagement, this may appear to be somewhat obvious or simplistic. However, creating and providing the environment in which the client can begin to explore, discuss and resolve thoughts and feelings appears to be crucial in addressing the client's desire to take his/her own life. This hearing and understanding need not be regarded as a form of sophisticated counselling, but is more a matter of attending to the client, encouraging him or her to explore thoughts and feelings, and providing the opportunity for the client to express painful emotions without being judged or condemned. The value and importance of this most fundamental of interpersonal processes is described by and alluded to throughout the limited research into care of the suicidal client. Talseth et al (1997) have described how nurses caring for suicidal clients ensured they listened to the clients. Davidhizar & Vance (1993) stated the value of hearing the clients when they are ready to talk. Long & Reid (1996) and Long et al (1998) have similarly pointed out the therapeutic value of hearing and empathising with the suicidal client. Talseth et al (1999) reported the value of listening without prejudice.

Similarly, the findings of Cutcliffe et al's (2006) study indicate that suicidal clients need to talk about their experiences and feel understood – understood by their nurse. The participants in this study were adamant that they needed to feel that someone understood their experience, their plight. Additionally, when they felt they were being listened to and understood, this had a profound therapeutic effect on them. Participants were very clear about how they often just needed someone to talk to during their 'recovery' from their suicide attempt and/or ideation. The importance and value of listening to the clients was not lost on the P/MH nurses. Participants described how the nurses would make specific attempts to listen and communicate that they wanted to understand. They were interested in the client, in their stories, in their experiences, and heard these narratives without passing judgement or condemning the clients' behaviour.

In addition, the participants explained how, in talking about their experiences and gaining a sense that they were being understood, they encountered a cathartic release, a feeling of emancipation and liberation. They were somehow 'lighter' emotionally having had this catharsis; their sense of 'psych-ache' was lessened. It is also of particular note that these interpersonal transactions were not personified by erudite sentences or cleverly constructed, deeply analytical insights into the clients' psyche. The transactions were personified by the 'normalness' of the interactions, and was most commonly described as 'just chatting'. As a result of the talking, hearing, being listened to and feeling understood, the participants also gained a sense of feeling less isolated, less alone. They began to experience this sense of reconnecting with another person. There were some clients who described another therapeutic process (or outcome) of talking about their experiences and feeling understood. The effect of this experience was to counter or combat their previous experiences of *not* being listened to. Whereas, in the past, clients had wanted to talk and to feel listened to, they had not experienced this, and one result of this was the growth of their suicidal ideation (and resulting increase in risk). Consequently, their experience within this therapeutic relationship was directly what they needed in order to begin to reduce their suicide ideation and related risk.

Inspiring hope

There is an abundance of evidence indicating that hopelessness is a key element in determining whether or not a person will commit suicide rather than merely considering it (see, for example, Motto et al 1985, Weisharr & Beck 1992, Prigerson et al 1995). Therefore, it is clear that suicidal people need hope, and P/MH nurses are ideally placed to be one such source of hope. However, recognition of the importance of hope in P/MH nursing is a relatively recent phenomenon. Only now is it gaining recognition as being central to the therapeutic potential of the nurse–patient relationship, and to the quality of the person's life (Cutcliffe 2004). Despite this pivotal position, the indications are that the inspiration of hope is low on the clinical agenda, and consequently it should be noted that, prior to the recent study undertaken by Cutcliffe et al (2006), there was no specific theory or research that informed nurses of how to inspire hope in suicidal clients.

There is a large and growing body of evidence suggesting that the inspiration of hope, in a variety of clinical situations and for various specific client groups, appears to be a subtle, unobtrusive, implicit process (for a review of this evidence see Cutcliffe 2004). Hope inspiration appears to be bound up with the necessary and sufficient human qualities in the nurse/counsellor and the projection of these into the environment (and client). It has been purported that, even though hope appears to have such an important influence on some people's lives, the process(es) of hope inspiration need to remain subtle and implicit rather than overt (Cutcliffe 2004). According to Frankl (1959), one cannot be forced to hope: hope cannot be commanded or ordered. Such a view clearly resonates with inspiring hope in suicidal clients, where such clients cannot be 'forced' to become more hopeful, forced to feel less suicidal. Therefore, theories that suggest the inspiration of hope appears to be bound up with the presence of certain 'human qualities', and with the interpersonal (spiritual) connection between clients and P/MH nurses, appear to have resonance with Frankl's (1959) views.

A significant component of hope inspiration appears to be the relationship between hope and caring. Hope is inherent is caring practices. Research into the inspiration of hope in terminally ill individuals, critically ill coronary care clients, older adults with cognitive impairments, bereaved clients and terminally ill oncology clients highlights that the presence of another human being, who demonstrates unconditional acceptance, tolerance and understanding, as (s)he enters into the caring practice, simultaneously inspires hope (Cutcliffe 2004, Cutcliffe et al 2006).

It has long been recognised and acknowledged, at least in humanistic theoretical literature, that the ways in which people are treated ultimately have an influence on how they feel about themselves. Accordingly, the nurse's attitude, demeanour and approach communicate a wide range of messages. If the suicidal person senses that a nurse is disinterested, uncaring, condemning or judgemental, then the effect on the person's feelings of self-worth is likely to be negative. Additionally, there is the likelihood that a subliminal message of hopelessness will also be communicated. Given the emerging relationship between hopelessness and suicidal intent, the need for sophisticated, hope-inspiring care of the suicidal person becomes clear.

Vaillot (1970, p 273) made similar remarks when she described the link between caring and hope inspiration:

'There is no simple, possibly no satisfactory answer to the question, how does one inspire hope in patients? Knowledge, techniques, good planning and sound assessment of nursing care are necessary and indispensable, but they are the tools one has in order to nurse.'

However, the attitude of caring does go some way to answering this question. As Vaillot (1970, p 273) added:

'the nurse inspires hope by what she is more than what she does . . . it is a salutary effect on the patient from the fact that it is an expression of the nurse's caring.'

Therefore, it becomes evident that, where people at risk of suicide are concerned, the caring relationship must be developed as a 'hope inspiring' form of engagement. Effective nursing is predicated on effective engagement with the person. Only through engaging with the person will the nurse come to understand the nature of the person's needs, and what might need to be offered to address them. The nurse's engagement with the suicidal person must, therefore, be dedicated to understanding the nature of that hopelessness, and to developing the means to reinstil hope.

Criticisms of the 'engagement–hope inspiration' approach

Within the limited debate that has ensued so far, the criticisms of the 'engagement–hope inspiration' position appear to centre on the following points:

1 It is a laissez-faire approach, which would result in less vigilance on the part of the nursing staff and would therefore result in more inpatients taking their own life (Bowers 2001).
2 It represents a semantic exercise in that the 'engagement–hope inspiration' approach is nothing more than a rewording of close or special observations. Thus, close observations would remain, albeit in another guise.
3 Close observation should remain as the *modus operandi* for care of the suicidal client as it has always enabled P/MH nurses to work therapeutically with such clients.
4 Instead of refocusing the interpersonal aspects of care, energy and time would be better served by addressing the physical environment that the suicidal client lives in, and reducing the opportunities for the client to take his or her own life.

Response to criticism 1

It has been suggested that to argue for the replacement of 'special or close observation' with the 'engagement–hope inspiration' approach is virtually to encourage and authorise nurses not to carry out special observation as the policy dictates and, further, that this 'engagement–hope inspiration' position represents a laissez-faire 'laid back' approach to care of the suicidal client. Bowers (2001) adds that *'this is dangerous, as I fear it is exactly then that catastrophes occur'*.

In response to this argument, we would point out that there is no empirical evidence that supports Bowers' arguments. Neither can there be a wealth of empirical data to support or refute either view of the argument until the engagement–hope inspiration approach replaces special observations in a number of settings, which would enable the data to be collected and analysed. Interestingly, in the only published empirical work to date on replacing observations with the engagement approach (Dodds & Bowles 2001), no such catastrophes as Bowers predicted occurred; inversely, there were a number of corresponding improvements (see above). While acknowledging the limitations of the study, it serves as preliminary evidence that refutes Bowers' position and supports the introduction of the engagement–hope inspiration position.

Response to criticism 2

In an exploration of the merits of the engagement–hope inspiration approach in an international psychiatric nursing discussion group, it was suggested that the approach amounted to little more than semantics: as the approach contains a key component of ensuring the client's security, it is simply a renaming of close or special observations. The present authors would not dispute that there are similarities between special or close observations and the engagement–hope inspiration approach, none more so than that both processes include a vital component that is concerned with client safety. (See Barker (1999) for a more detailed explanation of the 'security' component of the engagement–hope inspiration approach.) However, it is the emphasis on engagement and the inspiration of hope as the primary focus of this approach that sets it apart from any approach that emphasises observation as the mode of care for the suicidal client. For example, an examination of the Standing Nursing and Midwifery Advisory Committee's (1999) practice guidance on safe and supportive observation of patients at risk shows that, of the eleven policy guidance statements for undertaking the highest level of observation, only one makes any reference to forming a therapeutic relationship with the client. Also, this is the eighth of the eleven statements. Furthermore, there is a complete absence of any reference to work that the nurse should engage in while observing the client that is concerned with helping the client understand and overcome why they feel suicidal in the first instance; neither is hope referred to. This is clearly a different emphasis and, concomitantly, a different process to the engagement–hope inspiration approach that we have described above.

Response to criticism 3

In a similar vein to the arguments regarding criticism 2, it has been suggested that observation and engagement are not incompatible practices (Bowers 2001), that close or special observation facilitates engagement between clients and the nurse who is observing them. The present authors do not doubt that, in some cases, nurses who are carrying out observations do indeed make attempts to engage with suicidal clients, and we applaud such efforts. Some anecdotal evidence and a limited empirical literature support such a position. Indeed, earlier in this chapter we pointed out (limited) service user feedback of observations that supported this point. The limited supporting empirical evidence indicates that some clients can benefit from the engagement and feelings of security that some experienced while being 'under observation' (Pitula & Cardell 1996, Cardell & Pitula 1999). Nevertheless, there is a growing body of evidence (highlighted earlier in this chapter) that repeatedly points out how such client experiences of observations appear to be in the minority. Again, the present authors would point out that because the premise – the very purpose – of engagement, hope inspiration, is completely different to that of observations, it is more difficult for P/MH nurses who are attempting to engage and inspire hope in suicidal clients not to be working in a therapeutic way. It would be far more difficult for the nurse to engage with the suicidal client 'from behind a newspaper' (as has been reported in anecdotal accounts of being observed), or when the nurses do not talk to the client at all, as was found by Jones et al (2000).

Response to criticism 4

Alternative ways to address the problem of suicide in mental health 'inpatients' involve placing the emphasis on considering the physical environment. For example, Professor Kevin Gournay has reiterated some of the recommendations arising from the 'Safety first' report (DoH 2001), and pointed out the value in working together with the 'Estates' department of National Health Service (NHS) Trusts. Consequently, 'interventions' such as collapsible curtain rails around the client's bedspace should be used in order to prevent clients from hanging themselves on curtain rails. Such environmentally focused 'interventions' appear to have much in keeping with previous attempts to reduce the suicide rate in the general population, such as the removal of toxic gas from household gas supplies. Further, such interventions did produce an initial reduction in suicide rates. Therefore, the authors of this chapter consider Professor Gournay's suggestions to be laudable and add their support to them. However, as the longitudinal evidence of suicide rates in the general population has indicated, these 'environmental' interventions on their own may not be enough, in that, although there was a reduction in rates following the removal of toxic gas, the rates began to increase again once alternative methods had been 'discovered'. Therefore, in the context of mental health care, although the present authors support the practice of attempting to minimise the risk posed by the physical environment, they suggest that these interventions do not remove the need to consider, also, the interpersonal aspects of care for suicide prevention.

Conclusion

Suicide represents a growing problem, particularly for the P/MH nurse. The two principal current forms of intervention for this client group can be categorised as 'close or special observation' and 'engagement as the means to inspire hope'. There are similarities between the use of observation and the use of engagement to care for suicidal clients, in that both have an element that is concerned with ensuring the client's safety. However, there is a crucial difference, and that is in the emphasis. Engagement is concerned with inspiring hope through the interpersonal relationship. It is concerned with exploring and attempting to understand the nature of the person's problems that led them to feel suicidal in the first place. It is concerned primarily with addressing the person's need for emotional and physical security, rather than serving the needs of the organisation, and it is concerned with reconnecting the person with humanity.

Criticisms have been levelled at this model, suggesting it is 'laissez faire' and lazy, that it is little more than a semantic enterprise, and that it does not differ much from close or special observations. However, when one considers the benefits as evidenced by the literature (see, for example, Dodds & Bowles 2001), and the failings of the current 'observation'-focused approach, the need to move away from observation to engagement becomes clear. For this reason, we advocate strongly that a new model of nursing *engagement* should replace 'observation', as a matter of principle.

Acknowledgements

This chapter has been adapted and reproduced with the kind permission of Blackwell Science Publishing Ltd, from a paper that originally appeared in the *Journal of Psychiatric and Mental Health Nursing* 9(5):611–619.

References

Barker P 1999 Developing the security plan. University of Newcastle, Newcastle.

Barker P, Cutcliffe J R 1999 Clinical risk: a need for engagement not observation. Mental Health Care 2(8):8–12.

Barker P, Walker L 1999 A survey of care practices in acute admission wards. Reports submitted to the Northern and Yorkshire Regional Research and Development Committee, University of Newcastle.

Bowers L 2001 Response to J Cutcliffe. Psychiatric Nursing discussion list. Online. http://www.city.ac.uk/barts/psychiatric-nursing/threads/spec_obs_engage.htm accessed 2001

Bowles N, Dodds P 2001 Dismantling formal observation and refocusing nursing activity in acute inpatient psychiatry: a case study. Journal of Psychiatric and Mental Health Nursing 8:173–188.

Cardell R, Pitula C R 1999 Suicidal inpatients' perceptions of therapeutic and non-therapeutic aspects of constant observation. Psychiatric Services 20(8):1066–1070.

Cutcliffe J R 2003 The differences and commonalities between United Kingdom and Canadian psychiatric/mental health nursing: a personal reflection. Journal of Psychiatric and Mental Health Nursing 10:255–257.

Cutcliffe J R 2004 The inspiration of hope in bereavement counselling. PhD thesis. Jessica Kingsley, London.

Cutcliffe J R, Stevenson C, Jackson S, Smith P 2006 A modified grounded theory study of how P/MH nurses provide care for suicidal people. International Journal of Nursing Studies. In Press.

Davidhizar R, Vance A 1993 The management of the suicidal patient in a critical care unit. Journal of Nursing Management 1:95–102.

Department of Health 2001 Safety first – five year report of the National Confidential Inquiry into Suicides and Homicides by People with Mental Health Problems. HMSO, London.

Duffy D 1995 Out of the shadows: a study of the special observation of suicidal psychiatric in-patients. Journal of Advanced Nursing 21:944–950.

Fletcher R F 1999 The process of constant observation: perspectives of staff and suicidal patients. Journal of Psychiatric and Mental Health Nursing 6(1):9–14.

Frankl V 1959 Man's search for meaning: an introduction to logotherapy. Harper & Row, New York.

Gournay K, Ward M, Thornicroft G et al 1998 Crisis in the capital: inpatient care in inner London. Mental Health Practice 1:10–18.

Gunnell D J, Frankel S 1994 Prevention of suicide: aspirations and evidence. British Medical Journal 308:1227–1233.

Jones J, Ward M, Wellman N, Hall J, Lowe T 2000 Psychiatric inpatients' experiences of nursing observation: a United Kingdom perspective. Journal of Psychosocial Nursing 38(12):10–19.

Long A, Reid W 1996 An exploration of nurses' attitudes to the nursing care of the suicidal patient in an acute psychiatric ward. Journal of Psychiatric and Mental Health Nursing 3:29–37.

Long A, Long A, Smyth A 1998 Suicide: a statement of suffering. Nursing Ethics 5(1):3–15.

Maris R W, Berman A L, Silverman M M 2000 Comprehensive Textbook of Suicidology. Guilford Press, New York.

Motto J A, Heilbron D C, Juster R P 1985 Development of a clinical instrument to estimate suicide risk. American Journal of Psychiatry 142:680–686.

Pitula C R, Cardell R 1996 Suicidal inpatients' experiences of constant observation. Psychiatric Services 47(6):6491–6651.

Prigerson H G, Frank E, Kasl S V et al 1995 Complicated grief and bereavement-related depression as distinct disorders: preliminary empirical validation in elderly bereaved spouses. American Journal of Psychiatry 152(1):22–30.

Pritchard C 1998 Psychosocioeconomic factors in suicide. In: Thompson T, Mathias P, eds. Lyttle's mental health and disorder, 2nd edn. Baillière Tindall, London, p 276–295.

Rawlins R P 1993 Hope–hopelessness. In: Rawlins R P, Williams X, Beck C, eds. Mental health nursing – a holistic life cycle approach, 3rd edn. Mosby, St Louis, p 257–284.

Standing Nursing and Midwifery Advisory Committee 1999 Practice guidance: safe and supportive observation of patients at risk: mental health nursing – addressing acute concerns. Department of Health, London.

Talseth A G, Lindseth A, Jacobson L, Norberg A 1997 Nurses' narrations about suicidal psychiatric inpatients. Nord Jour Psychiatry 51:359–364.

Talseth A G, Lindseth A, Jacobson L, Norberg A 1999 The meaning of suicidal in-patients' experiences of being cared for by mental health nurses. Journal of Advanced Nursing 29(5):1034–1041.

Vaillot M 1970 Hope: the restoration of being. American Journal of Nursing 70:268–273.

Weisharr M E, Beck A 1992 Hopelessness and suicide. International Review of Psychiatry 4:177–184.

Martin F Ward & Julia Jones

Close observations: the scapegoat of mental health care?

Introduction

Throwing the baby out with the bath water is a saying that implies a lack of forethought and a modicum of hindsight. Taken literally, it describes a situation where, having washed a small child, cared for it, pampered and preened it, both it and the tub of water are taken to the drain and discarded, leaving neither water nor child. Wasteful to say the least and, in today's enlightened times, also illegal. Of course, it was never meant to be taken literally. It is a prophetic expression warning against hasty and ill-conceived actions. It describes a situation where the needed is cast out with the unwanted; where good and bad are falsely perceived as one and the same thing; and where the end result is nothing of any substance whatsoever. In this chapter we present the case that close observations face a similar situation in the contemporary world of psychiatric/mental health (P/MH) nursing.

This chapter will explore close observations from three different perspectives, each of which is considered to underpin and undermine the way in which close observations are currently conducted in mental health settings. These perspectives are: nurse leadership (or its absence); the lack of nurses' confidence to challenge and take professional risks; and the detrimental effects of organisational risk-taking. At first glance, it could be considered that these three issues have little to do with the actual procedure of close observations. However, the ways in which these issues are initiated and undertaken play an important role, as they constitute some of the fundamental threads that weave the tapestry upon which P/MH nursing practice is conducted. We will argue that these three components represent the mental health care 'bathwater', with close observations the 'baby', and that it is these three components, and not the procedure itself, that act against the successful use of close observations. Either getting rid of close observations altogether, or attempting to initiate some other form of alternative practice without first examining what is wrong with the current one, only neglects to address the underlying problems and will ultimately lead to further clinical disappointment. In this chapter we will posit that close observations are being targeted as the scapegoat for inherent failures within mental health care as a whole, and the inability of the nursing profession to deal with them. However, before considering this position further we need to examine what we currently know about close observations.

What do we know about close observations?

Close observations is a commonly used P/MH nursing intervention for patients 'at risk', and involves the allocation of one nurse (or sometimes two) to one patient for a prescribed length of time in order to provide intensive nursing care. The main purpose of conducting observations is to keep people safe when they are acutely mentally ill and disturbed, particularly patients who are assessed to be at risk of harming themselves or others, or at risk of being harmed or exploited by others. Observations are typically used for patients who are suicidal or actively interested in harming themselves, patients who are aggressive and who pose a danger to staff or other patients, vulnerable patients, those who are prone to abscond, and patients who are sexually disinhibited (Bowers et al 2000, Bowers & Park 2001).

The present authors consider the therapeutic intention of close observations under four headings: (1) care based, (2) management based, (3) care team based and (4) patient-personal. Care-based intent includes the maintenance of intensive reality contact: acting as a helper and guide; protecting the patient from negative contact with others; establishing positive regard for the patient's values and beliefs whilst acting as a sounding board for the patient's ideas, thoughts and intentions; and protecting the individual from harming him/herself or others. Management-based intent includes providing targeted communication with the patient as per the individual care plan objectives, plus giving outcomes feedback to the rest of the care team. Care team-based intent includes the above elements of the management process, but also consists of monitoring patient progress generally and the patient's responses to targeted communication activities specifically. Finally, patient-personal intent includes 'being there' for the patient irrespective of the difficulty of their situation and embracing the concept that someone cares about them no matter what trauma they may be suffering, acting as a companion or confidant but, by and large, trying to make a difference to someone's life by generating a positive self-image.

Arguments about the practice of close observations are typically idiosyncratic and often dependent upon entrenched personal opinions. Unfortunately there is little concrete 'evidence' regarding how the procedure should be conducted effectively; existing research to date has been confined to small-scale studies, with findings that often suggest little more than 'common sense' and the need for nurses to conduct the procedure with human kindness and professional competency. The two most recent and comprehensive reviews of the literature come from Bowers & Park (2001) and O'Brien & Cole (2003). In addition, there are a number of studies that consider different aspects of close observation, including: the procedure with different client groups (Gournay & Bowers 2000); patient and staff opinions and experiences (Duffy 1995, Cardell & Pitula 1999, Fletcher 1999, Jones et al 2000, Svedberg et al 2003); organisational and policy issues (Nirui & Chenoweth 1999, Bowers et al 2000, Horsfall & Cleary 2000); and a growing number of papers calling for alternatives to the procedure (Dodds & Bowles 2001, Bowles et al 2002, Cutcliffe & Barker 2002, Barker 2003). So, what do we actually know from the current literature on the topic of close observations?

We know that the activity of close observations is called many different things, for example: special, close, continuous, formal, one-to-one, maximum, raised, risk, supportive or intensive observations. These are not all of the terms used; there is great variation and confusion, and; as Bowers et al (2000) have pointed out, the terminology used can vary even amongst staff on the same unit, as well as across different services. Patients, or service users, who experience this form of clinical intervention typically have a broad range of psychiatric diagnosis, specifically schizophrenia, depression, mania, dementia, personality disorders, alcohol and drug abuse, organic brain disorders and anorexia. Perhaps more relevant are the reasons cited for the prescription of close observations, which include: aggression (either to self or others); violence (usually towards others); a risk of suicide or self-harm; a risk of absconding and subsequent vulnerability; being acutely disturbed; and difficult to manage.

Patients who have experienced close observations can have very strong views about it, with most people expressing negative feelings and opinions about being on the receiving end of the intervention. A major complaint amongst patients who experience observation is that they are sometimes not even told that they are being observed. When patients are told, often it is not explained clearly to them and they rarely feel involved in the decision-making about this component of their care (Cardell & Pitula 1999, Fletcher 1999, Jones et al 2000). This situation is not helped by the fact that policies relating to the procedure rarely indicate how patients are to be involved in decisions, simply that they should be given a rationale for its implementation (Bowers et al 2000) However, it is important to provide a balance to this negative picture and stress that, when observation is conducted well, it can have positive outcomes for patients. Some studies have shown that some patients report positive experiences from being observed closely by nurses, particularly when the observers are friendly and supportive. Positive experiences reported included: feeling safer, respected, and more hopeful and less anxious (Cardell & Pitula 1999, Jones et al 2000). The findings from these two studies in particular suggest that patients' experiences are determined predominantly by the behaviours and attitudes of the staff. Thus, it is not the procedure *per se* that is the problem, but the way in which it is carried out.

To date there has been no research conducted to tell us who (qualified or non-qualified staff) is most effective in terms of providing the 'best' and 'safest' close observations. Bowers & Park (2001) provide a review of the existing literature regarding this issue, which shows that in different places a variety of different people perform the 'observer' role, including: qualified nurses, unqualified nurses, nursing and medical students, agency nurses, family members, friends and volunteers. It is apparent from the literature, and also from our own experience, that observation is often regarded as an unpleasant low-status and low-skill task and is frequently delegated to junior or untrained staff, or to agency and bank staff who may be unknown to the patient (Dodds & Bowles 2001). This runs counter to the small amount of evidence that exists which says that close observations should be the responsibility of proficient, experienced and specifically trained nurses, known to the patient and capable of developing a relationship of skilled companionship within the procedure (Department of Health 1999, Jones et al 2000, Meiklejohn 2003).

Close observations are undertaken predominantly in acute inpatient units of psychiatric services or in psychiatric intensive care units (PICUs). We know that staff report a growing number of close observations assignments and that more and more patients appear to receive such care (Dodds & Bowles 2001). We also know that a large proportion of surveyed qualified mental health nurses report professional dissatisfaction with, or a dislike for, undertaking the procedure (O'Brien & Cole 2003). Nursing staff also suggest that they are being used by other mental health disciplines to 'police' the risk elements associated with serious mental health problems and feel disenfranchised by the decision-making processes of these staff who have, in the nurses' opinion, assumed responsibility for an essentially nursing activity within the multidisciplinary team (Horsfall & Cleary 2000). Many nurse academics and practitioners feel that close observations are neither professionally nor philosophically appropriate to contemporary P/MH nursing, and argue that mental health care generally should be resculptured to provide more meaningful and therapeutic interventions (Dodds & Bowles 2001, Cutcliffe & Barker 2002, Svedberg et al 2003). Conversely, other authors argue that its use is the only real way to ensure patient and staff safety at times of extreme crisis or to provide a rubric for intensive patient–nurse interaction (Nirui & Chenoweth 1999).

Most organisations in the USA, UK, Australia and New Zealand have standards or policies covering the way in which clinical procedures should be carried out successfully and safely. Those relating to close observations appear to be lacking any evidence base and are primarily concerned with staff activities of assessment (of risk or suicidal intent), observation (for feedback to other health care disciplines) and maintaining patient safety (a ubiquitous term that has gradually come to mean little other than controlling the patient milieu) (Bowers & Park 2001, O'Brien & Cole 2003). These authors argue that descriptions of therapeutic actions to be undertaken during close observations are often absent from organisational standards, with phrases such as 'communicate with the patient', 'establish a relationship' and 'explain close observations' being the closest that the policy comes to separating it from a restraining order. Most policies, if not all, describe the different levels of close observations, anything from the nurse being at arm's length at all times to checking the patient's whereabouts every 15 minutes. They also detail operational orders, and many have checklists for ensuring that staff undertaking close observations can successfully assess, observe and maintain safety.

The implications of what we think we know

What does so much conflicting material tell us about the practical application of close observations? Well, for a start, it suggests that the whole process is in a mess – philosophically, organisationally and practically. It is clear that something is very seriously wrong when an activity so intrinsic to P/MH nursing care seems to lack a therapeutic focus. It is highly problematic that there is no real 'evidence base' for the effective practice of close observations, and that the written guidance that exists is hugely variable across different settings and localities. Careful reading of the literature will indicate similar critical scenarios concerning other interventions. In fact, the literature is strewn with papers that decry pretty much everything in mental health care. Does this mean that all developments and interventions in mental health care are flawed or wrong? Does it mean that practitioners who use these approaches or work within these structures actually cause more harm than good? Before we can answer this, let us first look at what is going on behind the scenes in P/MH nursing, to review the context within which close observations is currently operating.

The responsibility of nursing leadership

Leadership is not just about an individual acting as a role model for others; it is also about how the workforce is recruited, educated, supervised and supported. Within nursing, leadership is determined by the responsibilities attributed to nurses within an organisation, and also by the way in which these responsibilities are defined and controlled. Having direct responsibility for undertaking safe practice, monitoring professional progress and providing an environment in which nursing is allowed to express itself therapeutically are functions equally as important as representing the profession within multidisciplinary teams, determining conditions of employment and decision-making at senior management level. The primary role of nurse leaders, from staff nurses heading nursing teams through to nurse directors or those within national administration, is to ensure that nursing impacts on patient care in a therapeutically safe and positive fashion. Above all, the role includes the fundamental imperative that nurses should be provided with the requisite skills and support to be able to achieve this. Positive outcomes within P/MH nursing care are dependent upon the nurse being a skilled and effective practitioner, and nurse leaders at each relevant level of the organisational hierarchy have to assume responsibility for ensuring that this intensity of practice is achievable. However, the evidence from the literature suggests that this is not always the case. Consider the following example.

The survey conducted by Bowers et al (2000) found that in one-third of the Trusts that responded to the survey student nurses on placement were not allowed to undertake close observations; inversely, 24% of the Trusts allowed students to carry out all levels of close observations, and 43% at some levels. Although the survey did not ask questions about training or supervision for students during these placements, one would assume that classroom teaching on the theory and purpose of close observations would already have taken place. Therefore, conducting observations during their placement period would provide the practical experience to complement what was learnt in the classroom, thus bringing together the theory and the practice. However, if one-third of Trusts (if one takes this sample to be reasonably representative) exclude students from undertaking any form of close observations throughout their formative training, and a further 43% fail to provide the full spectrum of practical experience, this is of considerable concern. Furthermore, if students do not gain experience of close observations as a student, when do they begin to do so? Is it on the first day of registration, six months later, when supervised, or once a period of preceptorship has been finished? What if a student qualifies in one area that does not allow students to undertake close observations and then, on registration, accepts a post in another area where students are allowed to perform the procedure? Does anyone at interview ask whether close observations is part of the newly qualified nurse's experience? We doubt it! In fact, we doubt whether any of these questions is seriously considered by health care organisations. There is a worldwide shortage of qualified P/MH nurses and, with the exception of countries where preliminary preceptorship is undertaken (usually of a standard format to ensure clinical safety), a qualified nurse is expected to perform the roles and functions of the post, irrespective of years of experience. (This also begs questions about clinical supervision for qualified nurses and the involvement of nursing leadership in developing and safeguarding this vital resource. However, such a debate is beyond the scope of this chapter.)

We are not suggesting that careful experience screening at recruitment or ongoing provision for professional supervision is absent everywhere, but we are convinced that it happens in under-resourced inpatient acute mental health units a great deal of the time. The significant thing is not that it happens, but that nursing has not regulated itself sufficiently to ensure that it does not happen. If a cardiac surgeon turned up on her first day in theatre and told the surgical team that she had never actually carried out a heart bypass but had seen one performed, she would not be employed as a cardiac surgeon for very long. You might argue that there is a big difference between carrying out heart bypass surgery and developing and maintaining a relationship with someone who is so distressed that they wish to take their own life, but we argue that the principle is the same. They are both procedures that should be carried out by highly skilled and technically proficient professionals – not amateurs (Meiklejohn 2003). If nurse leadership is prepared to allow its practitioners to set foot into clinical areas with neither the proper background skills nor the support to develop hands-on personal technology, then it is with nurse leadership that we should be discussing close observations.

The reported world shortage of qualified P/MH nurses, and the effects this has had on the variety of care offered, has been noted in several reviews. Of these, the inner-London survey (Ward et al 1998) and the second national visit by the Mental Health Act Commission (Sainsbury Centre for Mental Health 2000) show that, in the UK at least, these shortages appear to have dramatically reduced the amount of therapeutic activity being undertaken by nurses. Moreover, the inner-London survey reported the apparent disparity between mixes of skill (what you are trained to do and capable of doing) and grade (what level you are in terms of nursing hierarchy) for those staff on duty at any one time. This survey described acute inpatient services as being devoid of routine therapeutic options, in effect reducing them to mere *holding pens* (our italics). It also noted the shortage of a crucial group of staff, namely junior staff nurses or those with middle-level experience and skills.

This finding is highly significant because, in the absence of the senior nurse in any unit, it would be expected that these mid-level nurses would take responsibility for the running of the unit. It would be presumed that these nurses would learn from their role-model seniors for the development of professional heuristic decision-making skills. In addition, senior nurses would be prepared to use their advanced skills only in the knowledge that they would be supported within the unit by the mid-level staff. In the absence of this group of staff (mid-level) the senior staff are less likely to demonstrate their expertise in advanced practice, reverting to 'safer' forms of care that do not demand challenge and risk-taking (Ward et al 1998). The knock-on effect is that mid-level nurses do not get to see how advanced practice can influence care quality and outcomes but, instead, role-model the sterile aspects of 'safe' practice. They, in turn, are incapable of role-modelling advanced skills for the benefit of the staff for whom they have responsibility, namely the very junior nurses and students on placements. Thus, not only do we have a situation where some students receive no experience of close observations during training, but those who do (and all the reviews noted that it was often the very junior staff who were more likely to be expected to undertake prolonged and even quite complicated close observations assignments) receive whatever supervision is available from staff who themselves may not be skilled in the procedure. It does not take a genius to realise that at some point or another in the future the skills base of these nurses will have been distilled to nothing more than that of paid carers, or worse, paid *keepers*.

Lack of therapy or lack of confidence?

If senior nurses and the nursing leadership cannot convince their own discipline that undertaking close observations is an advanced procedure that requires many years of supervised practice to perfect, then what, we ask, do nurses consider to be the core to their practice? A survey conducted in England and Wales by the Mental Health Act Commission, in collaboration with the Sainsbury Centre for Mental Health (2000) highlighted an absence of therapeutic activities within inpatient mental health units in the two countries (and the authors do not consider this situation to be any different elsewhere in the UK). These types of unit are staffed primarily by P/MH nurses. Perhaps these nurses feel so undermined by being asked to undertake activities for which the clinical intent is confused, and for which they have not been prepared, that their efficacy as practitioners is hampered while trying to carry them out? We would suggest that a lack of confidence in their own ability to carry out such work has a negative impact on their beliefs about the efficacy of the procedure itself. Thus, demoting the primacy of the procedure negates the necessity for experienced staff to perform it. It therefore becomes acceptable for the procedure (therapy) to be either ignored or (in the case of close observations) carried out by junior members of staff while their senior counterparts undertake more meaningful activities – which, from our observations, often seems to involve attending countless meetings and doing paperwork in the office, away from the clinical area. This, of course, does not suggest that the senior nurses actually want to be doing paperwork and attending meetings – the increasing bureaucracy of our health care organisations in part imposes this shift in priorities. However, it does provide one reason to explain the apparent devaluing of the activity of spending time with patients, with a suggestion that anyone can do it, and that the time of senior staff is better spent on 'more important' management (organisation) matters.

The centrality of the patient in P/MH nursing seems to have been lost. Nursing seems to have forgotten that the use of close observations should be reserved for the most acutely ill, who are assessed to be in need of this intensive form of care, and that they should be conducted by skilled and competent practitioners (Ward et al 1998). So why, as Meiklejohn (2003) and Ward et al (1998) have demonstrated, are there reported instances of the most junior staff carrying out such procedures? Surely logic tells us that it should be those with the most skills, not the least, who carry out the advanced activities, of which close observations is patently one? Why then has nursing not identified close observations as an advanced practice procedure, demanding from it the very things that the 'anti-close observations lobby' identify as being its current failings, namely its lack of *'intrinsic value of personal experience and the centrality of narrative in the development of contextually bound, personally appropriate, mental health care'* (Barker 2003, p 498).

Obviously low staffing and poor skill mix have a part to play here, but it seems to be more than this. It is about perception, the values and beliefs of P/MH nurses and about what they do, why they do it and what they see as being primary and secondary to their role. Fundamentally, it is also about how confident each individual nurse is in his or her ability to perform this role competently.

An underlying problem with close observations currently is that its original purpose as a therapeutic activity has shifted, apparently unchecked, to becoming a method of controlling 'difficult' patients. As noted by O'Brien & Cole (2003, p 172), there is a *'plethora of literature about control and restraint, seclusion and aggression but that this is seldom linked to the milieu in which it occurs: the close observation area'*. They also state that the clinical intent (or 'nursing skills and interventions') is aimed at *'assessment and risk assessment, management of aggression, prevention of violence, pharmacological management and collaboration'* (p 172). In effect, they reduce the procedure of close observations to a controlling one, with the so-called skills requiring defensive behaviours on the part of the nurse. Collaboration, presumably with the patient, is relegated to last place on this skills hierarchy. Yet surely it should be at the head of this list if the clinical intent listed at the beginning of this chapter were to be achieved? In Australia, which at that time had a relatively high reported suicide rate, research from the Health Outcomes Unit of South Eastern Sydney Area Health Service (Nirui & Chenoweth 1999) reported that health staff displayed a lack of diagnostic and management skills and a poor attitude towards suicide.

Once again, there was no mention of therapeutic values or the necessity for staff to have sensitive interpersonal skills. The paper is misleading because it implies that diagnostic activities are crucial to the management of suicide. Is this another example of the absence of therapy, or an absence of the ability to undertake therapy?

Contrast this to the alternative approach. Yonge & Molzan (2002) suggest that the most important *gift* (their word) a nurse can bring to patient interventions is that of time. In their research, they found that time spent in contact with the patient that showed caring and positive intent seemed to go beyond that normally expected by human being towards one another. In other words, it was a professional activity highlighted by a genuine sense of wanting to make a difference in someone's life.

In a UK study exploring patients' perceptions of being the recipient of close observations, Jones et al (2000) highlighted the importance of something very simple and straightforward – that nurses should communicate with patients and treat them with respect. This study found that it makes a positive difference to patients when they are observed by a nurse whom they know (compared with a nurse they have never met before, i.e. a complete stranger) and by someone who talks to them, rather than a nurse who doesn't introduce him/herself and just sits outside the room reading a book or newspaper. This finding is consistent with the study by Cardell & Pitula (1999), who found that observers' lack of empathy and lack of acknowledgement were perceived by patients to be particularly unhelpful. Indeed, Cardell & Pitula (1999) found that the very fact of not being communicative, of not 'going beyond' as Yonge & Molzan (2002) would say, of simply not demonstrating a sense of caring, had totally adverse or non-therapeutic effects during close observations.

If we consider close observations with other intrusive procedures that nurses are expected to undertake within a mental health environment, such as restraint and seclusion, we find a marked similarity between what patients say about these activities. In the USA, Mohr et al (1998) highlighted the necessity to involve patients in decision-making concerning the use of restraint, while in Australia Meehan et al (2000) identified five major themes that appear to have an over-riding impact on patients' perceptions of the use of seclusion. These themes – emotional impact, sensory deprivation, maintaining control and staff–patient interaction, plus that of patient involvement – appear time and again within nurse or patient research into the use of all difficult or intrusive interventions. The study by Fletcher (1999) adds yet another dimension to this issue, highlighting the fact that the lack of communication between those undertaking and those receiving close observations is recognised by both nurses and patients, yet this universally recognised problem is rarely acted upon.

Being in a situation where intensive contact between patient and nurse is anticipated has to be seen as an opportunity for the development of supportive and therapeutic conversation. Becoming a skilled companion to someone in serious threat of harming themselves or others requires time, skill and a sense of caring. We would argue that, if the nurse does not have the belief in their ability to undertake this work, they are less likely to attempt it. The consequence is that communication between patient and nurse fails, the clinical intent of close observations is negated, and patient management becomes the substitute for more professionally appropriate behaviours. Thus, it is the lack of confidence to carry out close observations properly, and not the procedure itself, that becomes the cause of it becoming a defensive intervention with no real therapeutic outcome. Is close observations a missed opportunity by P/MH nurses to demonstrate their much vaunted interpersonal capabilities, or have they simply altered their perception of who they are and what they are supposed to be doing?

Perhaps one answer (though by no means the only one) can be attributed to an apparent crisis in identity. We would argue that psychiatry, and in particular psychiatrists, have long mesmerised some (many?) P/MH nurses, using a process that has all the hallmarks of professional hypnosis, into believing that somehow care is secondary to treatment, for which they (psychiatry) are responsible. The implication of such a disjointed supposition is that sensitive and skilled caring is in some way less important, that developing a therapeutic relationship is both mundane and ancillary to the more important activities of diagnosing and patient management (including the management of real or perceived risk) – hence the concentration of literature around these areas within published nursing journals.

Subsequently, a procedure such as close observations, which requires high levels of skill and sensitivity to carry out effectively, receives the same level of personalised attention and priority as form-filling. This is a dangerous position from which to argue the necessity to withdraw close observations from care options, as it fails to recognise that good close observations requires intense personal technology from its practitioners, as does good P/MH nursing, and that this, and not management, is the primary function of therapeutic activities for which nurses see themselves as being responsible. It also fails to take account of the messages from patients receiving any form of intrusive or intensive mental health care; namely that they demand it shows that somebody cares! If therapy is absent, but the processes are available, then surely some other psychological processes, perhaps those of professional identity, are at work in the minds of P/MH nurses. It does not show that there is an absence of therapy, or interventionist opportunities. It does, however, suggest that shifting the emphasis away from the traditional skills of P/MH nursing has had a detrimental effect on the ability to perceive where those skills can be best put to use, with an ensuing reduction in confidence to deliver them when the situation arises. As a result, close observations is now viewed as merely a patient management function.

Paralysed by risk

'Risk thinking' increasingly pervades mental health care, with a growing culture of defensive practice (Rose 1998). Such an environment is viewed as a contributory factor in close observations becoming more about controlling patients than caring for them. As already discussed in this chapter, the purpose of close observations is to keep people safe and support them during a time of crisis. Thus, the process must be both safe and therapeutic, with the aim of maintaining positive engagement with the patient. However, as detailed in the review of the literature and from the authors' personal experience, it is clear that the practice of observation in many places has become diluted and compromised by all the many cultural and structural problems operating within acute mental health settings. We therefore find ourselves in a situation where nurses are not given the necessary opportunities to develop the therapeutic skills associated with close observations. Nurses are not being provided with strong professional leadership to develop the confidence to work therapeutically with patients and to feel valued when they spend time with patients, instead of doing paperwork. We believe that this is the crux of the matter: that the value of caring has been eroded by an institutional culture of risk reduction, tipping the balance between the concepts of patient care and public safety.

As with all health care professionals, P/MH nurses have a responsibility to maintain a safe environment – for their patients, themselves and society as a whole. Increasingly, however, in many parts of the world they are being expected to divert therapeutic practices in support of other priorities and/or public institutions in an attempt to demonstrate their effectiveness as health care providers. The authors' experiences over the last ten years suggest that risk has moved from being simply another factor within the care profile to number one on the list of clinical imperatives. Additionally, the lack of resources and the failure to develop the ability to deliver therapeutic interventions described in this chapter may have led to a general lack of confidence in mental health care services and its practitioners. Contracting these down further to ensure that 'nothing goes wrong' has increased the tendency to minimalise the value of caring and the perceived need for therapeutic intervention.

We would argue that this is the 'final nail in the coffin' for the effective and therapeutic practice of close observations. The need to provide intensive support and attention to patients who are acutely unwell seems to be neglected by health care organisations, which appear to have no confidence in their practitioners to be able to work in such a way. Moreover, this lack of confidence has gradually eroded practitioner efficacy in terms of their own abilities. This, linked to the issues of training and experience already discussed in this chapter, has brought us to a state of affairs where the concept of risk has effectively paralysed health care organisations to such an extent that their belief in themselves as caring agencies has all but disappeared (Raven & Rix 1999). Why else would they feel the need to invent observational levels, ranging from the nurse being constantly at arm's length, to checking where the patient is every 15 minutes (Bowers et al 2000)? We believe that a patient is either at risk or not! The mere fact that these policies exist shows that the organisation has no concept of what constitutes therapeutic need. Devising such policies merely puts additional pressure on the nurse because the implication is that, if something goes wrong, this is the responsibility of the nurse, not the organisation (O'Brien & Cole 2003). In other words, the blame culture has slowly infiltrated the therapeutic one, and high-risk mental health organisations are now the place where care staff are still expected to work miracles, but not at the expense of public safety.

Perhaps more alarming is that, within such a risk culture, individuals are not expected to make their own decisions – these are the domain of the policy, procedure or protocol, devised by the organisation to ensure standard practices and so reduce (in theory) risk. The result is that close observations assignments are often decided by other members of the multidisciplinary team, themselves guided by the hospital policies and the need to reduce the possibilities of 'untoward events'. Those who are to carry out the procedure, usually nurses, may find themselves undertaking close observations for patients for whom it is patently not necessary. This is not only a waste of valuable resources, but also disenfranchising for those expected to treat all levels of potential risk with the same degree of intensity. The risk culture fails practitioners because they are denied the opportunity to practise their traditional caring skills appropriately; it fails close observations because it has taken away the true purpose of the intervention, to provide intensive nursing care at a time of considerable need; and it fails the patients for whom close observations could be beneficial, because staff are not allowed to differentiate between patients who are acutely unwell and those who are difficult to manage. In such a 'draconian' environment, close observations ceases to be a therapeutic activity but a controlling and policing one, with those charged with carrying it out recognising its devalued state and therefore failing to commit themselves wholeheartedly to its undertaking (Duffy 1995).

Conclusion

In this chapter we have attempted to demonstrate that the apparent shortcomings of close observations are not the fault of the procedure itself, but a consequence of underlying problems within mental health care. There is, in our opinion, nothing wrong with the notion of spending an intensive period of time with a person suffering dramatic and potentially harmful distress. We would argue that this is what P/ MH nursing is meant to be about. Therefore, *throwing the close observations baby out with the bath water* will solve nothing, apart from replacing close observations with yet another scapegoat. This will simply prolong the process of actually sorting out the real problems in our mental health care system.

References

Barker P 2003 The tidal model: psychiatric colonization, recovery and the paradigm shift in mental health care. International Journal of Mental Health Nursing 12(2):96–102.

Bowers L, Park A 2001 Special observation in the care of psychiatric inpatients: a literature review. Issues in Mental Health Nursing 22: 769–786.

Bowers L, Gournay K, Duffy D 2000 Suicide and self-harm in inpatient psychiatric units: a national survey of observation policies. Journal of Advanced Nursing 32(2):437–444.

Bowles N, Dodds P, Hackney D, Sunderland C, Thomas P 2002 Formal observations and engagement: a discussion paper. Journal of Psychiatric and Mental Health Nursing 9(3):255–260.

Cardell R, Pitula C R 1999 Suicidal inpatients' perceptions of therapeutic and non-therapeutic aspects of constant observation. Psychiatric Services 50:1066–1070.

Cutcliffe J R, Barker P 2002 Considering the care of the suicidal client and the case for 'engagement and inspiring hope' or 'observations'. Journal of Psychiatric and Mental Health Nursing 9(5):611–621.

Department of Health 1999 Report by the Standing Nursing and Midwifery Advisory Committee (SNMAC). Mental health nursing: addressing acute concerns. HMSO, London.

Dodds P, Bowles N 2001 Dismantling formal observation and refocusing nursing activity in acute inpatient psychiatry. Journal of Psychiatric and Mental Health Nursing 8(2):183–188.

Duffy D 1995 Out of the shadows: a study of the special observation of suicidal psychiatric in-patients. Journal of Advanced Nursing 21(5): 944–950.

Fletcher R F 1999 The process of constant observation: perspectives of staff and suicidal patients. Journal of Psychiatric and Mental Health Nursing 6(1):9–14.

Gournay K, Bowers L 2000 Suicide and self-harm in in-patient psychiatric units: a study of nursing issues in 31 cases. Journal of Advanced Nursing 32(1):124–131.

Horsfall J, Cleary M 2000 Discourse analysis of an 'observation levels' nursing policy. Journal of Advanced Nursing 32(5):1291–1297.

Jones J, Ward M, Wellman N, Hall J, Lowe T 2000 Psychiatric inpatients' experience of nursing observation: a United Kingdom perspective. Journal of Psychosocial Nursing and Mental Health Services 38(12):10–20, 52–53.

Meehan T, Vermeer C, Windsor C 2000 Patients' perceptions of seclusion: a qualitative investigation. Journal of Advanced Nursing 31(2):370–377.

Meiklejohn C 2003 Nursing observations in a medium secure unit: a review of practice. Mental Health Practice 7(3):12–14.

Mohr W, Mahon M, Noone M 1998 A restraint on restraints: the need to reconsider the use of restrictive interventions. Archives of Psychiatric Nursing XII(2):95–106.

Nirui M, Chenoweth L 1999 The response of healthcare services to people at risk of suicide: a qualitative study. Australian and New Zealand Journal of Psychiatry 33:361–371.

O'Brien L, Cole R 2003 Close-observation areas in acute psychiatric units: a literature review. International Journal of Mental Health Nursing 12(3):165–176.

Raven J, Rix P 1999 Managing the unmanageable: risk assessment and risk management in contemporary professional practice. Journal of Nursing Management 7(4):201–206.

Rose N 1998 Living dangerously: risk thinking and risk management in mental health care. Mental Health Care 1(8):263–266.

Sainsbury Centre for Mental Health 2000 National Visit 2: A visit by the Mental Health Act Commission to 104 mental health and learning disability units in England and Wales: improving care for detained patients from black and minority ethnic communities. Sainsbury Centre for Mental Health, London.

Svedberg P, Jormfeldt H, Arvidsson B 2003 Patients' conceptions of how health processes are promoted in mental health nursing. A qualitative study. Journal of Psychiatric and Mental Health Nursing 10(4):448–456.

Ward M, Gournay K, Thornicroft G, Wright S 1998 Inpatient mental health in inner London: 1997 census. First Interim Report. Royal College of Nursing Institute, London.

Yonge O, Molzan A 2002 Exceptional nontraditional caring practices of nurses. Scandinavian Journal of Caring Sciences 16:399–405.

Commentary

Peter Campbell

There seems to be widespread agreement that there are significant problems with the practice of close observations. Concerns are shared at all levels of the psychiatric and mental health nursing discipline, from frontline workers to nurse leadership. Service users who have experience of the procedure have also voiced numerous criticisms. Although the perspectives and agendas of various groups and individuals inevitably differ and there is disagreement about how far we must go to achieve positive change, there is actually a good deal of common ground concerning what the major problems are. One of the most important of these is connected to the issue of therapeutic interaction.

Any consideration of close observations must acknowledge the increasing debate about acute ward care as a whole. Service user organisations have been criticising acute care and proposing improvements and alternatives since the mid 1980s (Good Practices in Mental Health/Camden Consortium 1988). For many years, a number of service users have felt that the acute ward often provides interventions that are as much unhelpful as helpful. In the past ten years, views of this kind have been more consistently recognised and have led to a series of reports, research articles and other literature from service providers, academics and voluntary organisations examining the nature and quality of the acute ward experience. These have frequently criticised in strong terms wide-ranging aspects of acute care including the physical environment, safety, staff–patient contact, provision of social and recreational activity, lack of patient involvement in care and treatment, and boredom. It is likely that many P/MH nurses have felt under attack as a result. It is possible that some have come to believe that the acute ward is indeed in some way an inherently non-therapeutic environment.

An assertion of this kind may be seen as both extreme and a counsel of despair. At the same time, the character and extent of shortcomings revealed by investigators suggest that fundamental problems may exist that cannot be addressed simply by 'piecemeal' improvements to procedures and practice. Improving guidelines and training around procedures such as close observations and seclusion can bring appreciable benefits, but positive change may not be sustained until underlying attitudes are addressed and consideration is given to what P/MH nurses think they should best be doing and are capable of doing.

In an era when service users are supposed to be at the centre of care, it is appropriate that a more detailed examination of the issues surrounding close observations should begin with their experience. Although very little research has been done on this topic, a number of broad reactions to close observations do begin to emerge and these are backed up by anecdotal evidence. Some service users find close observations supportive; however, more do not like it and consider it unhelpful. The practice of close observations is by no means alone in these latter respects. There are a host of acute ward interventions, carried out by nurses and other mental health professionals, that produce similar reactions. This does not necessarily mean they are completely useless and should be abandoned, although it does suggest they may be significantly overvalued in the professional's eye. Attempting to deny the opportunity to commit suicide through staying close to a person and watching over them may have saved their life, and that should not be discounted.

Close observation is inevitably intrusive and potentially oppressive. It is not surprising that many service users do not like it. Clearly the acceptability and helpfulness of the procedure is closely linked to the degree of interaction that takes place. Dr Diana Rose's experience of close observations illustrates one extreme and is by no means unique:

'It is possible for a close-observations nurse to have no interaction whatever with the patient during an eight hour shift. They read magazines'.

(Rose 2000, p 8)

While simply watching over someone to deny them the opportunity to commit suicide can increase a feeling of safety, it may do very little to reduce the desire to kill oneself – and might even increase it for certain people. Denying the ability without addressing the desire must be a major reason why service users find close observations unhelpful. Observation without interaction is a cold comfort.

It is important that service users be involved in the assessment and management of risk (Langan & Lindow 2004). This is not just crucial in terms of securing maximum effectiveness but is necessary if the service users' often repeated demand for respect and dignity (a demand that is expressed not only in regard to close observations but to all aspects of care and treatment) is to be answered positively. Informing the person that they are going to be observed closely and explaining what is going to happen would seem to be absolutely basic. However, the acceptability and benefits of close observations are likely to be, and perceived to be, greater if the person takes part in discussion about the need for observation, the closeness of observation necessary and the desirability of continuing close observations. Developing and agreeing a plan for close observations and wider aspects of safety, and revisiting it on a daily basis to discuss adjustments, must be a good way to ensure that involvement is meaningful and is maintained.

Anecdotal evidence that nurses or support staff carrying out close observations sometimes do not introduce themselves, or observe while reading newspapers and magazines, as mentioned above, suggests that common courtesies can be overlooked. Few people, whether service users or ordinary members of the public, would not be offended by such behaviour. Sharing one's personal space with another for a long period, even on friendly terms, is not easy for any of us. It is clearly an underlying reason why close observation is unpopular with service users and nurses. Carrying out such an intrusive intervention makes the need for courtesy even more important. Without common courtesies, respect and dignity must suffer.

A major dilemma for the practice of close observations revolves aroung the issue that an intervention declared by nurse leadership to require a high level of skill is usually carried out by students, transient or unqualified staff. On the face of it there seems to be little room to disagree that this is an unhappy state of affairs, although the fact that the situation continues to exist suggests that some P/MH nurses, along with other mental health professionals, may have come to accept, perhaps reluctantly, that close observations can legitimately be a low-skill activity. A number of causes are suggested for the gap between theory and practice, and seem largely convincing. They include: the absence of guidelines in some Trusts, the lack of emphasis on therapeutic interaction in guidance and guidelines, failure to give students sufficient practical experience of close observation, shortages of psychiatric/mental health nurses, and the growing preoccupation with controlling risk. It is unlikely that close observations or any alternative to it will achieve full potential without successfully addressing some of these problems.

Attitudes are critical and the growth of a risk and blame culture is cited as a major factor in emphasising the need for physical safety at the expense of therapeutic interaction. But has interaction ever been a major feature of the acute ward? Perhaps conversations with nurses and inpatients from the 1960s and 1970s would reveal that separation and 'non-reciprocal observation' have been longstanding realities (Podvoll 1991). My own memories from those days are that, although there was more interaction, qualified nurses were often not included in this and inpatients were left to their own devices much of the time. Staff talking only among themselves or concentrating on magazines in the day room happened then, as it does now.

The 'engagement and inspiring hope' approach may offer a way forward, in terms of both close observations and the delivery of care and treatment on acute wards more generally. In most ways, the engagement and hope approach seems to be an active rather than a laissez-faire approach, although fears that absence of formal observation might lead to more suicides is understandable. The effectiveness of close observations in preventing suicide needs to be increased, and it is too soon to make a good judgement on whether an alternative approach will lower or increase suicide rates. Nevertheless, by focusing more on interaction, as the engagement and inspiring hope approach appears to do, and by addressing the desire for suicide in a more sophisticated way, it is quite likely that the number of suicides will go down.

Observation does not necessarily rule out interaction. Nevertheless, there is a perception implicit in the general concept of observation that implies objectivity rather than subjectivity, a standing back, a diluted sense of being with. Such standing back is a feature of observation across many areas of human concern. It seems to have an even greater attraction when dealing with mental distress because of the complicated, alienating and challenging nature of the problems involved, particularly at an acute stage. The desire to provide clear information, to protect, to meet the observer's need for self-preservation, usually leads to a containing curtain being constructed around distressed individuals rather than getting in there with them. As has been suggested above, this can go only part of the way to meeting need.

Whether a proper emphasis on therapeutic interaction demands the relegation of observation to a position where it is no longer used in the headline description of the nursing practice involved is quite hard to judge. Many outsiders, including service users, might think this is of limited importance. Polarisation may suit the dynamics of the P/MH nursing discipline, may lead to stronger debate, can perhaps produce major change more rapidly, but whether mental health services are well served by polarisation is not obvious. Perhaps the only way really to change the landscape is for rival parties to set up camp on far-separated mountains and then work their way towards eventually meeting somewhere on the plains below.

The engagement and inspiring hope position is putting a helpful emphasis on the types of interaction that service users, or at least those we hear from most, seem to want. It is also likely to make sense to many P/MH nurses and people in other caring professions. Listening, understanding, caring, inspiring hope are clearly vital aspects of any sensitive way to attend to the wants and needs of people in mental distress. They are also likely to lead to more positive results. Nevertheless, there may be difficulties in actually pinning down the components of these qualities in such a way that practising nurses, students and support staff can learn to put them into day-to-day use. We seem to have been discussing for centuries what 'caring' actually means and implies. Some may feel that all this is mundane, involves experts talking in circles, and can actually be provided automatically if they have a genuine desire to help. While this may not be true, have we lost the plot slightly through over-elaboration?

Engagement is a useful concept because it puts a premium on closeness. Most service users and P/MH nurses want more closeness. They would probably opt for close, but not too close. Nevertheless, engagement can also have negative connotations (engagement as a battle), and can particularly have implications of closure and inflexibility (getting engaged, telephone/toilet engaged). The idea of 'bridging' has recently been put forward, and this might be more liberating (Barker & Buchanan-Barker 2004). Inspiring hope is obviously important in both reducing the desire for suicide and increasing the motivation to pursue recovery in the longer term. Caring must be a component of this process, but challenging the underlying hopelessness conveyed by most mental health services and society's preconceptions about 'dangerous, mysterious and incurable illness' is essential. Hopelessness affects the quality of life of P/MH nurses as well as that of people with mental distress. More hope could have a snowballing effect, eventually producing happier service users and more and better nurses.

Paying better attention to people in acute wards who are suicidal is not in itself going to transform the world for service users or P/MH nurses. It can cut down the number of suicides and have an impact not only on care for the suicidal but for all those in acute ward care, even if more widespread changes in the delivery of acute care do not materialise. Better close observations or greater use of the engagement and inspiring hope approach will both move us towards these objectives to some degree. Cynics might suggest that the present debate is about packaging as well as content, and there could be some truth in this. What is certainly clear is the need to do something practical now and to test out the effects of the alternatives available.

References

Barker P, Buchanan-Barker P 2004 Bridging: talking meaningfully about the care of people at risk. Mental Health Practice 8(3):12–15.

Good Practices in Mental Health/Camden Consortium 1988 Treated well? A code of practice for psychiatric hospitals. Good Practices in Mental Health, London.

Langan J, Lindow V 2004 Living with risk: mental health service user involvement in risk assessment and management. The Policy Press, London.

Podvoll E 1991 The seduction of madness: a compassionate approach to recovery at home. Century, London.

Rose D 2000 A year of care. Openmind 106(Nov/Dec):8–9.

The standardisation of psychiatric/mental health nursing: eliminating confusion or settling for mediocrity?

CHAPTER 16

In support of standardisation

Susan McCabe

CHAPTER 17

Against standardisation

Gary Rolfe

Commentary

Wendy Austin

Editorial

In an ever-changing world the possibility of form, shape and continuity can sometimes seem like a safe harbour on a stormy night. Yet not everyone wants, or indeed needs, to take refuge within the realms of a guarantee. One of the main reasons for choosing this debate was that we noticed the extent to which those who supported, and those who did not support, the need for standardisation within P/MH nursing would go to sustain their chosen position. As with all decent debates, the polemics of this one are completely at variance with each other. On the surface there appears to be no common ground, no linear continuum and certainly no point at which the two camps are able to compromise. You might think that we have reached a stand-off. However, dismantling the two sets of arguments does provide us with a clearer view of their respective rationales.

Depending on which 'side of the fence' you stand, the lines of reasoning for standardisation range from an acceptable way of ensuring quality of care, to a method of reducing P/MH nursing to the level of automatism. Similarly, some argue that standardisation would enable practitioners to provide equality of care for all their patients, irrespective of geographical situation, while others see it as a reductionist puzzle that denies P/MH nurses the opportunity to express themselves freely within the care process.

These arguments reflect the positions of humanism versus organisationalism, with the notable exception of those who choose to ignore all debate and do their 'own thing' irrespective of what is going on around them. However, if one considers the stance of the pro-standardisation lobby, there are some irresistible arguments concerning the necessity to ensure that high level, complex interventions are delivered by experienced, confident and well prepared practitioners, for every patient with whom they have contact. The converse of this, for the anti-standardisation group, is that making each practitioner comply with preordained interventionist practices actually works against the notion of the individuality of each patient, and that care quality can be ensured by having a more professional and better educated workforce. This notion of individualisation, the Deon of contemporary Western mental health care, is the cornerstone of this debate, as for many it is the one thing that separates *adequate* care, from *good* care. Such meaning is not the sole prerogative of either of these two camps but, in fact, of them both. Therefore, the debate is not about the nature or quality of care, but the route by which it is achieved. If the two protagonists are unwilling to establish a truce and compromise on the method of achieving this, we are in danger of reaching an entrenched position, i.e. *non-instructive interaction* (Fruggeri 1995), totally at odds with what we expect of modern mental health care, namely, the power to change using every tool at the discipline's disposal. In other words, P/MH nursing stagnates because it cannot deconstruct itself sufficiently to generate new ways of applying itself to the therapeutic process.

Of course, nothing is ever that simple, for as the following chapters will show, even the concept of standardisation means different things to different people. If we are to move this debate through what Wittgenstein (1953) described as *restoring positions through negatives*, it is important that readers spend a few moments exploring their own positions prior to reading the debate. An open mind to this debate ought to produce an enlightened appreciation of how it can be used to further the effectiveness of P/MH nursing.

References

Fruggeri L 1995 Therapeutic process as the social construction of change. In: McNamee S, Gergen K, eds. Therapy as social construction. Sage, London; Ch. 3 p 40–53.

Wittgenstein L 1953 Philosophical investigations. Investigations 1. Trans. G E M Anscombe. Blackwell, Oxford.

In support of standardisation

Introduction

Psychiatric disorders, craziness, lunacy and emotional disturbance: mental illness. These are powerful words connoting powerful emotions. The images, assumptions and beliefs embedded in these words have power to move us, touch us, make us respond as human beings, and ultimately frame the professional lives that we as P/MH nurses live. We are both proud of and confused by the power inherent in our professional domain. Our confusion is mirrored in our role and identity struggles and the lack of unity of focus within our discipline. Standardisation of care is arguably the most seminal issue demonstrating that confusion.

The paradigm within which we practise assumes that P/MH nursing is a unique and distinct subspeciality of the nursing discipline. As the nursing speciality most interested in emotions, feelings and perceptions, we have believed, and still believe, that we are the nurses closest to the 'humanness' of patient experiences. Our espoused epistemology highlights this assumption. Historically, all things pertaining to communication, to anxiety, to grief, to development, to emotional reactions have been seen as the purview of P/MH nursing. Steeped in history and myth, P/MH nurses have believed that our path to professional efficacy and respect ran through the humanisation of care practices, one patient at a time. We have believed that the more we humanise our practices, the more effective and more purely 'psychiatric' is our nursing care.

The problem with our belief lies at the heart of the storm surrounding standardisation. The problem is with our implementation of the notion of humanised care. Many P/MH nurses view interpersonal individualisation of care as the best way to humanise the experiences that bring individuals into and out of the health care arena. The more we could individualise care practices through interpersonal means, we believed, the closer to pure P/MH nursing, and the closer to quality care, we came. Our modern history as P/MH nurses is a history of the interpersonal. Almost all of our common care practices are practices that have arisen, like the phoenix from the ashes of science, from the one-to-one nurse–patient relationship. The 'interpersonal' has become the single, solitary, most critical element of P/MH nursing epistemology. At a time before genetic understanding, before awareness of the structure and function of the brain, at a time of mind metaphor not brain metaphor (McCabe 2002), it was our so-called science. Our roles of advocacy, of supporter, of teacher are historically drawn from Freudian terms, predicated on surrogate roles as parent-protector that enable replication and redemption of the roles of the patient's interpersonal family of origin. How then, many of us wonder, can we standardise care and still be P/MH nurses?

Standardisation of care practices has been viewed by some as the antithesis of P/MH nursing care. It has been seen as the imposition of non-individualised, impersonal care on to the most personal of nursing practices. The issue of standardisation of care practices for P/MH nurses is contextually structured within both emotion and power. Pressures to standardise care surround us. From issues of fiscal control, to promotion of effective health outcomes, almost all nursing practice is becoming 'standardised'. Yet for P/MH nursing, it remains an issue that is contentious, confusing, and whose outcome may well decide the future of the discipline.

This chapter will argue that many of the assumptions that underpin our current strong resistance to the notion of standardisation of care are based on vacuous nonsense. We have seen individualised care as synonymous with non-standardised, interpersonal care and have therefore assumed that standardising practice would impinge on individualised care, be highly impersonal and be distinctly unpsychiatric. Pursuing dreams of the interpersonal and beliefs of individualisation, we have even fought the notion of 'disease' and 'symptom clusters' as aspects of standardisation, settling instead for a comforting blanket of 'touchy feely', non-scientific nosology and the concomitant closeness with patients as a substitute for a real, scientifically grounded system of care practice. This chapter will contend that this is the stuff of ignorance and the path to professional suicide. The time to standardise P/MH nursing care has come and is almost gone. If we delay further, we will 'individualise' ourselves out of existence, we will fail to be meaningful in the health care arena and we will be the generation that squandered the legacy of the giants of our discipline. In avoiding standardised care, we will lose the very heart of P/MH nursing and will lose all chance of making the rich, imperative impact on our patients' lives that we potentially could.

Standardisation: what it is and is not

Emotional and psychiatric disturbances are personal. They are deeply felt. They sting, throb for years, hurt, incapacitate, and can be some of the most debilitating health conditions known. Individuals will construct very private, diverse meanings from their experience of mental illness. One of the most basic and cherished tenets of P/MH nursing is to provide individualised care that matches the needs of the patient and is congruent with a person's beliefs, values, culture and needs. So the obvious question becomes, how can individualised care ever be standardised? The answer lies in understanding the differences between these two related, yet often misunderstood concepts.

Examination of the etymology of the word 'standardisation' is perhaps the best way to begin to see the conceptual differences from 'individualised' care. Coming from Middle English, the root derivation 'standard' means something established by authority, custom, or general consent as a model or example. Standards are set up and established by authority as a rule for the measure of extent, quality and value. A standard tells us what something is and, by comparison, is not. Standards function as a yardstick, a criterion against which to measure. Standards are a critical element of being professional and all established professions, including nursing, have identified standards. Professional nursing emerged in the late 19th century mainly because of the adoption of standards. Standards provide a common language for discussing what is elemental to a profession and a frame for the identification of complex or abstract actions by its professionals. Standards do not control specific nursing actions, but rather create a boundary for those actions, guiding nurses as they define and develop care with and for their patients.

Standardised care is the hypothetical, the abstract, the criterion of what constitutes the scope and best practice of the professional. One knows what to expect from a nurse as opposed to a dietitian because of standards. One knows that nurses give an intramuscular injection while laboratory technicians do not because of standards. Standards protect and preserve scope of practice by identifying who is, and by comparison who is not, expected to perform certain responsibilities. Standards provide authoritative statements by which the nursing profession describes the responsibilities for which its practitioners are accountable (American Nurses Association 2000) and, in so doing, standards also reflect the values and priorities of the nursing profession.

'Individualised' on the other hand is a word derived from Medieval Latin 'individuus', meaning related to or distinctively associated with the individual (Barnhart 1995). Individualised care is the care delivered to the person. Nothing about it is hypothetical or abstract. It represents the humanness, the attention to the unique person, all the while reflecting the standard of what role and responsibilities should be undertaken. Individualised care is relational and contextual. It is how care is delivered; it is process, it is thinking, it is the praxis of caring enough to tailor care to a person not an illness. It is the decisions undertaken by the nurse to adapt care, to contextualise care, to meet the diverse needs of the individual patient. It is not incompatible with, nor the antithesis of standardised care, but rather the inescapable, requisite correlate of humanness enabling us to live up to our standards as nurses. Efficacious P/MH nursing care must be consistent with identified standards, delivered in an individualised, nurse–person relationship. Standards are the science, are the content of our professional knowledge. The interpretation, i.e. the translation of the science to the person, is the individualisation of our care and therefore the interpersonal. Individualised care, our epistemological heart, is not a sufficient substitute for the science any longer. Individualised care is the process through which a P/MH nurse translates science and personalises care for a specific patient. Standardisation without individualisation decontextualises the science from the person, just as individualisation without standardisation decontexualises the person from the science.

Professional elements of standardised care

Practice or clinical standards are emerging to give boundaries to the daily clinical decisions made with respect to the specific health states treated by nurses. These standards are time related, detailed, measurable and actionable; they change as knowledge changes, research accumulates, and professional clinical roles expand and contract. Clinical practice guidelines, clinical algorithms, practice standards, protocols and clinical pathways are largely synonymous terms describing systematically refined parameters that can function to guide clinical decision-making (Institute of Medicine 1992). These algorithms and clinical practice guidelines were developed to address growing concerns that individual patients were not getting the most current and efficacious care, were suffering needlessly and longer than necessary, and that the quality of care received by patients was difficult to measure when some aspects of patient care were not standardised. The clinical standard movement was born to provide a sequential framework for clinical decision-making, to translate research to practice, to improve quality of care, to increase patient safety, to control costs and, quite simply, to provide standardisation of care.

Practice standards are intended to assist patient and nurse decision-making about health care practices and are attempts to distil a vast amount of health care information into a digestible, usable format. As the practice standard movement has progressed, many of the standardised approaches are increasingly subsumed under the rubric of evidence-based care. Practice standards are intended to be consensus statements from clinical experts aware of the knowledge in the field and, in definition and intention, also from patients as consumers of care and experts in their own health (Titler et al 1999, Clingerman 2000, DiCenso et al 2003).

The attempt to bound P/MH nursing practice by the science of practice standards has raised howls of protest, focusing mainly on the threat that practice standards might impinge on individualised, personalised care. Although we undertake care practices because we believe that they will make a difference to the quality of the individual's life, we struggle with the standardisation of those practices. Care can be, should be, must be, both standardised and individualised. Proficiency with technical procedures and a depth of scientific knowledge are both necessary but not sufficient for P/MH nursing. The ability to talk with the patient, to form meaningful relationships and attend to the interpersonal is necessary but not sufficient for P/MH nursing. Technical competency is the standard and the science, while interpersonal competency is the individualisation, the art, the translation and application of the standard. Knowledge of practice standards applied through therapeutic interpersonal interaction provides the patient with the best practice, matched to their individual need, and protects the subdiscipline of P/MH nursing by demarcating who is a P/MH nurse and what actions constitute P/MH nursing. Without the blend of standard and the interpersonal, science and art, quality suffers and the continued development of knowledge in the subspeciality is impossible.

The relationship of standardisation to quality and research: why we must standardise

What is a P/MH nurse? Who can and should call himself or herself a P/MH nurse? Can anyone with a modicum of empathy, an interest in helping people, a focus on the general health needs of a person diagnosed with mental illness, or the ability to form strong interpersonal relationships be considered a P/MH nurse? What is quality P/MH nursing care? What is the appropriate P/MH nursing action to achieve a clinical outcome? Why hire or reimburse a P/MH health nurse instead of a paediatric, obstetrical or generic nurse? To what standard should P/MH nurses be held accountable? What should patients, supervisors and peers expect from P/MH nurses?

These questions are central to the discipline's existence. If we distinguish ourselves as separate, as a unique discipline, as a speciality of 'professional' nursing, P/MH nurses must be able to demonstrate to other health care providers, to the patient, family and to the public how we are special. We must be able to articulate succinctly and measure directly what we do that is unique, and to determine the impact of what we do on the health of those we care for.

These questions matter and are almost impossible to answer without the yardstick and role protection provided by practice standards. Without standards anyone can, and increasingly many do, teach P/MH nursing content in educational programmes and provide traditional psychiatric care without the requisite educational and experiential background to be P/MH nurses. In many places patients experiencing emotional problems and psychiatric illness are receiving care from individuals with no formal education or training as P/MH nurses (McCabe 2000, 2002) and with little interest in this population. In the USA, patients with anxiety, substance abuse and other common psychiatric illnesses are increasingly being mainstreamed to non-psychiatric professionals for care. Some of this relates to economic pressures, some relates to the decline in the numbers of P/MH nurses, but mostly it relates to our inability thus far to identify clearly and succinctly the practice standards of the subspeciality of P/MH nursing. If we have not identified what we do, if there is no safety from the boundaries of practice standards, then we are open to anyone believing they can 'do it', and we leave the door open to anything done with a psychiatric patient being called P/MH nursing. We do not allow a nursing aide to perform the responsibilities and functions of a professional nurse. We do not allow a non-nurse midwife to give routine prenatal or birthing care. Why do we allow non-P/MH nurses to teach and to practise P/MH nursing? It is because we have not identified the territorial boundaries of our discipline. Our failure to establish and embrace practice standards and our own territorial boundaries, has and continues to limit severely the quality of the care our patients receive, whilst dramatically limiting the growth of our science. Although this may seem an abstract issue for many P/MH nurses whose hearts and souls are found in interactions with individual patients, it is an issue threatening to engulf us. It is the 'canary singing in the mine' of our professional future and is the single largest issue that has the potential to render us invisible as a subdiscipline.

Nursing as a discipline believes that quality matters. We strive for quality in our application of knowledge and skills to assist patients towards health, either by assisting with change, or with understanding what it means not to change, or by adapting life patterns to health states. Since the 1960s our extant literature has been ripe with discussions of quality nursing care and the centrality of nurses' individual and collective accountability for professional care. Moving from quality assurance programmes to outcome measures and evidence-based nursing practice, nursing's modern history is the history of the pursuit of quality. Practice standards, and determinants of the absence or presence of quality that flow from them, are increasingly being accepted as the main way to identify the contributions of nursing, including P/MH nursing, to quality health care (King 2000).

Quality is measurable and objective. It is the proof that P/MH nursing interventions matter, and are efficacious in meeting outcome objectives, and that there is indeed a body of science to support our practice. The ability to identify quality measures proves we are a distinct subspeciality, and failure to accept practice standards means a failure to identify these quality measures. Without the practice standards we have no yardstick, no comparative data, which allow us as P/MH nurses to identify and measure what we do, and especially what we do well. If we cannot say what we do and do well, we severely limit the professional power, status and growth of P/MH nursing practice.

Research is the accepted doorway to the development of knowledge and the growth of a body of science such as P/MH nursing. If there are no practice standards that demarcate the discipline, how do we know what research agenda is best suited for our science to grow? If we have no consensus agreement about what we are and what we do, how do we apply for financial support for important P/MH nursing research, focused on the populations and phenomena of most concern to us? Without boundaries our discipline is increasingly becoming diluted and watered down in discouraging and disconcerting ways. As an example of the growing dilution of P/MH nursing science we need only look to recent extant research reports. A check of the database Cumulative Index to Nursing and Allied Health Literature (CINAHL), using the search terms 'research findings' and 'psychiatric and/or mental health nursing' reveals 2430 citations. At first glance, this number should bring joy to the hearts of all P/MH nurses. It appears that we are active and prolific in our research and that the body of our P/MH nursing science should be growing by leaps and bounds. Appearances, however, can, and in this case do, lie. The broad spectrum of so-called 'psychiatric research' foci ranges through multiple aspects of cancer care, the emotionality of breast feeding, emotional reactions to HIV-positive status, multiple aspects of dealing with chronic medical conditions, diabetes mellitus (most notably), with enormous volumes on stress and adaptation in otherwise mentally healthy individuals. This is valuable research, no doubt, but it is psychosocial research at best, not P/MH nursing research. While touching on being human, the greatest amount of the identified 2430 citations deal with research conducted on subjects with no mental or psychiatric disorder, but rather with individuals experiencing, quite simply, being human. It is research done by nurses who are not P/MH nurses and is largely reported in non-psychiatric journals most commonly read by non-P/MH nurses.

So why are non-P/MH nurses doing 'psychiatric nursing research' and does it really matter? Where, or what, is the legitimate agenda for P/MH nursing that will truly cause our science to grow? We cannot find it because we do not know it. The lack of practice standards propels the lack of focus of the boundaries of our subdiscipline, which in turn allows any and all others interested in emotions to usurp and to bastardise our legacy in any way they wish. What is a P/MH nurse? What are the boundaries of P/MH nursing? If you were to base judgement of these questions on the body of 'psychiatric nursing' research, it would be any nurse the least bit interested in emotions, caring for patients who display the normal reactions of being human. Does this protect or develop us, or bode well for the survival of our subprofession? I fear not. Does this advance accountability and quality? I fear not. To fail to identify standardised care practices is tantamount to wholesale abdication of our professional legacy, and constitutes the first of the three most compelling reasons why we must standardise our practice.

Giving away our birthright: the first compelling reason for standardised care

Without practice standards to define care, what is the justification for our assumption that we are a distinct subspeciality? Hildegard Peplau, revered as the 'mother of psychiatric nursing' (Haber 2000), is accepted as a founding giant of our discipline. Her contributions are innumerable but most consider her development of the Interpersonal Relations Theory, with its emphasis on the nurse–patient relationship, as her most influential and important contribution to our discipline. Based on her work, we have inculcated the nurse–patient relationship as perhaps the most essential role for a psychiatric nurse. Because of the obvious contribution of this role to patient outcomes, she has allowed every P/MH nurse to feel and believe that we were a distinct and unique discipline of nursing. At a time before discussions of quality measures and practice standards, she gave every P/MH nurse a standard of practice that has become universally accepted. Every P/MH nurse was educated and trained to establish, nurture and then terminate the nurse–patient relationship. We believed it mattered, we standardised this practice role, claimed this practice territory as our own and had a single, focused, practice standard that still resonates with us today.

So what went wrong with this picture? What happened was that, arguably, all other nurses recognised the centrality of the interpersonal role, and we gained volumes of knowledge regarding the physicality of psychiatric illness. Because of P/MH nursing it became clear to all of nursing that attention to the individual within the context of the nurse–patient relationship was important, and it became apparent that emotional, psychosocial care was holistic care. The notion of attending to the individual slowly spilled into other nursing specialities. While this gift to nursing is one legacy of our profession, it cannot be allowed to be the final legacy of P/MH nursing.

As P/MH nurses we are diluted when others are performing and beginning to claim that which has been our central role, all at a time when we are failing to embrace new territory. Our failure is not in continuing to embrace the relational but in failing to expand, to develop from the initial contributions of our giants. P/MH nurses have yet to arrive at a consensus definition or operationally applied extraction of our roles and responsibilities for a new century (Keen 2003). We have not defined the interpersonal within the context of people with emotional and psychiatric disturbances or within neuroscience. We have not developed or implemented practice standards that say how and in what way the relational role is performed differently by P/MH nurses – differently with patients experiencing schizophrenia, for example, than with patients with cancer. We have not extended the basic Peplauvian standard of establishing a therapeutic relationship to standards of establishing a one-to-one relationship with the child of alcoholic parents who is homeless and at genetic risk for developing major depressive disorder. We have failed to define our discipline and in so doing are risking our relational birthright as P/MH nurses. If we do not soon claim our birthright it will slowly, inexorably and imprecisely slip away from us and be taken over by other health care providers and other subspecialities of nursing.

The power drain: the second compelling reason for standardised care

The advance of the evidence-based practice movement gives insight into the link between practice standards and power. Evidence-based practice has been embraced by almost every westernised country over the past two or three decades, fuelled by an ever-rising demand on limited resources. The clash of rising demands for health services and limited resources, including personnel, will ultimately be decided on the basis of power and it cannot be forgotten that knowledge is power. Practice standards reflect the current state of knowledge about best practice for a particular state of health. Nurses with clear practice standards, built on solid science and patient involvement, will be able to demonstrate economic impact and quality and therefore be able to broker resources for the health of individual patients (Sitzia 2001). The more that P/MH nurses reflect knowledge in practice standards, the more influential our subdiscipline will become. To date, P/MH nursing has few if any practice standards, and few evidence-based models of care (Stuart 2001).

The results of the power drain are evident all around us. P/MH nursing was once one of the most powerful of the specialities of nursing. This power translated to strong psychiatric content in curricula, representation at the table during discussions of research funding, programme and policy development, and new nurses wanting to go into P/MH nursing. This power is now being siphoned off by others. Without this power base, how do we collect and sustain power for political and professional advancement? How do we ensure that every psychiatric patient receives the best care, the most efficacious care, the best quality care, and that nursing students be exposed to the potential of P/MH nursing careers for themselves?

Rage and ethics: the third compelling reason for standardised care

The final compelling reason to develop and implement practice standards involves issues of rage and ethics. How much longer are we willing to accept the injustice of substandard care endured by most individuals with psychiatric disorders? In the USA, how much longer are we willing to accept that the majority of patients with psychiatric disorders receive their care from a non-mental health specialist, if they receive any care at all? When will we as a speciality group feel the rage that is ethically appropriate as a response to the present state of psychiatric care?

Why rage? We are acutely aware that psychiatric disorders constitute some of the most common, most expensive and most debilitating disorders known. There is a growing body of knowledge about the brain-based nature of these disorders, yet jails have become the largest mental health treatment centres. Criminalisation of mental health illness goes on unchallenged in any organised way by our discipline and continued acceptance of suboptimal care practices for the mentally ill goes on too, with no strong voice being heard from the P/MH nursing community. Known high levels of physical health illnesses still go unrecognised, underassessed and undertreated. Nursing curricula continue to cut out P/MH nursing content, or integrate it in such a way as to dilute it beyond recognition, all at a time when we are beginning to know more than ever about such states of health. In many schools of nursing in the USA, psychosocial experiences and content are seen as analogous to exposure to traditional P/MH nursing clinical experiences. Basic scientific content such as genetics, immunology and neuroanatomy continues to be lacking in our nursing programmes, making the utilisation of new knowledge unlikely for another generation of patients. The information for developing practice standards lies scattered at our feet. Uncollected and unstructured, it forms an ethical quicksand that indicts us as guilty of knowing, but not using, knowledge and of extending patient suffering needlessly. It is time to rage. Practice standards are inescapable and constructive, and we ignore their implementation at the risk of ethical pain.

Conclusions

It is time – almost past time – to standardise the practice of P/MH nursing. Of course, we need to be careful about non-individualised, 'cookie-cutter' care. Of course, we need to be sceptical and inquisitive about the source of the evidence that constitutes evidenced-based care. Of course, we need to know in advance that the practice standards of this year will either grow or constrict next year, as we know more or realise we now know less (Asplund et al 2002). Of course, we risk practice guidelines that are so vague or so rigid that they fail to provide useful boundaries for our practice. Of course, practice standards take a great deal of time, effort and political influence to develop, which may affect their relevance in an age of time-sensitive informational growth. Of course, different standards can be drawn from exactly the same information. Nevertheless, none of these factors looms large enough to obscure the reality that it is time to standardise practice. We need to define our speciality's area of practice. Our challenge is to have the courage to name the issues that confront us and prevent a move to standardisation. Our challenge is to own the problems we have; to identify, realistically, the size of the problems we confront, but to do this while rejecting the tendency to dismiss and shut out those with whom we disagree. We must find ways to be inclusive and incorporate the growing body of knowledge about psychiatric disorders as we move, together with our patients, to solve the problems we face.

P/MH nurses are uniquely positioned to play a fundamental role in delivering measurable, standardised, up-to-date quality care, whilst acting as advocates for our patients in an increasingly complex health care environment. The professional pressures on us will only increase and it will never get easier to standardise our practice. Dark clouds loom on the horizon, ominously signalling challenges to come from reductions in reimbursement and insurance coverage, ageing populations, decreased numbers of P/MH nurses, and expanded demands for electronic data collection and retrieval (Kirkman-Liff 2002). It will never get easier. If we do not do it, someone else will. The knowledge that encompasses P/MH nursing will migrate into the practice standards of other nurses and other health professionals. Our birthright, science and future are drifting away. We need to gather them back to the shelter of P/MH nursing practice standards.

References

American Nurses Association 2000 Scope and standards of psychiatric mental health nursing practice. American Nurses Association, Washington, DC.

Asplund K, Alton V, Norberg A, Willman A 2002 Vard I Norden. Nursing science and research in the Nordic countries 20(1):46–49.

Clingerman E 2000 Nurses in the new millennium. Michigan Nurse 73(8):20–22.

DiCenso A, Ciliska D, Cullul N, Guyatt G 2003 Evidence-based nursing: a guide to clinical practice. Mosby, St Louis.

Haber J 2000 Hildegard E Peplau: the psychiatric nursing legacy of a legend. Journal of the American Psychiatric Nurses Association 6(2):56–62.

Institute of Medicine 1992 Guidelines for clinical practice: from development to use. In: Field M J, Lohr K N, eds. National Academy Press, Washington, DC, p 45–64.

Keen T M 2003 Post-psychiatry: paradigm shift or wishful thinking? A speculative review of future possibles for psychiatry. Journal of Psychiatric and Mental Health Nursing 10(1):29–37.

Kirkman-Liff B 2002 Keeping an eye on a moving target: quality changes and challenges for nurses. Nursing Economics 20(6):258–265.

King I M 2000 Evidence-based nursing practice. Theoria Journal of Nursing Theory 9(2):4–9.

McCabe S 2000 Bringing psychiatric nursing into the twenty-first century. Archives of Psychiatric Nursing 14(3):109–116.

McCabe S 2002 The nature of psychiatric nursing: the intersection of paradigm, evolution, and history. Archives of Psychiatric Nursing 16(2):51–60.

Sitzia J 2001 Barriers to research utilization: the clinical setting and nurses themselves. European Journal of Oncology Nursing 5(3):154–164.

Stuart G 2001 Evidence-based psychiatric nursing practice: rhetoric or reality? Journal of the American Psychiatric Nurses Association 7(4):103–114.

Titler M G, Mentes J C, Rakel B A, Abbott L, Baumler S 1999 From book to bedside: putting evidence to use in the care of the elderly. Joint Commission Journal on Quality Improvement 25:545–556.

Against standardisation

Standards, standardisation and norms

The difficulty with arguing either for or against standardisation of care is that we need to agree what it is we are talking about. We need to standardise our understanding of the term:

'**Standardise** *verb trans* to make (things) conform to a standard; to test (a substance, etc) or ascertain the properties of (it) by comparison with a standard'   (Allen 2001, New Penguin English Dictionary)

Standardised care therefore conforms to certain standards:

'**Standard** *noun* a level of quality or achievement; a requisite level of quality; a norm used for comparison; a flag or banner

Standard *adj* denoting or conforming to a standard; sound and usable but not of top quality; denoting the smallest size of a range of marketed products; regularly or widely used, available or supplied'
                                       (Allen 2001, New Penguin English Dictionary)

The first problem with standards, then, is that they are just that: *standard*. This can be seen most clearly when we use the word as an adjective. Nobody wants standard (that is, average) care when they could have top quality care; nobody wants a standard (smallest size) hospital room when they could have a large or mega-sized room.

Clearly, however, when we talk about standardised care we are not using the term in a detrimental way. In fact, the word 'standard' derives from the Old French *estandard*, meaning a rallying point, usually a flag or banner on the battlefield. In its more typical and modern meaning, this banner around which we rally is usually metaphorical rather than physical. A standard is therefore an imaginary flag that we hoist as a sign of agreement about a requisite level of quality that we all find acceptable. One meaning of standardised care, then, is care that conforms to certain agreed standards of quality.

However, there is little point in standardising care if only a few are ever able to meet the standards, and so standards are usually set at a level that is potentially achievable by all, that is, at the *norm* for a particular group. As the earlier dictionary definition stated, standardised care is care that conforms to certain norms:

'**Norm** *noun* an authoritative standard, a model; a principle of correctness; a set standard of development or achievement, usually derived from the average achievement of a large group; a typical pattern of a social group'

(Allen 2001, New Penguin English Dictionary)

The word 'norm' derives from the Latin *norma*, literally a carpenter's square. To adhere to norms is therefore to ensure that everything 'squares up', that it is all the same. The carpenter who works with a square ensures that all of his cabinets are identical and, in a sense, perfect (or at least, perfectly square). However, more skilled craftsmen often eschew standards and norms and make judgements by eye, producing work that might not be perfectly square or 'normal', but which is nevertheless excellent. Clearly then, standardisation does not necessarily equate with excellence; what is being aspired to is not a level of *quality* that only a select few might achieve, but rather, a level of *conformity* potentially attainable by all.

Thus, standardisation of care refers to an agreed process that results in certain agreed standard outcomes. Indeed, standardised care more or less *guarantees* the agreed outcome. If we follow the standardised care procedures, then the standard care outcomes will inevitably be met, just as if we agree to use a square, all of our furniture will be of predictable shapes and sizes. If all P/MH nurses are following standardised procedures in their caring, then all of their patients can expect the same treatment and essentially the same outcome wherever and whenever they need it.

However, we have seen that standardisation might well be a guarantee of predictability and conformity, but it is not necessarily a guarantee of high quality. Standardised care aspires not to excellence, but to acceptability. In this chapter I will focus on the work of three theorists from fields other than P/MH nursing to emphasise this schism between standardised care and quality care. First, I will borrow from the work of the literary theorist Bill Readings (1996) to argue that standards and standardisation are concerned primarily with improving the health *service* rather than health *care*, and with administrative rather than therapeutic goals. Second, drawing on the work of social scientist George Ritzer (1993), I will argue that the drive towards standardisation is a form of 'McDonaldisation' that is primarily of benefit to the organisation rather than the consumer. And third, I will employ the work of philosophers and computer experts Dreyfus and Dreyfus (1986) to argue that standardisation might actually be *detrimental* to the patient, since it stifles creativity and expertise. These arguments will be presented with examples drawn from a UK P/MH nursing perspective, although I suspect that they will apply equally to other health care settings in other countries.

Standardisation and the administration of the health service

Readings (1996) has observed how, in recent times, notions of excellence in large organisations and institutions have become tied to standardisation, and has suggested that the selection of the criteria for standardisation has little to do with improving the quality of the service, and everything to do with its smooth administration. Although Readings was writing primarily about the institutions and discipline of higher education, his arguments can be applied equally to health care in general and P/MH nursing in particular. Even a cursory glance at recent UK Department of Health (DoH) reports and documents will reveal that most of the standards imposed on hospitals in the name of excellence by the UK government relate to health *service* improvements rather than directly to health *care* improvements, and can be achieved through more efficient *administration* rather than by more skilled *practice*.

This can be seen clearly in the National Health Service performance ratings (NHS 2002), in which stars are awarded for achievements such as reduced waiting times, improved discharge times and increased record keeping. The irony is that the stars are supposed to reflect *quality*, when in fact they are awarded almost solely for *quantity*. Where quality *is* considered, it is only to the extent that it results in faster throughput of patients and shorter waiting lists, and even then it is largely irrelevant whether short waiting lists and high throughput are the result of successful treatment leading to discharge or unsuccessful treatment leading to death. Hospital managers are therefore forced into directing resources away from care towards administration, and the role of the nurse, at least in the UK, is thus increasingly concerned with facilitating the smooth flow of patients through the system in the most efficient way rather than with providing the most effective care. Patients might well be seen by the service more quickly, in keeping with government standards, but the relocation of limited and finite resources in order to shorten waiting times and bed occupancy is likely to mean that the quality of the service that they receive is diminished.

This is a clear example of the way that the imposition of standards simply replaces issues of quality with those of quantity. My own local NHS Trust scored zero stars in 2002, and the new chief executive was quite explicit in stating that his primary aim was to *'build on the recent hitting of waiting list targets, to improve our all round performance,* so we can significantly improve our star rating' (Portsmouth Hospitals NHS Trust 2002, my emphasis). This he did (from zero to two stars in just one year), but there is little to suggest that the quality of care is any *better* (nor, indeed, that there was anything wrong with the quality of care in the first place); it is simply more *efficient.* It is perhaps churlish to complain about an improved star rating; after all, that is why the new chief executive was appointed, and he has clearly achieved his managerial objective. However, the danger is that management objectives are beginning to take precedence over health care objectives and patients are becoming the means to the end of government targets and standards rather than the end itself.

This same argument, that a political agenda of efficiency has replaced a clinical agenda of excellence, is apparent in the standards set in the National Service Framework (NSF) for mental health (DoH 1999), where we can see the same shift in focus from means to ends and from excellence to efficiency. Take, for example, the standard of preventing suicide (Standard 7), whose aim is:

'. . . to ensure that health and social services play their full part in the achievement of the target in Saving Lives: Our Healthier Nation *to reduce the suicide rate by at least one fifth by 2010'*   (DoH 1999, p 76)

What is seen to be of primary importance is the endpoint of a reduction in suicide by 20%. This is a managerial objective rather than a clinical one, concerned with meeting targets rather than with providing best care. There is no discussion in the document of whether it is always in the best interest of the patient to prevent suicide attempts, of the quality of life of those who survive attempted suicide, nor of the impact on that quality of life by the treatment intervention. The qualitative experience of the patient is not considered at all, only the quantitative outcome.

The only mention of quality (as opposed to quantity) in the entire section on Standard 7 is that suicide could be prevented by *'delivering high quality primary mental health care (Standard 2)'.* However, Standard 2 is concerned purely with the delivery of *effective* care to be measured by such instruments as the *National Psychiatric Morbidity Survey,* the roll out of NHS Direct (explained below) and *'the extent to which the prescribing of antidepressants, antipsychotics and benzodiazepines conforms to clinical guidelines'.*

It might seem self evident that we should aim to employ the most effective treatment methods, but this supposes that the *end* of suicide reduction is more important than the *means* by which such a reduction is achieved. Taken to its extreme, this position would advocate amputation of the arms to prevent a patient from cutting her wrists, or ECT to stop a patient from remembering why he wanted to die. These interventions would certainly be effective and efficient, and would perhaps help to achieve the target of suicide rate reduction. Furthermore, they are only different in degree from sanctioned interventions such as involuntary detention and forced administration of medication under the UK Mental Health Act (DoH 1983). In both of these cases, the means of denying the human rights of the patients is seen as justifying the end of preventing them from trying to kill themselves.

Perhaps the problem is with the notion of standards themselves. Standards have to be seen to be achievable, that is, they have to be measurable – and what could be simpler to measure than suicide rate? Indeed, one reason for selecting suicide rate reduction as a target from the myriad of other mental health issues might be the ease with which it can be assessed. Seen in this light, the driving force of mental health policy is political rather than therapeutic.

A better aim than the reduction of suicide might be to address the *causes* of suicide. Indeed, the NSF document clearly outlines many of these, including poverty, poor housing, unemployment and imprisonment. However, these are identified not in order to tackle them, but merely to identify those individuals most at risk of suicide so that they can be monitored and treated through risk assessment strategies, involuntary medication and admission to hospital for 'one-to-one' observation. This is rather like using a CAT scan to identify brain tumours so that those at risk of dying from them can be given painkillers. Furthermore, there is little consideration of whether the intervention might exacerbate the suicidal feelings; the only consideration is that those feelings are not translated into action.

To extend the point made by Readings about university lecturers, P/MH nurses are increasingly being employed not as healers or carers, but as administrators. That does not necessarily mean that they spend their time filling out paperwork (although many do), but rather that their role is to administer the patient through the system in such a way as to facilitate the achievement of government goals and standards rather than to address the mental health needs of the patient. In the case of suicidal patients, this entails merely ensuring that they do not have the opportunity to kill themselves, rather than addressing the psychological, social and emotional causes of suicide.

The 'McDonaldisation' of psychiatric and mental health nursing

I referred earlier to the definition of standardisation as conformity to certain procedures and norms. This approach has famously been referred to as 'McDonaldisation', which George Ritzer (1993, p 1) described as:

'The process by which the principles of the fast-food restaurant are coming to dominate more and more sectors of American society as well as of the rest of the world'.

The principles of McDonaldisation have been applied to many aspects of society, and relate well to the current state of the health service in general and P/MH nursing in particular. The concept of McDonaldisation is based on the principle of standardisation and offers the promise that the experience of buying a burger from an outlet in, say, New York will be identical to the experience of buying one in Moscow or Delhi. For McDonald's, this is a quality issue; the quality of the burger is defined not on a continuum from poor-tasting to good-tasting, but rather on a continuum from nonconformity to conformity to the McDonald's recipe, taste and presentation. The definition of a good quality McDonald's burger is one that looks and tastes the same as every other McDonald's burger. It may be possible to obtain burgers that taste better than McDonald's burgers, but ironically, unless they conformed to McDonald's standards, these would be deemed of unacceptable quality.

We might draw parallels here with the UK National Health Service. For example, the National Institute for Health and Clinical Excellence (NICE) sets standards for prescribing medication in the UK that are based on its definition of excellence as:

'. . . both clinical effectiveness and cost effectiveness. By focusing on the most clinically effective and cost-effective treatments, healthcare professions can deliver the best possible healthcare' (NICE 2003)

For NICE, excellence entails a consideration of cost, and some effective drugs are therefore *pro*scribed because they are too expensive to dispense on a regular basis. This, in effect, means that physicians can prescribe a drug in private practice that they cannot prescribe in the NHS, even though that drug might, in the physician's opinion, be the drug of choice for a particular patient. Thus, although it is possible for a patient to obtain better treatment privately than is available on the NHS, this treatment will, *by definition*, be of poorer quality as it does not conform to the standard of cost-effectiveness set by NICE; in other words, it is not a clinically excellent treatment. How does this affect P/MH nursing? Ritzer outlined four themes within the McDonaldisation process.

Efficiency

The first is efficiency, which entails reaching a predetermined end as quickly as possible and with the least amount of cost or effort. We have already seen from the NICE definition that efficiency in the NHS is usually justified as the most effective use of limited resources. However, for Ritzer, the real point of efficiency is that it is always in the interests of the service *provider*, but is promoted as of benefit to the service *user*. In the case of McDonald's, this includes persuading the customer to collect her own food, eat it from the box with her fingers, and clear away her own table. Not only does the customer end up doing work that was previously done for her, but she also pays for the privilege through having to queue, by getting ketchup all over her fingers and by taking on the role of an unpaid waitress.

In terms of P/MH nursing in the UK, the cynics among us might regard the entire 'care in the community' initiative of the 1990s (DoH 1990) as an exercise in efficiency and cost-cutting rather than as improving the care of service users. Indeed, care in the community was often cynically paraphrased as 'care *by* the community', emphasising the McDonaldisation strategy in which the customer performs tasks that have traditionally been carried out by the service providers. Similarly, more recent developments in the user/carer movement could be seen in much the same light, with the 'customers' (primarily the relatives of the service users) providing much of the care formerly delivered by paid P/MH nurses.

Calculability

Ritzer's second element of McDonaldisation is calculability, which *'involves an emphasis on things that can be calculated, counted, quantified'* (Ritzer 1993, p 19). Standardisation and calculability go hand in hand, since in order to verify that standards are being met, we need to be able to measure output. We have already seen that the NHS performance ratings reward achievements such as improvements in waiting times, discharge times and record-keeping rather than quality of care (NHS 2002), and I further suggested that targets such as suicide rate reduction (DoH 1999) might have been selected because they are relatively simple to measure rather than because they are the most pressing issues for mental health care. The concern for mental health nursing with this emphasis on calculability is that *quality* of care becomes a euphemism for *quantity* of care, so that, for example, the performance of community mental health nurses is judged according to the size of their caseloads rather than on the more ineffable and unmeasurable qualities such as their skills and expertise as practitioners.

Predictability

The above concern with valuing only qualities in the P/MH nurse that are measurable in a quantitative way is linked to Ritzer's third aspect, predictability. As we have already seen, predictability is a cornerstone of the McDonald's experience, and it is becoming equally important and valued in P/MH nursing. Clinical guidelines, evidence-based practice, care pathways and national service frameworks are all premised to some extent on the idea that care should be predictable; that the same situation should always be dealt with in the same way and that there is a single 'best' intervention for any given clinical problem, and a simple 'gold standard' methodology for judging competing interventions. Standardised care is, to a greater or lesser extent, predictable care. I will return to this issue later in the chapter when I discuss expertise.

Control through the substitution of non-human for human technology

For Ritzer, the fourth aspect of technological control is closely linked to the previous issue of predictability:

'Specifically, replacement of human by nonhuman technology is often oriented towards greater control. The great source of uncertainty and unpredictability in a rationalizing system are people – either the people who work within those systems or the people who are served by them.'

(Ritzer 1993, p 148)

To some extent, Ritzer's vision has been realised in the UK by the introduction of the NHS Direct telephone information scheme. When they telephone NHS Direct, patients are confronted with a disembodied voice on the end of a telephone, which dispenses advice based on predetermined computer algorithms, and it is surely only a matter of time before the system is fully automated and can dispose of human beings altogether.

However, P/MH nursing will always depend to some extent on mental health nurses, that is, on people. The point that Ritzer is making is not that people will disappear from service industries such as nursing, but rather that their role will be dehumanised. As Keel (2001) has observed, in a McDonaldised service:

'the human employee is not required to think, just follow the instructions and push a button now and then', such that 'the skills and capabilities of the human actor are quickly becoming things of the past'.

We have already seen how the telephone counselling service of NHS Direct has largely fulfilled Ritzer's criteria for a standardised or McDonaldised service by requiring human employees to 'just follow instructions and push a button now and then'. The advice given by NHS Direct workers clearly follows the trend for evidence-based practice, and therefore offers a model of clinical decision making for nursing and health care as a whole. It is again, perhaps, only a matter of time before all health care practitioners, including P/MH nurses, will have palmtop computers containing the same algorithms that are used by NHS Direct so that standardised solutions to standard problems are available to all at the touch of a button.

Such a system represents the 'holy grail' of standardised practice, since it ensures that all customers of the health services, like all customers of McDonald's, receive the same treatment and have essentially the same consumer experience. Furthermore, they are arguably receiving the intervention which scientific research tells us is the *best* for their particular problem. However, Ritzer points out that while such evidence-based practices might be more *rational*, they are nevertheless *unreasonable*, because '*they deny the basic humanity, the* human reason, *of the people who work within or are served by them*' (Ritzer 1993, emphasis added). Not only are mental health nurses dehumanised by such a rigidly technological approach to practice, but the service users are likewise dehumanised by the systematic application of a particular 'gold standard' of care regardless of the unique qualities of the individual recipient.

I have argued that Ritzer's analysis of the standardisation of the fast food industry has a number of resonances within the NHS and P/MH nursing, and suggests that health care is regarded as a commodity to be bought and sold rather than a caring or healing interaction between two individuals. In particular, there is a move towards the recipients of care providing many of the services previously considered to be the responsibility of the nurse (efficiency), towards the quality of care being judged in terms of crude numerical measures (calculability), towards the valuing of care interventions that are standardised and rigidly predetermined (predictability), and towards a dehumanising process in which care is based on predetermined computer algorithms rather than on the skills and expertise of the practitioner. This suggests that standardised care is in many ways the very opposite of expert care, which is seen as the domain of skilled and highly qualified nurses, is based on the experiential knowledge of those experts, and which cannot be measured or encapsulated by crude quantitative measures of output.

Standardisation and expertise

This brings me to my final objection to standardised care, which is that it is the antithesis of expertise. I have already mentioned expertise in relation to calculability, when I suggested that the expert who just knows the right thing to do is devalued because the rationale for her actions cannot be expressed in quantifiable and/or measurable terms. Thus:

'*In reality, a patient is viewed by the experienced doctor as a unique case and treated on the basis of intuitively perceived similarity with situations*

previously encountered. That kind of wisdom, unfortunately, cannot be shared and thereby made the basis of a doctor's rational decision.'
(Dreyfus & Dreyfus 1986, p 200)

Similarly, expertise is also devalued where (as Keel observed above) the human employee is expected simply to follow predetermined instructions. In the case of nursing, this might be to practise according to the recommendations from a meta-analysis of randomised controlled trials or according to an algorithm rather than according to her own body of experiential knowledge.

Dreyfus & Dreyfus (1986) have labelled such research-based care as novice practice and contrast it with expert practice that is based on an entirely different and non-rational (but nevertheless reasonable) process of 'pattern-matching'. According to Dreyfus & Dreyfus, we all start out as novices, having nothing on which to base our clinical decisions except what we have read in books or heard at lectures. As a novice P/MH nurse, my encounters with psychotic patients are determined by my theoretical understanding of psychosis and my procedurally oriented 'textbook' practice interventions. I have read that delusions should not be reinforced and have been told that I should respond to delusional behaviour in a non-judgemental but neutral way. I might even have been given a list of statements with which to respond to certain delusional remarks. In a perfectly standardised world, I could simply type the patient's remark into my palmtop computer and be presented with the ideal standard response.

However, Dreyfus & Dreyfus point out that expert practitioners do not operate in this way. Expert practice is intuitive, it is unpredictable (even by practitioners themselves) and it is tacit; the rationale for acting in a certain way to a certain situation cannot easily or readily be put into words. The expert will respond to the unique context in a unique way, and will almost certainly act differently each time, even in seemingly identical situations. Patricia Benner, who based much of her early work on the Dreyfus model of expertise, cites an expert P/MH nurse attempting to describe her practice:

'When I say to a doctor "the patient is psychotic", I don't always know how to legitimise the statement. But I am never wrong. Because I know psychosis from inside out. And I feel that, and I know it, and I trust it.'
(Benner 1984, p 32)

Expert behaviour, as described here, is the very opposite of standardised care. Indeed, we have seen that, for Dreyfus & Dreyfus, standardised care is novice care that the practitioner quickly grows out of.

Thus, a standardised process produces care outcomes that are standard in both definitions of the word. They are standard insofar as they are all the same and also in that they are *'sound and useable but not of top quality'* (Allen 2001, New Penguin English Dictionary). But, you might argue, why can't we have standardised care that is excellent rather than standard; why does standardisation necessarily result in mediocrity? The answer is to be found in the Dreyfus model's most important point about expertise. Although it presents a graduated five-stage path from novice to expert, it is not seen as a smooth continuum. Rather, there is a clear and fundamental break between the competent practitioner (Stage 3) and the proficient practitioner (Stage 4). As Benner (1984, p 37–38) points out:

'There is a leap, a discontinuity, between the competent level and the proficient and expert levels . . . formal structural models, decision analysis, or process models cannot describe the advanced levels of clinical performance observable in actual practice.'

In other words, the difference between novice practice and expert practice is qualitative rather than quantitative, a difference in kind rather than degree. An expert is not simply a more advanced novice; experts practise in a way that is fundamentally different. Novice practice is standardised practice based on formal models and decision analysis, but expertise is not achieved simply by raising the standards or improving the process. In order to become experts, we have to abandon the standardised procedures of novice practice for something fundamentally different. Just as McDonald's burgers might never be great if their cooks have to suppress their tacit knowledge and follow a standard recipe in a standardised way, so the very highest standards of care can only be achieved through non-standardised processes.

But, clearly, non-standardised processes produce non-standard outcomes, that is, outcomes that are neither predictable in advance nor of a uniform quality. Just as non-standardised practice can result in excellence, it can also result in poor or even dangerous outcomes. This is one of the reasons why standardisation was introduced in the first place; the point of standardisation is that it aims to guarantee safe practice by controlling and monitoring what practitioners do. Excellence is traded for safety; it is considered better to have everyone eating the same standard burgers than some eating 'cordon bleu' and others dying of food poisoning.

Perhaps this is only to be expected in today's litigious culture where individuals, organisations and governments are called into account for each and every mistake, and where far-reaching policy decisions are made in response to single isolated incidents. For example, the tragic case of Christopher Clunis, a diagnosed schizophrenic who killed a stranger without apparent provocation, prompted a media-driven characterisation of all schizophrenics as axe-wielding homicidal maniacs. This in turn, at least in part, resulted in the government introducing the care programme approach (CPA) to community mental health care in an attempt to prevent the recurrence of similar incidents through a standardisation of practice. As Dernedde (2003) argues, *'risk contain-*

ment (through improved communication) rather than improving provision for patients' needs is the vested primary objective of introducing CPA'.

But we have seen that, at least for Dreyfus & Dreyfus (1986), standardised practice will never result in true expertise. If we want all practitioners to aspire to excellence rather than mediocrity, then we must encourage expertise rather than standardisation. In other words, we must encourage them firstly to 'reflect-on-action', to explore their decision-making processes after and away from the practice setting, and then to 'reflect-in-action', to experiment reflexively in the midst of practice (Schon 1983). Rather than imposing novice practice on nurses, we should be facilitating them to make the qualitative leap from procedural to reflexive practice; rather than insisting that all nurses follow the same standardised patterns of care, we should be encouraging each nurse to practise creatively and uniquely in response to each unique clinical encounter; rather than attempting to control and monitor practice through procedures and algorithms, we should be encouraging and preparing nurses to monitor and control their own practice through reflection in and on action.

Conclusion

In my argument against standardisation in P/MH nursing, I have drawn on the work of three theorists. First, I took Bill Readings' (1996) critique of the American University and applied it to the current state of the UK National Health Service. In particular, I used his argument that practitioners are becoming increasingly concerned with administration, and argued that the government's agenda is with the improvement of health care *services* rather than health care *practice*. Seen in this way, the role of the practitioner is with the smooth facilitation of the patient through the service, and standardisation of practice is seen as a way of enhancing the *means* of service provision, often to the detriment of the *ends* of care. For example, the length of the wait to see the health care practitioner becomes a more important goal than the quality of the care received when the practitioner is eventually seen.

Second, I applied George Ritzer's (1993) analysis of the fast food industry to the health service. Unlike Readings, who observes that the means of facilitating the customer through the service has become more important than the outcome, Ritzer sees ends and means as inextricably tied together. Whereas for Readings the indicator of quality was the smooth administration of the patient through the system, the indicator of quality for Ritzer is the regularisation of the care process and outcome. Standardisation is therefore the means by which a standard outcome is achieved, and the fact that the outcome is predictable and controllable becomes more important than the quality of that outcome. So, for example, an assessment of risk of a suicidal patient is only of high quality if it is performed in a regularised way using a standardised risk assessment tool.

Finally, I drew on the work of Dreyfus & Dreyfus (1986) to show how this association of standardisation with quality is not only spurious, but is actually detrimental to the advancement of expert practice. I showed how, for Dreyfus & Dreyfus, standardised care is the antithesis of expert care, and that true expertise entails the rejection of practising 'by the book' in favour of intuition and reflection in and on practice. While this clearly entails a degree of risk, I argued that practice can never be entirely safe, and that the penalty to be paid for attempting to maximise safety is the loss of creativity, spontaneity and expertise.

Whereas standardised care implies controlled and predictable interventions, experts are erratic and unpredictable; they act according to tacit, internal and intuitive knowledge rather than public, propositional knowledge. That is not to say that they are unregulated or unaccountable, but rather that they regulate themselves. As we have seen, this entails risk, but in my opinion it is a risk worth taking. Moreover, it is a risk that we *must* take if we are serious about high-quality care. In order to impose external regulation on expert practice we must reduce it to measurable procedures and outcomes, and as soon as we do that, it is no longer expert practice. Rather than dragging experts back down to the level of novices by attempting to standardise what they do, we should be devising ways to raise novices to the level of expertise by freeing them from standardised practice and the achievement of standards that have little to do with quality care. That, surely, must be the challenge for P/MH nursing for the 21st century.

References

Allen R, ed. 2001 New Penguin English Dictionary. Penguin, Harmondsworth.

Benner P 1984 From novice to expert. Addisson-Wesley, Menlo Park.

Department of Health 1983 Mental Health Act. HMSO, London.

Department of Health 1990 National Health Service and Community Care Act. HMSO, London.

Department of Health 1999 National Service Framework for Mental Health. DoH, London.

Dernedde C 2003 Mental health: is the desire for safety driven by the needs of the mentally ill, by fear of litigation, or by bad press? Online. Available: http://www.critpsynet.freeuk.com/Dernedde.htm accessed 2003

Dreyfus H L, Dreyfus S E 1986 Mind over machine. Blackwell, Oxford.

Keel R O 2001 The McDonaldization of society. Online. http://www.umsl.edu/-rkeel/010/mcdonsoc.html accessed 2004.

National Health Service 2002 Performance. Online. http://www.nhs.uk/performanceratings accessed 2003.

National Institute for Health and Clinical Excellence 2003 Welcome to NICE. Online. Available: http://www.nice.org.uk accessed 2003.

Portsmouth Hospitals NHS Trust 2002 Welcome to our New Chief Executive. Online. http://www.portshosp.org.uk/text/news/chiefexec.html accessed 2002.

Readings B 1996 The University in ruins. Harvard University Press, Cambridge, MA.

Ritzer G 1993 The McDonaldization of society. Pine Forge Press, Sherman Oaks, CA.

Schon D 1983 The reflective practitioner. Temple Smith, London.

Commentary *Wendy Austin*

The debate about standardisation within psychiatric and mental health nursing is an intense one – so intense that one of the authors suggests that 'standardisation' is viewed by some as the 'antithesis' of psychiatric nursing. The strong language of the authors as they articulate the 'for' and 'against' stances suggests what may be at stake: the loss (or dilution) of power, birthright and future; the dehumanisation and the 'McDonaldisation' of care; the trading of excellence and expertise for safety and predictability. Dire consequences are seen by each if the opposing position is enacted. The fervency of the debate is a good indication that some foundational issues are at stake.

Within the debate, the positions taken tend to be all-encompassing, embracing not only the use of standardised clinical care plans but also standards of nursing practice for the speciality. It is the very idea of *standardisation* that is at issue: acceptance of common criteria, common language, and common trajectories and boundaries for action. *Common*, in fact, captures the essence of the disagreement over standardisation and P/MH nursing practice.

Common can mean *ordinary* and bear a derogatory connotation of *low class, vulgar, inferior* (Barber 1998). Common can imply a pulling down, a regression to the mean (with the emphasis on regression); it is movement away, not toward, innovation. It connotes mediocrity. Common stifles creativity. Yet, it is argued by the 'against standards' author, innovation and creativity are exactly what P/MH nurses need, for they must strive for excellence and view no patient's care as basic and ordinary. To allow nurses' expertise to be appropriately tapped, their professional autonomy must be protected, not reduced. Standards, as norms achievable by all, are like a carpenter's square, a tool that ensures predictability. Services conceived and delivered with a 'one size fits all' mentality rather than adapted to each 'customer' may be more cost efficient and easier to control, to measure and to evaluate, but are they more effective?

Concurrently, common also means *occurring often* and *belonging to the whole community* (Barber 1998). We share knowledge *in common*. Articulating, exploring and advancing the richness of this common knowledge offers enormous potential for the advancement of practice. Uniformity of care is a good thing, if it means that all patients are ensured that best practice is used in designing and evaluating their care, that expertise has shaped its basic design and delivery. All P/MH nurses, including novice ones, have the shared knowledge of the profession grounding their efforts to achieve safe, competent care and to make good clinical decisions. Identifying the common competences and understandings of P/MH nursing is a way to declare the scope of our speciality's practice and to focus the direction of our research. Failing to do so, the pro-standardisation author argues, puts our legacy and our professional authority in jeopardy.

Standards of practice

Standards of practice do have significant influence on the development of a discipline. They are the explicit expectations that a professional group holds for its members and comprise the claims the group makes to the public regarding its specialised knowledge and skills. Nursing practice standards clarify nurses' accountability and serve as a basis for performance evaluation. These are important functions. They are, perhaps, particularly important when designating an area of speciality within a discipline.

About a decade ago, I was involved in the development of the first Canadian standards of practice for psychiatric and mental health nursing (Austin et al 1996). As a required component for national certification as a designated speciality by the Canadian Nurses Association, P/MH nursing practice standards had to be created. To achieve designation, the Canadian Federation of Mental Health Nurses (CFMHN) also had to identify their unique knowledge within the field of nursing, define the population for which they provide care, and the specific techniques and measures that they use.

I became, through a flurry of circumstances, the Chair of the CFMHN committee created to develop the standards. It was in facing this responsibility that I realised how cavalierly I had, up until then, viewed nursing practice standards. They were on my bookshelf, but I seldom referred to them. They seemed so obvious to me; I took them for granted. The challenge of articulating the standards of our speciality, however, changed that attitude of indifference forever. My involvement in the identification of competences essential to P/MH nursing practice and in the challenging process of stating clearly the roles and functions that are based on our specific knowledge and skills made the power of standards visible to me.

Standards of practice are a declaration we make to ourselves, our colleagues and the public. Our assumptions about our practice are made evident; for example, our practice is situated in the therapeutic relationship and the primary intervention is 'therapeutic use of self'. Our standards differentiate us from other professional groups and can be used to call us to account. As such, they must be realistic and attainable within the context of our current health care system, yet directed by our aspirations for future possibilities. In the Canadian standards of practice, the autonomy of the individual nurse had to be acknowledged and it was made explicit that each nurse would meet the practice requirements according to their chosen nursing model.

It was not possible to create such a document without accessing a wide range of P/MH nursing expertise from across the country. Once created, an opportunity arose for the competencies to be sent to randomly selected Canadian P/MH nurses (practitioners, administrators, educators and researchers), who were asked to rate each competency in terms of significance and frequency of use. The results of this survey indicated that the competencies captured our practice: no competencies were removed and none added.

The CFMHN keeps their practice standards current by continuing to revisit, revise and republish them as our knowledge and skills evolve. They have been used as a basis for the blueprint of the Canadian P/MH nursing credentials examination, as a foundation for P/MH nursing curricula, as the criteria for performance evaluations, and as a document that informs staffing requirements. I personally know that they were used to defeat a challenge to the holding of a therapist position by a nurse rather than a member of another health discipline. There is power in having declared standards. Acknowledgement of that power means that we need to be highly attentive to the processes of their development and use.

Standardisation and the mapping of care

Our suspicions about the ways in which standardisation can be implemented, however, are well grounded. They come from our experience. In the mid-1990s in my part of the world, 'care maps' were promoted as a means of reducing costs and of improving quality of care. It seemed to many of us that the former, not the latter, was the primary focus for their use. Although care maps enabled the development of typical clinical pathways based on research evidence and clinical experience, some contained generalisations too broad to be of real use. The most extreme example of this for me was nursing documentation proposed to support a care map for the inpatient care and treatment of a person with a major depressive disorder. It had a box for 'insight' that was to be checked (or not) by the patient's nurse during each shift. For me, this component revealed a serious lack of insight into the concept of 'insight'! This potential for reductionism is what concerns opponents to standards of care.

They foresee standardisation of practice used as a means to restrict ingenuity, resourcefulness and sensitive responsiveness to patients. Insight becomes a 'yes' or 'no' state on a checklist; treatment day ('Is it Day 1 or Day 4?') determines nursing actions; the patient's score on an assessment rating scale identifies their 'problem'. With standardisation, the care journey becomes a fixed tour.

Viewing standards as 'maps of care' can be useful when we reflect on the up and down sides to their use. Consider the metaphor of a map. What is a map? A map is a representation of some aspect of reality that serves as a tool for navigation, as a guide to journeys and travel, as a marker of territories and boundaries. As representations, maps necessarily contain distortions. Choices have to be made regarding what will and will not appear on a map. It is vital to recognise the use for which a particular map was designed. I would not attempt to drive across Canada using a flight map, nor a map of the world: what I would need to know would not appear on them. I would want a road map (maybe several as Canada is a big country), one designed to scale and indicating the roads I can choose to take. I *could* attempt the journey without a map. There would be road signs along the way and I could stop and ask others for directions. On the whole, however, I am more likely to complete my journey safely if I have the information provided by a good, up-to-date, accurate and suitable map.

Maps, however, are not only travel tools; they are political statements of a kind. Maps show our boundaries, for example: 'If I cross this road, I enter a foreign land; my status changes'. Maps show claims to territory, revealing power and relationships. When I was a child, Commonwealth countries were coloured pink on our classroom maps. These were the areas of the earth with which Canadians had an alliance; pink indicated our friends. A Chinese child's classroom map, no doubt, looked different at that time. It is important to understand whose view of the world a map reflects.

If we understand standards as maps, as shared visions of our current, evolving reality, marking territory (scope of practice), relationships (accountability) and agreed-upon best routes (best practice), we may be able to develop and use them well. The recognition that they are only guides must stay before us. That nurses will need to take 'the road less travelled' at times must also be recognised and strongly defended. We need to stay conscious of the political and power issues that are encompassed in any standards and what they signify about our accountability to the public, colleagues and one another. We must be attentive to who is designing our standards, attentive to the values that are used to colour them. Standards should support and protect those values, not subvert them.

Aristotle (1996), writing about ethical action, said that '. . . *agents themselves have to be able to consider what is suited to the circumstances on each occasion, just as is the case with the art of medicine or navigation* (II-ii, 5)'. Nurses, when choosing how to act, bring the shared knowledge of nursing (reflected in standards) and their own personal knowledge (acquired through lived experience) to the context of practice. Their professional freedom to choose how to act in the context of each particular circumstance must be safeguarded. Standards can only be guides to that choice.

Conclusion

In the standardisation debate, foundational issues are at stake. Yet we are not, it seems to me, in an either/or situation. The 'pro-standards' argument shows us the power of shared standards that can facilitate best practice and support accountability. The 'against standards' side warns us what can happen if that power is misused, applied rigidly or oppressively: non-individualised care, lacking in sensitivity to each unique patient. The commitment to nursing excellence shown by both sides of the debate suggests that the debate itself can serve as a means to revitalise our understanding of practice in our speciality. It can contribute to our evolution toward excellence.

References

Aristotle 1996 The Nicomachean ethics. Wordsworth Classics, Ware, UK.

Austin W, Gallop R, Harris D, Spence E 1996 A 'domains of practice' approach to the standards of psychiatric and mental health nursing. Journal of Psychiatric and Mental Health Nursing 3:111–115.

Barber K 1998 The Canadian Oxford Dictionary. Oxford University Press, Don Mills, Canada.

An appropriate, useful and meaningful research paradigm for psychiatric/mental health nursing: the qualitative–quantitative debate

CHAPTER 18

Qualifying psychiatric/mental health nursing research

Chris Stevenson

CHAPTER 19

'Pro' quantitative methods (on being a good craftsperson)

Nigel Wellman

Commentary

Philip Burnard

Editorial

This debate will have appeal for a variety of individuals, not least because, in the true style of good debating, the chapters raise as many questions as they answer. What is certainly interesting is that the huge shift towards the evidence-based mental health care movement has imposed serious limitations on the old style 'freelance' P/MH nurse meandering through his or her clinical day doing a little of this and a little of that, without there ever being any checks or balances to establish the efficacy of such practice. Well, that's a good thing, isn't it? Possibly, say our authors, but while agreeing with the principle of position they also posit alternatives to what this clinical *free spirit* ought to be doing instead. This should come as no surprise as it is but a microcosm of the debate that has raged within many of the nursing journals over the past few years.

Yet, notably, if one steps outside of the world of P/MH nursing, one finds that few other disciplines are even considering such a debate. Indeed, in the USA, Hysong et al (2005) saw no problem in defining the nature of guideline development (historically the quantitative icon of evidence-based medicine) by undertaking a large piece of qualitative research. In the UK, this would probably have been seen as heresy by some sections of the professional community, with calls for Hysong and colleagues to be burnt at the stake! The principal pessimism concerning the others' chosen method appears to be a construct based upon likes and dislikes, with some individuals expressing vehemence akin to 'kill the viper and the contents of the nest will die also'. In itself this is a strange position because we are, after all, talking about people whose core discipline is nursing. It is strange that such strong feelings should be generated by an approach to undertaking research, presumably designed to enhance nursing actions.

But, herein lies a clue to solving this puzzle. Most P/MH nurses did not become members of the caring discipline because of their mathematical abilities. As such, their natural inclination is towards organic, human and nominally humanistic activities, caring being one of them and, presumably, 'people-oriented' research being another. The formulation of a defence for qualitative approaches has to take this into consideration if it is to justify fully the not insignificant research of this type that has been undertaken by the profession over the years. Similarly, exponents of the quantitative approach cannot simply adopt the pseudo-political stance of decrying the position of their qualitative counterparts as a suitable defence for their own position. The absence of any real cohort of quantitative researchers within the ranks of the practitioners suggests that they have carried the qualitative banner because of their natural preference for an approach that fits better with their way of thinking, not necessarily their educational preparation. We must explore the approaches adopted by other professional groups and the fit that is produced when comparing this to the nature of the work they do.

Our three authors explore all of these options and argue them in their own inimitable style. At the end of the day it is our decision as to which approach, or combination of approaches, is most appropriate, but the debate itself makes for very interesting reading.

Editorial footnote

Apropos Chris' remarks on page 315, the editors note that for some, qualitative research *does* produce scientific knowledge/evidence.

Apropos Nigel's remarks on page 324, the editors note the well established and crucial differences between nomothetic and idiographic generalisability. Further, the reader is directed to relatively recent developments in qualitative meta-synthesis, for example the workshops undertaken under the auspices of the Qualitative Research Methods group of the Cochrane Centre, http://www.cochrane.org (see Booth A. 2005 (recovered 2006) Minding the qualitative and feeling the width: identifying qualitative research for inclusion in systematic reviews).

References

Hysong S J, Best R G, Pugh A J, Moore I F 2005 Not of one mind: mental models of clinical practice guidelines in the veterans health administration. Health Service Research 40(3):829–847. http://www.cochrane.org

Mills E, Wilson K (recovered 2006) Systematic reviews of qualitative studies: heresy or necessity. http://www.cochrane.org

Noyes J, Popay J (recovered 2006) Methods for synthesising qualitative data. http://www.cochrane.org

Qualifying psychiatric/mental health nursing research

History is not destiny

In this chapter I am taking a strong position on the nature (useful) of knowledge in nursing. Why? Formal nursing is a new discipline compared with the classical sciences, medicine, the arts and humanities. Understandably, it has been a practice in search of a theory that would progress its identity. In its newness, nursing has in many respects borrowed the ideas of positivism, of linear, scientific progress towards a disease-free state found in medical research and practice. This is consistent with modernity (Rolfe 2001), wherein knowledge is seen as being encapsulated by science; the production of knowledge by means of systematic and objective study of phenomena which subsequently leads to nomothetic generalisable laws.

The laws are logically linked together as theory. The positivist paradigm entails a strong definition of realism as:

'. . . the position that reality exists, can be discovered by people in an objective way and thus strongly determines what we know'

(Stevenson 1996, p 104).

In short, the assumptions of science-based (modernist) nursing are that there is a correct (real) practice that can be detected, represented and theorised about, and then offered as a foundation for (evidence-based) practice. The love-children of this relationship are the randomised controlled trial, experimental and quasi-experimental design, large-scale survey, etc. These are seen as *'the highest forms of evidence'* (Rolfe 2001, p 39) and something that researchers should aspire to, according to Gamble & Wellman (2002). Many such studies are related to the effectiveness of psychological therapies as practised by therapists or nurses. The research 'evidence' has encouraged nurses to ally themselves to psychological therapies and to become specialists, for example, as cognitive behavioural therapists or in psychosocial interventions. In adopting the evidence base of the specialism comes the status from owning legitimate knowledge, that which is authorised by its scientific underpinnings. However, the degree to which such specialist practice can be considered nursing remains an area of debate.

It may seem that this is research 'game over'. But history is not destiny. Alongside the proliferation of quantitative studies is the recognition that nurses still fail to use such evidence in practice (Stevenson 1996). Why? Although formal nursing is a new discipline, the craft of caring (Barker 1999) has been around for centuries. Caring is a complex concern and it is not readily exposed by research methods that manipulate and control events in order to establish cause-and-effect relationships. This may be why some psychiatric nurses have rejected it:

'I think that psychiatric nurses have found research irrelevant because it has been conducted through an objectivist process and been concerned with measures that simply have not reflected nurses' own needs in relation to practice. Psychiatric nurses want to understand more about the complex dynamics of their work . . . [such] understanding could not solely be achieved by quantitative, objectivist/realist methods that reported outcomes'
(Stevenson 1996, p 105).

If nursing is a contested arena with contrasting camps of specialists (therapists) and crafters of care, it is not surprising that there is difference in the kinds of research interest. In that knowledge and power are intimately linked (Foucault 1980), some nurse researchers can be described as engaging in a political struggle in relation to the dominant ideas about evidence-based practice. In a sense, qualitative research is a resistance to the authorised version of what constitutes nursing knowledge and how that knowledge is achieved. Rather than trying to apply scientifically driven evidence across care settings, the qualitative researcher furnishes the nurse (often one and the same person) with theory that is embedded within local practice and with a low level of generalisability. Modernist nursing research is anchored in the possibility of objectivity. This excludes practitioners themselves from undertaking research into aspects of their own practice, as this would be open to the criticism that objectivity had been compromised. Yet, as Reed & Proctor (1995) point out, insider researchers have an informed perspective on their practice area and know what questions need to be answered. They can contribute to *'the body of nursing knowledge'* (Reed & Proctor 1995, p 30). But the conduct of insider research usually creates concerns amongst more modernist colleagues. It is seen as subjective, biased, unreplicable and ungeneralisable. However, this lack of appreciation may be more to do with a fear of practitioner research as resistance to the dominant paradigm than concern over its legitimacy per se. To a great extent, qualitative nursing research discourses do not describe reality but *'systematically form(s) the objects of which they speak'* (Foucault 1974, p 49):

'To be in control of your own discourse means that you have power over what you want [your discipline] *to be rather than accepting what others say it is; this consequently empowers you, not them'*   (Jenkins 1991, p 71)

As well as offering more pragmatic theory in relation to 'going on with' practice, qualitative research reports that touch the clinical soul of nurses may lead to the re-authoring of nursing knowledge, threatening the research and practice status quo. I return to writing and rhetoric as a means of challenging the dominant discourse of science later in the chapter. First, I look at how nurse researchers can create meaningful theory.

Making meaningful theory

Let us begin with a story . . . CS has a patch of eczema on her left foot:

'I have no other patches on my body. Irrespective of the medical facts about the skin condition, I have a narrative about it. It goes something like this. My eczema is intelligent. It 'knows' that it can survive so long as it stays somewhere where it is not highly visible. It has chosen the left foot because my right foot already has an injury. It limits its site and significance. It acts as a barometer for my more general and mental health. We live together'.

Now consider how we might apply research to the individual with eczema. The quantitative researcher might be interested in:

- How frequently patches of eczema only on the (left) foot occur in the general population. This would tell the researcher how typical or atypical CS is.
- What is the nature of the eczema (as determined by comparison with standard descriptions of eczema 'forms' already established through previous research)? This would tell the researcher what kind of eczema CS has and how common or rare it is in relation to incidence and prevalence.
- What is the preferred treatment (as determined by reference to a systematic review of existing studies – Cochrane Library)? This would be the basis of evidence-based intervention.

CS says:

'No amount of information about diagnosis/treatment will persuade me to act against the eczema. My story works (is real) for me'.

Blumer (1986) noted that when we believe something to be real or true then real consequences flow from the belief. From another perspective, CS might be seen as 'treatment resistive'. However, such an analysis makes two assumptions:

- That the researcher/practitioner knows what is best for the person
- That the evidence regarding diagnosis and treatment is 'real'.

The first assumption is an account based in medical hegemony. In other words, the dominance of medical over other explanations of the world is assumed. But this is not meaningful or helpful in this case. What are the implications of this?

'Human beings live "in language" in the same way that fish live in water' (Anderson & Goolishian 1988, p 56). In order to connect with the person in care, the nurse cannot apply preformed theory/evidence that has no meaning for the individual. Nurses seem to need 'peculiar' knowledge. Cronen & Chetro-Szivos (1998) suggest that the 'findings' from qualitative research operate in a similar way to case law, where a new principle of law is developed from a single case. However, the law is reviewed in relation to its continued applicability in the light of each new case to which it is applied. By presenting the nursing community with a rich set of possible understandings (gained from experiential accounts, ethnographic study, etc.) there is the possibility of finding a story that (partially) fits for the person in physical or psychiatric distress. This story can be modified *in vivo* in order to make it more relevant. In other words, if we want to understand complex human action, we need to explore the reasons (narratives) people have as causes of meaningful behaviour and be prepared to engage in dialogue towards reaching a shared understanding.

Such action is possible because the world is not represented in our language in a straightforward way. de Saussure (1916/1983) notes that there is always a gap between the signifier (the word or act) and the signified (the concept to which the signifier refers). Together, the signifier and the signified make up the sign that points to an object of reference (Stevenson & Beech 2001). For example, cat is the signifier (word) that *I choose to use* when communicating about what *I believe* is animal, four legged, furry, purring, clawed, etc. Together, the word and concept help me to refer to an object in the physical world. However, I could equally well use the word 'coral' instead of 'cat', to refer to my conceptualisation. The word does not in any way embody the concept. For this reason, language is always ambiguous. It has a meaning in use, which accrues through the willingness of people to support it. The 'meaning in use' is sustained so long as it is helpful in carrying on with our forms of life.

An example of the problems of trying to represent the world in words is found in the Diagnostic and Statistical Manual IV (American Psychiatric Association 1994). In this version of the taxonomy of psychiatric distress, a wider range of biopsychosocial factors is incorporated in arriving at diagnostic categories that are said to represent an illness state. The function of this has been to expand the territory of psychiatry and psychology *'invading that behavioural area once differentiated as "healthy" or "normal"'* (Holmes & Warelow 1999, p 167). The flip side of such inclusiveness is the removal of previous categories, for example homosexuality, masturbation and some types of intellectual disability. If diagnoses in some way represent an 'illness reality', then it is difficult to account for why such reclassification occurs. Once delimited, a category should hold good for all time for a critique of diagnosis, science and power. A more tempting explanation is that DSM in all its versions embodies socially constructed categories relevant to particular contexts and circumstances (Holmes & Warelow 1999). If this view is accepted, a different order of conversation about illness can occur. The conversation does not focus on assessment of symptoms (often through an inventory) in order to match them up to a category and/or measure severity, but seeks to understand the individual illness experience. Of course, this is the domain of qualitative research as well as clinical practice.

The second assumption rests on the belief that scientific knowledge is possible, in scientific or epistemological hegemony. Put simply, how we know about the world is thought to be best achieved by scientific method. To explore this further, I turn to the issues of diagnosis and treatment in postnatal depression. Positivist research may tell us what the incidence of postnatal depression is, what 'type' of woman is more likely to exhibit symptoms and what treatments are deemed to be most effective. The outcome measures improved by treatment are predetermined by the researcher and are allegedly amenable to objective measurement. However, what this scientific research cannot do is illuminate the experience of women who are labelled as having postnatal depression. An appreciation and understanding of such experiences is of equal (if not greater) value to psychiatric nurses working with women than more scientifically derived knowledge that a particular drug is likely to reduce depressive symptoms.

The quality of qualitative research

In this section of the chapter I want to deal with the problems that arise when qualitative research is compared to quantitative research, drawing on the work of Lyotard (1984). I am treating quantitative and qualitative approaches as discourses. Discourse is defined as *'a loose network of terms of reference which* construct [original emphasis] *a particular version of events and which* position *subjects in relation to these events'* (Willig 1999, p 160). According to Rolfe (2001), Lyotard describes a dispute *within* a particular discourse, for example qualitative research, as a 'litigation'. The dispute can be settled with reference to the rules of that discourse. For example, a disagreement as to whether an ethnographic description is more useful than a grounded theory can be settled with reference to whether the approach is 'fit for purpose' (in generating rich description rather than substantive theory) without implying *general* inferiority or superiority. However, this does not apply when two positions are incommensurable – when like is not compared with like, as occurs when quantitative and qualitative approaches are compared.

'Lyotard (1984) described this impasse as "le différend". Put simply, there are no rules equally applicable to each position which would allow a comparison between the positions' (Stevenson & Beech 2001).

Quantitative and qualitative research are underpinned by different paradigms. Put more simply, when the scientific tradition is brought to bear in evaluating the contribution of qualitative research, an inappropriate evaluative assessment is made, and vice versa. Such evaluations are political, in the sense that they serve to power or disempower. Shotter (1993) notes that when conversations become formalised into a particular discourse ideological processes are likely to benefit some groups over others. Cooper and Stevenson (1998: 484) have pointed out that '. . . *scientific knowledge in our society is seen as legitimate and disciplines adopting scientific methods as respectable'*. Referring to psychology, they argue that the desire to be *'squeaky clean'* as a discipline '. . . leads to a *'tidying away'* of discrepant forms of knowledge, by overlaying them with science.

Lather (1991) points out that traditional ways of knowing and of being known necessarily involve a political dimension that includes some self-serving bias. Thus, when there is an orthodox, legitimated approach to knowing about the world, other approaches become subjugated. For example, ethical committees are firmly attached to the idea of scientific research. They lack understanding in relation to qualitative approaches, because they do not value the kind of knowledge that would be generated. They work from a position of epistemological hegemony, as described above – scientific knowledge is better than all other knowledge (which is seen as not really being knowledge at all). This inequality has given rise to a number of questions including those of Stevenson and Beech (2001):

'Do traditional ideas about truth become a normative imperative for all researchers? Who are the authentic voices in knowledge production? What benefits do they gain? How do non-traditionalist researchers establish their authority?' (Stevenson & Beech 2001, p 144).

Cutcliffe & Stevenson (2001) suggest strategies for ironing out *le différend* in relation to conflicts between qualitative researchers, ethical committees and grant-awarding bodies. Their advice is to use *'weasely words'* to engage with the grammar or language game of the committees, or to use a structure that will not seem too alien to the assessors. For example, the sacred cows of quantitative research, validity and reliability, can be recast as 'rigour'. This is a pragmatic approach, yet it may not go far enough.

An alternative is to engage the sceptic in a dialogue about validity, for example: *'What aspects of validity are particularly important to you and why do you think they should be emphasised?'* Such an inviting question allows the knowledge or assumptions underpinning the quantitative language game to be exposed, allowing for a dialogue to begin and the qualitative researcher to engage the quantitative in a different way. Because of *le différend*, simple argument will not be convincing. Instead, I think that challenging the authorised voices of research means convincing people through the power of rhetoric, the beauty of writing, the creativity of metaphor, the cutting up of previously accepted textual structures (Rorty 1989). Such devices invite people to think about something in a different way, to create a 'third' story, which 'connects' the conflicting grammars, even though the receiver may be challenged in adopting a different perspective. Thus, the quantitative researcher may be moved to resite her/himself within the qualitative paradigm in order to make an assessment of qualitative work rather than sniping from the 'quantitative sidelines'.

Faith, hope but no charity

My concern in this chapter is that critiques of qualitative research in nursing may serve to conserve a particular dominant paradigm. By explicitly favouring quantitative approaches, they are *'a self-descriptive, externalising of the ideology of the day'* (Rorty 1982, p 1–2), in that they foreground science over art, diminish the contribution of non-standard methodologies, etc. Rolfe (2001) argues that the meta-narratives of modernity (including quantitative approaches to knowledge production) justify a particular story about the world (as something external that can be represented objectively), but simultaneously justify a story about modernity itself. Thus, modernity's ideas are true simply because it says they are true. This is an irrational argument, based in faith and hope, and the more paradoxical because modernity itself entails a belief in the importance of rationality.

Yet, living in faith and hope does not seem to impact much on modernist, quantitative researchers. Why? In order to answer this question, we turn to the issue of authority. It may be the case that we live in a decentred universe, as Derrida (1974) claimed. In our postmodern world, battered by information, it seems to be the case that there is no final and absolute authority by which to judge competing ideas or knowledge claims, as argued above. Szasz (2000) suggests that the authority of the church in relation to deciding right and wrong was overtaken by the state when Enlightenment thought came to the fore. The power of the state was intimately related to rationalism as an important underpinning of science. Thus, the power of the state and scientific knowledge went hand in hand, as Foucault (1980) pointed out. This legacy has given the people in power the scope to decide what counts as knowledge, and they have foregrounded modernist science.

Thus far, the hegemony of modernist nursing research has had far-reaching effects. The expert researcher presides over the practitioner, who is superior to the patient. Qualitative research opens up the opportunity for a more democratic research arrangement. To some extent, this already is happening – in emancipatory and participatory and feminist research (Lather 1991).

In conclusion: possibility not probability

Given my arguments about the social construction of knowledge, it would be self-contradictory for me, the author, to suggest the definitive answer in relation to how nursing research and the production of knowledge might be undertaken. How we know will be emergent from particular sociocultural–political contexts. To present my accounts as something special would be to:

'. . . present another authorised version (grand narrative) of the nature of knowledge, from the academy. To do so would be to present a different marginalising discourse. According to Lyotard (1984), what counts as knowledge is less important than an analysis of how the decision is made about what is classed as real, and of whom has the authority. For what is classed as not real becomes second class'

(Stevenson & Beech 2001, p 144).

In the spirit of reflexivity invited by the quote, I note that the context set by the commission for this chapter has positioned me as a champion of qualitative research, and so, understandably, I have made the case for its authenticity in the field of nursing inquiry. However, I prefer to think that I have offered some accounts that can be placed alongside the critiques of qualitative research/knowledge in order to allow you, the reader, to make your own judgement.

References

American Psychiatric Association 1994 Diagnostic and statistical manual IV. APA, Washington.

Anderson H, Goolishian H 1988 Human systems as linguistic systems: evolving ideas about the implications for theory and practice. Family Process 27:371–393.

Barker P J 1999 The philosophy and practice of psychiatric nursing. Churchill Livingstone, London.

Blumer H 1986 Symbolic interactionism. University of California Press, Los Angeles.

Cooper N, Stevenson C 1998 'New science' and psychology. The Psychologist 11:484–485.

Cronen V, Chetro-Szivos J 1998 Pragmatism as a way of inquiring with special reference to a theory of communication and the general form of pragmatic social theory. In: Perry D, ed. American pragmatism and communication research. Erlbaum, New York.

Cutcliffe J, Stevenson C 2001 The long and winding road: obtaining funding for qualitative research proposals. Nurse Researcher 9(1):52–62.

Derrida J 1974 De la grammatologie. Minuit, Paris [English translation: Of grammatology (trans. G. Chakravorty Spivak). Johns Hopkins University Press, Baltimore].

de Saussure F 1916/1983 Course in general linguistics (trans. Roy Harris). Duckworth, London.

Foucault M 1974 The archaeology of knowledge. Tavistock, London.

Foucault M 1980 Power/knowledge: selected interviews and other writings 1972–1977 (edited by Colin Gordon). Harvester, London.

Gamble C, Wellman N 2002 Judgement impossible. Journal of Psychiatric and Mental Health Nursing 9:741.

Holmes C A, Warelow P 1999 Implementing psychiatry as risk management: DSM-IV as a postmodern taxonomy. Health, Risk and Society 1(2):167–178.

Jenkins K 1991 Re-thinking history. Routledge, London.

Lather P 1991 Getting smart. Feminist research and pedagogy with/in the postmodern. Routledge, London.

Lyotard J-F 1984 The post-modern condition: a report on knowledge. Manchester University Press, Manchester.

Reed J, Proctor S 1995 Practitioner research in health care. Chapman & Hall, London.

Rolfe G 2001 Postmodernism for healthcare workers in 13 easy steps. Nurse Education Today 21:38–47.

Rorty R 1982 Consequences of pragmatism. University of Minnesota Press, Minneapolis.

Rorty R 1989 Contingency, irony, and solidarity. Cambridge University Press, New York.

Shotter J 1993 Conversational realities. Sage, London.

Stevenson C 1996 Taking the pith out of reality. Journal of Psychiatric and Mental Health Nursing 3:103–110.

Stevenson C, Beech I 2001 Paradigms lost, paradigms regained: defending nursing against a single reading of postmodernism. Nursing Philosophy 2:143–150.

Szasz T 2000 Psychiatric power. In: Barker P J, Stevenson C, eds. The construction of power and authority in psychiatry. Butterworth Heinemann, Oxford.

Willig C 1999 Introduction: making a difference. In: Willig C, ed. Applied discourse analysis: social and psychological interventions. Open University Press, Buckingham.

Nigel Wellman

'Pro' quantitative methods (on being a good craftsperson)

Introduction

The quantitative versus qualitative debate in P/MH nursing research has been going on for many years, often driven by seemingly irreconcilable ideological differences about the nature of P/MH nursing and thus about the nature of the research that P/MH nurses should or must undertake. Pragmatically, the nature of a research question being asked will often determine the appropriateness of the methodology to be used in attempting to answer that question. Some types of question can be answered only by using qualitative methods, whereas other types of question can be answered only by using quantitative approaches, and this remains true regardless of *who* carries out the research (i.e. professionals and/or service users), and regardless of *why* the research is being carried out. Some types of question require mixed quantitative and qualitative methods, and there are other questions that are potentially open to either qualitative or quantitative approaches but which may be answered more efficiently, effectively or reliably by one approach than by the other. There are numerous textbooks that will set out at length the nature, strengths, weaknesses and appropriateness of different research approaches under a wide range of conditions. This chapter will not seek to emulate those texts, and also does not seek to denigrate qualitative approaches to P/MH nursing research. This chapter aims to set a broad context in which the strengths and weaknesses of both approaches can be appreciated and in which both approaches may find their rightful place.

Well conducted qualitative research can provide a different kind of evidence to that of quantitative approaches such as cross-sectional or cohort studies, or randomised controlled trials (Williams 2002). In Williams' (2002) view, the types of questions that qualitative approaches can best address include questions about what exists, i.e. about people's beliefs, experiences, expectations and attitudes to and about all aspects of health care and health-related behaviours. Qualitative approaches are especially useful in elucidating the 'insider perspective' on health issues and can be enormously useful in generating new concepts and precise definitions of key issues. Qualitative research can also help illuminate processes of change and decision-making through the systematic collection and analysis of people's accounts of why they do the things they do. Qualitative studies that help to define the nature of particular problems may precede quantitative methods in programmes of research, and may also be employed to help explain or make sense of the findings of quantitative studies. Despite these many benefits, qualitative studies are highly vulnerable to personal biases (Watson 2003). When carried out inappropriately, qualitative studies tend to have small sample sizes, do not produce generalisable findings, and generally do not produce reliable findings in areas such as the proportion, or number, of people who do X or who do X because of Y. Gournay (1999) argues that they do not produce reliable findings with regard to questions such as whether particular approaches to training, or to the organisation or delivery of care, that may be popular with their recipients in the short term actually help or harm them in the longer term.

For several decades mental health researchers from all disciplines studying reports of clinical trials have worried about publication bias, particularly that small studies and studies with negative or equivocal findings tend not to get published. However, with qualitative research, small studies abound and sometimes receive a level of attention completely unjustified by their size and lack of methodological rigor. In the field of qualitative research, unlike with quantitative data, there are also no agreed methods of meta-analysis, with some theorists arguing against the possibility of developing meta-analytic approaches on theoretical grounds.

The nature of psychiatric/mental health nursing research

P/MH nursing is relatively young as a discipline; P/MH nursing research is younger still. The current state of P/MH nursing research reflects the immaturity of both the profession and of nursing academia. Until comparatively recently in the UK, career progression for P/MH nurses generally meant leaving patients behind and becoming either a nurse manager or an educator, and there are still only very restricted career pathways for nurse researchers or nurse clinician-researchers. Until the arrival in the UK mainstream of the consultant nurse role in the year 2000 (Department of Health 1999), the clinical career pathway for most nurses petered out at clinical nurse specialist level. Historically, only a relatively small percentage of nurse educators have been trained in research or research methods, and fewer still have been research active and publishing on a regular basis. In my opinion, most current nurse researchers conduct and publish qualitative rather than quantitative research studies and it is apparent that many active nurse researchers have a poor understanding of the strengths and flexibility of a full range of quantitative methodologies.

One aspect of the immaturity of nursing as a discipline has been a long-drawn-out identity crisis, marked by repeated attempts by various commentators to define the 'essence of nursing', to produce definitive statements of what P/MH nursing is or should be, or conversely what it is not or should not be, and to define what nurses do, should do or should not do. This enterprise of attempting to construct a core identity for nursing, separate from other health and social care disciplines (in this case psychiatry, psychology, social work, etc.) has resulted among other things in the production of numerous 'nursing models' and growing amounts of 'nursing theory'. This growth in theories of nursing and attempts to describe, define or perhaps petrify nursing has included attempts from various quarters to define on ideological grounds the kinds of question that nurses should research and the methods they should employ in their research.

Repeating previous findings, the most recent Research Assessment Exercise or review of the quality of university-based academic research in all subjects undertaken by the UK's Higher Education Funding Council failed to identify any world-class (five star) P/MH nursing research departments in the UK (Higher Education and Research Opportunities 2001). Research conducted by P/MH nurses has so far had only a very modest impact on clinical practice, and less impact still on health policy and resource allocation at the governmental level. A number of senior figures from psychology and psychiatry have privately remarked to the author that they have difficulty conceptualising what world-class P/MH nursing research would look like and that nurses need to adopt research methods (i.e. quantitative research methods) that produce reliable and generalisable findings, and seek opportunities for multidisciplinary collaboration if they are to compete for research funding – a view that has been echoed by some senior P/MH nurse academics (Gournay 1999, Watson 2003). This issue, that of lack of confidence in the robustness and reliability of nursing research, is undoubtedly one of the reasons why P/MH nursing research has so far attracted only very low levels of financial support from statutory, charitable and other research-funders in the UK.

Feeding into and exacerbating this problem is the lack of training in research methods, particularly in quantitative approaches and statistics, in the education of nurses, including UK P/MH nurses. This educational deficit leads to poor confidence and ability on the part of P/MH nurses in understanding and interpreting research studies, systematic reviews and meta-analyses that use quantitative data (Parahoo 2000). The difficulty that many nurses have in understanding quantitative/ numerical data stands in marked contrast to the ease of reading of the reports of many qualitative studies. In my opinion, it needs to be pointed out that ease of reading of research reports does not necessarily correlate with the quality of the research reported. Poorly conducted qualitative research will tell the reader much more about the prejudices of the researcher than the feelings, views and experiences of the research participants, and nursing is cursed by the uncritical acceptance of poor-quality and unreliable qualitative research (Watson 2003). Further complicating the issue is the fact that the randomised controlled trial evidence which many nurses most commonly encounter is that from trials of psychiatric drugs. Most of these trials are conducted by pharmaceutical companies for regulatory or marketing reasons. These drug company-sponsored trials are often subject to spin, for example through the use of inappropriate comparators, through utilising large numbers of outcome measures and reporting only those outcomes that appear favourable to the sponsoring company's product, or through multiple publication (Marshall 2002). This issue – that of the fundamental ability to understand and critically evaluate numeric data (Parahoo 2000) – is undoubtedly more acute in nursing than in many other health disciplines. This has arisen, in my view, because of serious deficits in contemporary nurse training and education, and particularly because most contemporary nurse educators are not statistically literate and lack confidence and enthusiasm in handling and teaching the analysis and critical appraisal of numerical data.

The nature of psychiatric/mental health nursing practice

P/MH nurses are the largest single group in the UK mental health workforce. There are many different views and ideological perspectives of what nursing is, what it is about, and of what nurses should or should not do. Despite this, it seems undeniable that in all health systems P/MH nurses work closely with individuals experiencing mental distress and who are seeking relief from that distress. Nurses also work closely with individuals whose thoughts, feelings and behaviours are felt to be disturbed or abnormal by those around them, or whose unusual conduct causes conflict, distress or danger to others.

When dealing with distress, we live and practise in a world of choice. For every action that we take in good faith, that is, every action taken in the hope or anticipation that our work will relieve the distress of our patients, there is an infinite number of alternative actions that we could take. That we practise in a world of choice remains true regardless of whether we describe the things we do with patients, and how we do those things, as care or treatment, or nursing or interventions or conversation . . . or any other term at all.

We also live in a world of cause and effect, or, at the very least, of action and reaction. Our actions produce effects, real effects – good and bad for our patients. Those patients think about, reflect on and are influenced by the things we say to them, the ways in which we interact with them, and the respect that we show to them. Our patients are also influenced by the medications we administer to them or the supportive observations we conduct to try to keep them safe and supported through times of crisis. Some of the courses of action we take are more effective than others in relieving the distress of our patients and in helping them to recover their hope and autonomy. Some actions we take will directly or indirectly harm our patients, and may even on occasion contribute to their untimely death. Indirect harm includes harm caused to patients by squandering limited resources on ineffective interventions or organisational patterns – thus wasting their (and our) time and denying them use of those resources for potentially beneficial approaches. Actions and health interventions that have the potential to harm patients include all nursing interventions, all psychological and 'psychotherapeutic' interventions, as well as all drug therapies and other somatic treatments.

We also live and practice in a world where resources are, in almost all cases, limited and often inadequate, and where mental distress is painfully real and at times may seem almost overwhelming. In this world in which we practise, populated as it is with human individuals in mental distress, we have a duty to use our limited resources wisely, to take the approaches most likely to help our patients through their distress while reducing to a minimum the harm that we cause them. In seeking to do more good and less harm, evidence from well conducted research studies can help give us guidance as to the approaches most likely to benefit our patients. In fact, I argue, much of the evidence that we need to help guide our practice can come only from research studies that use objective quantitative methods, including experimental and quasi-experimental approaches such as that of the randomised controlled trial. In the UK, evidence from well conducted randomised controlled trials has become the 'gold standard' of evidence in health care, because the randomised controlled trial is a highly flexible, powerful and robust tool (Thornicroft & Tansella 2002). The value of this tool lies in the fact that it can be used to test and measure the efficacy of virtually all imaginable health-related interventions or ways of organising the delivery of health care, including almost all aspects of nursing care. The major limitations to what can be tested in this way lie mainly in the imagination of potential trialists rather than in the method(ology) itself. The randomised controlled trial is also an excellent tool for detecting short- and long-term damage caused by health-related interventions, including psychological interventions, and can produce robust, generalisable conclusions with regard to both the likely help and the likely harm that may result from any particular approach to care.

In working with patients we proceed by trial and error. Every attempt we make to keep a patient safe through a suicidal crisis, or to help them manage their hallucinations or reduce their feelings of depression and despair, or to reduce the impact on the life of their obsessional symptoms or improve their social skills and self-esteem damaged through stigma and hospitalisation, is in effect a clinical trial with one participant. In this view, nursing is a pragmatic discipline. It is concerned not only with how patients and carers feel about their problems, but also and fundamentally with improving their clinical and personal outcomes through the things that we as nurses do with our patients and the ways in which we do those things. It is possible to adopt a 'lowest common denominator view', i.e. that mental health nursing is simply concerned with providing patients with fairly low-level psychological support and with ensuring that they stay safe, eat and drink adequately, take prescribed medications, receive welfare benefits, etc. In this view, P/MH nurses simply maintain patients while it falls to others such as psychiatrists, psychologists, occupational therapists or psychotherapists to work with the patients in systematic, deliberate and focused ways to help them overcome their problems. In this lowest common denominator view, nurses may assist in monitoring the effects of treatment but take little active role in it beyond administering medications and ensuring that patients get to therapy appointments on time. This type of view also implies that nurses who undertake training in specific psychological therapies cease to be nurses and become therapists instead. If you take the view that nursing, as a pragmatic discipline, should be concerned not just with basic patient maintenance, but also and fundamentally with the relief of distress and the promotion of change and personal growth in our patients, then it becomes impossible not to be concerned with outcomes and the measurement of outcome, i.e. with knowing whether your practice helps or harms your patients.

The history of mental health care is a history in which almost every generation has tried to do its best to help people afflicted with mental health problems, and almost every generation has been condemned by its successors for the inadequacy and/or the brutality and/or the sheer absurdity of the approaches to helping adopted (Porter 2002). Against this background we also know that over the decades patients suffering from mental distress have often been extremely grateful for the care, interventions, treatments and 'therapies' that they have received, regardless of whether or not those approaches have actually had any beneficial effects at all. We also have good reason to believe that patients have often expressed gratitude in the face of manifest harm caused by these approaches, including harm caused by milieu and talking therapies (Masson 1989). Against this background it seems likely that many of the things we do today with our patients may also be harming them in a range of ways, some obvious and direct, and others more indirect or more complex, subtle or long term and difficult to detect. The wisdom of hindsight is cheap, but if we are to do better in future, if we are to move on as a profession, we have to use the full range of qualitative research methodologies to describe more fully what we do and how we do it. Further to this, it is also vital that P/MH nurses come to be able to judge the real effects of their work with unique individuals, in the complex environment of practice on their long-term health and social functioning. According to Gournay (1999), to accomplish this it is essential for P/MH nursing to adopt robust quantitative approaches to the measurement of the effects and outcome of nursing, including the use of a range of experimental methods such as the randomised controlled trial, as well as cohort and correlational studies.

The place for quantitative studies

When well conducted, quantitative research methods, including randomised controlled trials, cohort and correlational studies, provide information that allows us to determine whether and by how much the actions we take in our professional lives are likely to help or harm our patients. From the service user's perspective, these approaches help to determine how much the available treatments, care or systems are helpful or harmful to service users as a group. As with qualitative research, quantitative research work can be undertaken by service user researchers and by professionals in collaboration with service users. Although there is not yet much of a tradition for this, it seems certain that in the future clinical trials and other quantitative studies will be conducted in ways that empower mental health service users and include them as full partners in the research process. Compared with the use of quantitative methods, in my view, qualitative approaches generally cannot answer these types of question, or would be highly expensive and inefficient in generating relevant data, although qualitative approaches can certainly add explanatory richness to quantitative outcome data.

These types of study again help us determine what types of intervention are most likely to help our patients and which ones to avoid if we do not wish to harm them. These types of study can guide us when faced with practical day-to-day clinical questions. An example of such a question would be that of how a community P/MH nurse working with a patient with a relapsing psychotic disorder can best help the patient to avoid future relapses. One aspect of this work, additional to the nurse's work on psychological symptom management, arises from the knowledge that taking antipsychotic medications promotes a better outcome for the majority of patients with relapsing psychotic disorders. There are now trials in the nursing literature that demonstrate ways of working with such patients to help them achieve optimal symptom control with minimal side-effects through the use of concordance promotion (see, for example, Gray et al 2003). Another example of this would be that good-quality quantitative research can help guide the ward manager or senior nurse of an acute psychiatric inpatient unit as to what type of support, debriefing or other intervention they should offer to patients and colleagues who have been distressed or traumatised by a serious violent incident on their unit if they want to maximise the chance of their coming to terms with the incident and minimise their chance of developing post-traumatic stress disorder (PTSD). The answer to this type of question is not immediately obvious, cannot be answered reliably by qualitative methods, and recent research has demonstrated that some types of intervention, which until very recently were commonly delivered to victims of trauma, and often delivered by nurses to other nurses, are at best ineffective and at worst may actually increase the risk of later developing PTSD (Nhiwatiwa 2003, Rose et al 2003).

Research and nursing models

P/MH nursing suffers from a severe shortage of high-quality quantitative data in almost all areas of contemporary practice. A good example of this would be in relation to the use of nursing models in psychiatric inpatient units. Over the past two or three decades a number of nursing models, including those produced by Peplau (1988), Neuman (1982), Roy & Andrews (1991), Orem (1995) and others, have been introduced into clinical practice, and subsequently adopted by various providers of mental health services and taught to nursing students in their colleges and universities. Despite the fact that very considerable resources have been devoted to their implementation, there is currently absolutely no reliable evidence that demonstrates whether or not the adoption of any specific nursing model improves the quality of mental health nursing care in inpatient units and thus improves patient outcomes, or whether the use of these models harms the interest of patients by squandering limited health resources on systems that produce no clinical gains (Gamble & Wellman 2002).

Library shelves groan under the weight of textbooks describing nursing models, and there are many articles in the nursing journals written by devotees of particular nursing models. The enthusiast authors of these articles seem often to have put huge efforts into qualitative exploration of the apparent benefits accruing from their introduction into various clinical areas. The only way genuinely to test whether the introduction into practice of any nursing model makes a real difference to patient outcomes would be to use both qualitative and appropriate quantitative measures in a carefully planned and fairly large-scale clinical trial (Gamble & Wellman 2002). Such a trial would need to compare two or more different models head to head against one another, and perhaps also against alternative or adjunctive approaches such as the use of care pathways or other control conditions. Such a trial would specify the outcomes of interest in advance, agree how these outcomes would be measured and by whom, and have a planned sample size, calculated to ensure that adequate statistical power would be achieved at predetermined levels of statistical significance for the estimated effect sizes. Possible confounding factors including unit size, staffing and demographic variables would also need to be controlled in the study design.

The measurement of outcome would also be conducted by research workers without any vested interest in any particular approach or model. It is worth noting that despite massive criticisms of the corrupting influence of the vested interests of the pharmaceutical industry, who conduct and report clinical trials of their own new products, the authors of many studies of nursing models, like the authors of a lot of the reports of innovations in care found in the literature, generally fail to disclose, discuss and report their own vested interests, including financial interests in the success of particular models or approaches. The inherent subjectivity of qualitative methods, their lack of controls and the fact that it is enthusiasts for particular models who produce studies confirming their value highlight their limitations in these areas. To paraphrase Watson (2003), when did a Marxist researcher ever not conclude that their work demonstrated the reality of class oppression, or a feminist researcher find that patriarchal oppression was not at work?

Crucially, if the evidence base of P/MH nursing is to move forward in this area, the design of such a trial would also need accurately to measure, and where possible control for, variables such as staffing levels, skill mix, and the training and educational inputs given to nursing staff. This latter point is vital, for it is possible and perhaps even likely that it is the non-specific motivating effects of increased education and training that lie behind most, if not all, of the benefits for the introduction of nursing models to units found in the literature, rather than anything intrinsic to any particular model (Gamble & Wellman 2002). With appropriate data collection, the control for most of the possible confounding variables could be done statistically, reducing the need for very tight matching of participating wards and units, and mental health nurses would finally have reliable data on whether there is anything intrinsic to the use of nursing models that improves patient care and promotes better clinical outcomes.

Research and supportive observations in inpatient care

Another example drawn from UK practice, in which good clinical trials using quantitative or mixed methodologies are urgently needed, relates to the use of supportive observations in acute inpatient areas. Currently, in England, the government, through the Standing Nursing and Midwifery Advisory Council (SNMAC), advises the use of four levels of nursing observation; these are:

'• *Level I:* General observation
  • *Level II:* Intermittent observation . . . [this] *means that the patient's location must be checked every 15 to 30 minutes (exact times to be specified in the notes). This level is appropriate when patients are potentially, but not immediately, at risk. Patients with depression, but no immediate plans to harm themselves or others, or patients who have previously been at risk of harm to self or others, but who are in a process of recovery, require intermittent observation.*
  • *Level III:* Within eyesight
  • *Level IV:* Within arm's length'   (SNMAC 1999, p 3)

However, if you step north over the border from England into Scotland, official recommendations with regard to the use of intermittent observations change. The Clinical Resource and Audit Group of the Scottish Executive in their document entitled 'Engaging people, observation of people with acute mental health problems' (ScotCRAG 2002) recommend three levels of observation:

  • *General: the staff on duty should have knowledge of the patients' general whereabouts at all times, whether in or out of the ward.*
  • *Constant: the staff member should be constantly aware of the precise whereabouts of the patient through visual observation or hearing.*
  • *Special: the patient should be in sight and within arm's reach of a member of staff at all times and in all circumstances.*
                                                        (ScotCRAG 2002, p 2)

The ScotCRAG (2002, p 7) document went on to say that:

'After much discussion the group agreed that timed observations do not contribute to the safety of the observation process although being aware of a patient's whereabouts contributes to good general nursing practice.'

So, within the UK, whether the use of timed intermittent observations is considered good practice and is recommended by government differs completely depending on which side of the English/Scottish border you stand! Despite the worldwide prevalence of formal observations in acute inpatient practice, despite the enormous financial cost of formal observations, and despite widespread and growing concerns about the use of formal observations, in the whole mental health nursing literature there is only one small and uncontrolled trial of any serious alternative to the use of formal nursing observations (Moran 1979). Despite growing claims that certain patterns of ward organisation reduce the need for the use of formal observations (see, for example, Dodds & Bowles 2001), there are no controlled studies, let alone randomised controlled studies, to test whether there are alternatives to formal observations that can be used safely and effectively, or whether certain patterns of ward organisation actually do reduce the need for formal observations. This is a core and fundamental area of inpatient nursing practice that cries out for the use of quantitative approaches, particularly in the shape of large multicentre controlled trials, to enable the science of mental health nursing and the practice of mental health nursing care to move forward together.

Aids to effective decision-making

Another way or area in which quantitative research is valuable is in the use to which the results of such research can be put in everyday clinical practice. Understanding the results of controlled trials, epidemiological and cohort studies helps us to give valid answers to questions from patients about how likely drug X or therapy Y is to help with their difficulties. This kind of information, when pitched at the right level and made available in understandable ways, empowers patients to evaluate the possible risks and benefits of proposed courses of action so that they can make informed choices about their treatment and lifestyle. These benefits accrue not just in relation to actions and interventions proposed or undertaken by nurses and other health care practitioners, but also and very powerfully in relation to lifestyle choices. An example of such choices would include the choice for a patient who has experienced several psychotic episodes as whether or not to continue to smoke cannabis. In working through such choices, motivational approaches including the construction with the patient of a cost–benefit analysis of the 'good' and 'not so good' aspects of cannabis use, informed by reliable quantitative information about the percentage risk of relapse for users and non-users of cannabis, may have a powerful influence on future health-related behaviour and thus on personal and clinical outcomes.

Conclusion – using the appropriate tool for the job at hand

I believe that most research published by P/MH nurse researchers in recent years has employed qualitative approaches, and this seems likely to continue for the foreseeable future. Nonetheless, as has been emphasised above, there are many questions about core areas of P/MH nursing practice that urgently need answers and that either cannot be answered at all, or cannot be answered sensibly and efficiently using only qualitative methodologies. Currently, however, in my opinion there are signs of an upsurge of interest in the use of quantitative research methods in P/MH nursing research and there are growing numbers of nurse researchers conducting high-quality studies that employ quantitative methods, including that of the randomised controlled trial. These studies may at last begin to address some of the yawning gaps in our knowledge of what helps and harms in our daily practice and in service planning.

There is an old saying that if the only tool you have is a hammer then everything begins to look like a nail. Contrary to this, a good craftsperson will generally have a range of tools in his or her toolbag and will use whatever tools are most appropriate to get a job done and done well. In this chapter I have argued that P/MH nurse researchers need to be less like the person with only a hammer and more like the good craftsperson, keeping a range of tools in their toolbags. I fear that purist researchers from either the qualitative or the quantitative camp would have us throw out many valuable tools on ideological grounds and that P/MH nursing will be the poorer if this happens.

References

Department of Health 1999 Making a difference. Department of Health, London.

Dodds P, Bowles N 2001 Dismantling formal observation and refocusing nursing activity in acute inpatient psychiatry: a case study. Journal of Psychiatric and Mental Health Nursing 8(2):183–188.

Gamble C, Wellman N 2002 Judgement impossible. Journal of Psychiatric and Mental Health Nursing 9(6):741–743.

Gournay K 1999 The future of nursing research will be better served by a shift to quantitative methodologies. Clinical Effectiveness in Nursing 3:1–3.

Gray R, Wykes T, Gournay K 2003 The effect of medication management training on community mental health nurse's clinical skills. International Journal of Nursing Studies 40(2):163–169.

Higher Education & Research Opportunities 2001 Online. Available: http://www.hero.ac.uk/rae/index.htm accessed 2004.

Marshall M 2002 Randomised controlled trials – misunderstanding, fraud and spin. In: Priebe S, Slade M, eds. Evidence in mental health care. Brunner-Routledge, Hove, p 59–71.

Masson J 1989 Against therapy. HarperCollins, London.

Moran J C 1979 An alternative to constant observation: the behavioral check list. Perspectives in Psychiatric Care 17:114–117.

Neuman B 1982 The Neuman systems model: application to nursing education and practice. Appleton-Century-Crofts, Norwalk.

Nhiwatiwa F G 2003 The effects of single session education in reducing symptoms of distress following patient assault in nurses working in medium secure settings. Journal of Psychiatric and Mental Health Nursing 10:561–568.

Orem D E 1995 Nursing concepts of practice, 5th edn. Mosby, St Louis.

Parahoo K 2000 Barriers to, and facilitators of, research utilization among nurses in Northern Ireland. Journal of Advanced Nursing 31(1):89–98.

Peplau H E 1988 Interpersonal relations in nursing. Macmillan Education, London.

Porter R 2002 Madness: a brief history. Oxford University Press, Oxford.

Rose S, Bisson J, Wessely S 2003 Psychological debriefing for preventing post traumatic stress disorder (PTSD). (Cochrane Review). In: The Cochrane Library, Issue 4, John Wiley, Chichester.

Roy C, Andrews H A 1991 The Roy adaptation model: the definitive statement. Appleton & Lange, Stamford.

Scottish Executive Clinical Resource and Audit Group (ScotCRAG) 2002 Engaging people, observation of people with acute mental health problems. A Good Practice Statement. Scottish Executive, Edinburgh. Online. Available: http://www.scotland.gov.uk/library5/health/opmh-02.asp and http://www.show.scot.nhs.uk/CRAG accessed 2004.

Standing Nursing and Midwifery Advisory Council 1999 Practice guidance. Safe and supportive observation of patients at risk. Department of Health, London.

Thornicroft G, Tansella M 2002 Mental health services research. In: Priebe S, Slade M, eds. Evidence in mental health care. Brunner-Routledge, Hove, p 81–100.

Watson R 2003 Scientific methods are the only credible way forward for nursing research. Journal of Advanced Nursing 43(3):219–220.

Williams B 2002 The role of qualitative research methods in evidence-based mental health care. In: Priebe S, Slade M, eds. Evidence in mental health care. Brunner-Routledge, Hove, p 109–125.

Commentary

Philip Burnard

In the 'pro' qualitative chapter (Ch. 18), the writer offers a postmodern critique of the (perceived) quantitative research position. In setting out to critique it in this way, it is, perhaps, inevitable that a very *particular* and strong view of qualitative research is set up – to be knocked down. Arguably, most qualitative researchers are much more cautious about their findings and their analyses than might be understood from this chapter. I doubt, too, whether many quantitative researchers make claims to having elicited any sort of 'truth' from their work. As with other forms of research, the researcher is normally merely offering a view of his or her findings, a tentative model of what *might* be going on. What that researcher cannot, of course, be responsible for, is what others make of his or her research.

Clinical decisions, both nursing and medical, are never made purely on the basis of recorded evidence of best practice. The skilled practitioner has to juggle many factors: what the patient is saying, what he or she is doing, how he or she appears to be, the patient's preferences, the patient's life situation, what the practitioner's experiential knowledge tells him or her *as well as* what the research literature says. Similarly, the medical practitioner, like the pharmacist, will always be on the look out for idiosyncratic reactions to any drug treatments. In some cases, too, based on experience, the practitioner will choose to *ignore* the research findings. If treatment was simply a case of applying the knowledge base to a particular patient, we could employ a clerk to search a database and prescribe accordingly.

Instead, clinicians act as scientists (Kelly 1955) – and pragmatic ones at that. They pose the question: 'What can I do to help this person?' They then identify the options, apply one, and later evaluate the effectiveness of that decision. If the 'treatment' has worked, the clinician may stop it, do more of it or, if it has not worked, change the prescription. The point, of course, is that all clinical work involves *judgement* and not simply the application of research findings. And that rule of 'judgement' applies to any interpretation and use of research findings. In deciding whether or not to accept and use a particular research finding, we are all likely to make a range of judgements about its suitability in *this* case. Clearly, those who use research findings are not robots trained *only* to pay attention to the research evidence base.

I confess to having some misgivings about what some psychologists do. They often take an abstraction (e.g. 'mind'), reify it (or treat the abstraction as if it had concrete reality), develop another abstraction (e.g. 'self-esteem' or 'self-awareness') and develop a questionnaire to test the degree to which people 'exhibit' that abstraction. Similar examples of the 'turning an abstraction into a thing and measuring it' are: empathy, hardiness and even stress. This approach is, of course, fraught with problems. People are wondrously variable. Because I am a certain way today does not mean that I will be that way tomorrow. Similarly, the way I fill in a questionnaire today is not indicative of how I might fill it in tomorrow. Psychological research of the type that attempts to 'measure abstractions' seems to me to be disingenuous at best, and dishonest at worst. The scope for compounding errors in this process seems immense.

Similarly, in nursing research, of recent years, we have seen attempts to explore and even to define abstract concepts such caring and suffering – mostly through the use of qualitative approaches. One of the writers in these two chapters is cautious of the concept sometimes discussed: that of the 'essence of nursing'. Of course, such an 'essence' (even if we accept that it is possible to have such a thing) will always be dependent on how we *define* nursing. We cannot assume that we all share a defined nursing in which, somewhere, is buried this essence. Thus exploration into essences of this sort are likely to be explorations into the researcher's own view of what nursing might be. Others, of course, might argue that 'nursing is what nurses do' and not attempt to posit an 'essence' for it.

The point also needs to be made, perhaps, that, given that humans are so variable and that the physical world of our environment may be less so, we must exhibit great caution in applying quantitative methods to a study of human behaviour. However, there seems to me no reason why we cannot use such methods in a more general way. For example, it seems reasonable to do some counting of people if we are planning a new hospital and want to know what the bed complement should be. On the other hand, really to understand other people seems to be out of reach of pure quantification. However, that should not lead us to the view that qualitative methods *will* take us to such an understanding either! In some debates about quantification and qualification, the debate seems to take on an almost *moral* edge, with both parties claiming they are 'right', in the ethical as well as the rational sense.

The rather slippery position adopted by the writer of the 'pro' qualitative chapter leads her to the unsatisfying (but inevitable) position of 'I cannot offer a definitive ending to this piece: I merely raise these issues to allow you to decide for yourself.' And, of course, if the reader (or the writer) *does* decide, then that reader (or writer) is guilty, too, of taking a strong position! The problem with postmodern debates, in my view, is that, while they undermine any strong position, they also leave the commentator unable to take any position for him or herself. Or, rather oddly, the reader can take *any* view. The writer's *own* view can, of course, always be undermined by another reading of that view. And so it all goes on, in a never-ending spiral, that ultimately takes us nowhere particularly useful.

The point, I suppose, is twofold. First, research methods can be decided by research questions. The data collection and data analysis methods that are chosen can be determined by the question: 'What do I need to do to answer my research questions?' There should, I think, be no attempt to set oneself up as a 'qualitative' researcher – as if qualitative methods are going to help answer all research questions. This is as blinkered a view as the view that the *only* research worth doing is quantitative.

Second, we need to be able to get on and *do* research. If all we can offer is a general undermining of any particular position, we may reduce the impetus to do anything. No piece of research is in any sense perfect. All we can do, perhaps, is to be as systematic as we can and attempt to represent the people we are engaging in our research as honestly as possible. That we will never find a means of undertaking an ultimate analysis of people and their work is a given. But, we can, at least, make an attempt at an understanding of them. The person who constantly quotes that the 'perfect piece of research is yet to be done' is likely to be right, but is also likely not to attempt any him or herself. Research is a messy business that never produces definitive answers, only further questions for further exploration.

In my view, while we cannot offer nomothetic generalisations from qualitative research, its findings do offer us an illumination or a description of some aspects of the human situation. However, qualitative researchers should also be careful that they do not, subtly, include nomothetic generalisations from their findings. It is not uncommon for such researchers to end their research reports by stating that their findings 'should help inform practice/teaching/assessment' and so on. Although their findings may be of interest to such practitioners and teachers, it is something of a leap of faith to assume that the findings will inform.

The mistake sometimes comes when the two approaches (quantitative and qualitative) are compared. They are different sorts of things and probably do not bear this sort of comparison.

The writer of the 'pro' quantitative chapter tends to use features of the quantitative approach to argue against the qualitative. This is, perhaps, a little like arguing that a bicycle is not as good as a car as it does not have the features of a car, the point being that approaches are different, their methods are different, their outcomes are different and their use is different.

The 'pro' quantitative writer also tends to adopt the position that 'quantitative methods are better, so we should adopt them in mental health care research'. Again, they are likely to be better for some things and not at all useful for others. Simply to state that a particular position is best, is not, itself, an argument for adopting it.

My overall point, then, having considered these chapters, is that, having used both approaches in my own research over the past twenty years, the only way to address the issue of what approach to use is to identify which one is going to answer the research question. If we start with a particular research approach in mind, we are likely to write our research questions accordingly. Better, perhaps, to state the questions first and then allow those questions to determine what we should use: a quantitative or a qualitative approach. Nor, in the end, can we allow rather arcane, postmodern arguments to distract us from doing research. In P/MH nursing, as in other fields, there is a real need to find out what helps patients, how they experience mental illness, and what skills we ought to be teaching students. It would be a shame if we were side-tracked from that project.

Reference

Kelly G 1955 The psychology of personal constructs, vols 1 & 2. Norton, New York.

"The proper focus: should psychiatric/mental health nursing have a humanistic or biological emphasis?

CHAPTER 20

Psychiatric/mental health nursing: biological perspectives

Kevin Gournay

CHAPTER 21

Biological psychiatry versus humanism: why taking meaning seriously in mental health practice is not inferior

Michael Clinton

Commentary

Bryn Davis

Editorial

The chances are that anyone who has been involved in psychiatric/ mental health (P/MH) nursing during the past three decades will have some familiarity with this debate. The ubiquitous nature of this issue might indicate, to borrow a phrase from qualitative research parlance, that it has reached 'saturation' – that there is nothing new to be discovered. If this were the case there would be little utility in continuing the debate. However, as Bryn Davis eloquently points out in his commentary, despite the recognised vintage of the debate it is still highly relevant and pertinent to the contemporary P/MH nurse. If the sheer number of papers published in the *Journal of Psychiatric and Mental Health Nursing* that focus on this matter is indicative of the concomitant level of interest, then this is one of the most 'talked about' debates of the last decade.

Interestingly, this debate, albeit manifest in a variety of forms, has been a feature of P/MH nursing, and the associated care of the person with mental health problems, since the early 1900s. For some, this not only denotes the cyclical nature of the history of P/MH nursing, but within this recurring context it also signifies that the current prevailing orthodoxy represents a return to 1930s perspectives of the person (Dawson 1997, Barker 1999, Cutcliffe 2000). During the 1930s, the perceived wisdom regarded the mind as an extended function of the brain. As Kevin Gournay highlights in his chapter (Ch. 20), this orthodoxy may have been superseded for some by the so-called 'antipsychiatry movement' in the 1970s, which eschewed biological explanations for mental health problems. In no more than 40 years, then, we may have come 'full circle' and returned to neo-Darwinian perspectives of the mind within contemporary psychiatry and mental health care. Which, as Michael Clinton notes in Chapter 21, results in humanistic perspectives in mental health practice being thought of as a poor relation to scientific psychiatry.

Drawing on Michael Foucault's notions of dominant discourses, it can thus be seen that, throughout the history of formal care for the person with mental health problems, the biological and humanistic 'stance' have, arguably, both held the position of the dominant discourse in this debate. In each case this resulted in the discounting of the value of anything related to or arising from the non-dominant discourse. Such reductionalistic and anachronistic approaches can only serve to impede our understanding, restrict our academy to certain questions, limit the range and value of the care/treatment that we offer, and constrain the very ways in which we view people with mental health problems.

References

Barker P 1999 The philosophy and practice of psychiatric nursing. Churchill Livingstone, Edinburgh.

Cutcliffe J R 2000 Fit for purpose? Promoting the human side of mental health nursing. British Journal of Nursing 9(10):632–637.

Dawson P J 1997 A reply to Kevin Gournay's 'Schizophrenia: a review of the contemporary literature and implications for mental health nursing theory, practice and education'. Journal of Psychiatric and Mental Health Nursing 4:1–7.

Psychiatric/mental health nursing: biological perspectives

Introduction

When I sat down to write this chapter, I became aware that there was a great deal that I wished to say about the biological underpinnings of mental health nursing. However, at the same time, I became aware that I could be unwittingly drawn into a polarisation of the biological and humanistic approaches to our subject, in the same way that I have been unwillingly, and sometimes unwittingly, drawn in to the quantitative versus the qualitative debate regarding research. On this latter point, I would like to take the opportunity to say that my position is, as ever, that, while I believe that quantitative approaches should be central, qualitative research has an invaluable part to play in providing evidence. I would also add my view that researchers with different skills need to work together to provide research methods that truly fit the particular question that requires an answer.

In a similar way, I need to say at the outset that, while I believe that biological approaches are important and should be one of the central features in the consideration of the education, training and practice of psychiatric/mental health (P/MH) nursing, this in no way reduces the importance of approaching our work in the most humane way possible. It is, of course, clear that understanding a biological dimension is in no way incompatible with a humanistic approach. Some years ago (in the days when antipsychiatry as an approach was fashionable, and R D Laing and Thomas Szasz were venerated by many), I worked in a 'radical' mental health service where *every* presentation to our mental health service was seen as being a mixture of social, psychological and political factors, with all biological explanations discounted. This formulation was also applied to patients with dementia, and I can recall a psychiatrist discussing a woman of 50 as 'play acting' when she became confused, forgetful and angry with her husband. The psychiatrist and his social work colleague spent a couple of hours assessing the 'crisis' in the patient's home and formulating an analysis of her presentation. This analysis boiled down to her confusion and anger being caused by an unhappy marital situation (which did definitely exist). Any biological explanation was, at that time, discounted. The patient was thence returned to the care of her general practitioner (GP) with a recommendation that the couple undergo marital therapy. Sad to say, it was several months before any physical investigations were carried out and the diagnosis of presenile dementia was eventually made. In the meantime the family endured months of distress during which time they received no specialist services. The woman died shortly afterwards.

Fortunately, the days of seeing Alzheimer's disease and other forms of dementia as being sociopolitical phenomena have passed, and we are now all aware of Alzheimer's disease as a neurological problem rather than a psychiatric one. Which leads me to the question: Does this change in our understanding of the condition lead us to treat people with dementia in a different way? I sincerely hope not. Recently I have had the personal experience of seeing an elderly relative with dementia being cared for by nursing and social care staff with the greatest compassion and skill. Indeed, because of this person's dementia and the resulting behavioural and psychological disturbance, I would argue that the person is probably most appropriately cared for by a registered P/MH nurse, rather than any other professional.

I also think that it is worth noting at this point that Alzheimer's disease and other neurological problems have important psychological and social dimensions, as social and psychological factors can certainly modify the impact of the condition on the particular individual. Because of the biochemical consequences of stress, social and psychological factors may have an impact on the biology of the condition and, once the condition has presented itself, social and psychological facts are obviously important in its maintenance. Finally, it is also worth noting that Alzheimer's disease, of course, has political dimensions. One of the greatest current injustices is that in the National Health Service (NHS), patients with Alzheimer's disease are often denied NHS-funded nursing care, for the obvious problems caused by the psychological and behavioural manifestations of the condition and, as a consequence, have to pay for the care and treatment they may receive in residential care.

I think that I have now made the point regarding the need to consider all dimensions of the problem, not just the biological. Having made this point, and for avoidance of any doubt, I wish to state clearly that a humane approach to all patients, regardless of problem, must be paramount.

Having offered this initial position, in the remainder of this chapter I will provide observation and comment on a number of areas where it is essential that the P/MH nurse appreciates the importance of the biological perspective. In the UK there are something in the order of 60 000 P/MH nurses who practise in areas directly relevant to their qualifications, and a further 30 000 P/MH nurses who work in other areas of nursing or general health care. Much of the debate in journals concerning the philosophical underpinnings of P/MH nursing has focused on the work of P/MH nurses with people with serious and enduring mental health problems, such as schizophrenia and major affective disorder. However, P/MH nurses work in a very wide range of areas, and with people of all ages. In this chapter, I will therefore focus on six particular topics and demonstrate the importance of appreciating the biological perspectives in each of these areas. I do not for one moment pretend that these topics are, by any means, an exhaustive list. I am, of course, constrained by the length of the chapter, and have selected some areas that may provide food for thought, and indeed further debate.

These areas are:

- Attention deficit hyperactivity disorder
- The immune system
- Suicide
- Psychological treatment and its effects on brain activity
- Drug-induced psychiatric problems
- Serious and enduring mental illness.

In addition, it is worth noting that there are some excellent texts that set out for the undergraduate student of nursing, and indeed for qualified nurses, some of the biological aspects of P/MH nursing (see, for example, Rinomhote & Marshall 2000). Such texts provide useful background to some of the more important biological perspectives but, importantly, highlight the need for all nurses, including P/MH nurses, to understand physiological and biochemical processes as they relate to, not just activities of daily living, but to specific psychiatric problems. Texts such as this underline the importance of appreciating the fact that P/MH nurses, often being the primary health professional involved in the patient's care, need to appreciate basic processes of living such as nutrition, elimination and sleep. In turn, nurses also need to understand how these are affected by various mental health problems. Rinomhote & Marshall (2000) draw attention to the concept of homeostasis, which was probably first adumbrated by Claude Bernard in his central statement: *La fixité du milieu intérieur est la condition de la vie libre* (translated as *The constancy of the internal environment is the condition for free life*). This statement describes the essence of the human condition, that is, a state of equilibrium that is maintained by a complex of self-regulating processes within the human body. Indeed, it can be argued that Bernard's major contribution was to challenge the Cartesian philosophical position, which in essence stated that the mental and physical worlds were separate. My own position is far from unique in that I subscribe to the position that has been, rather inelegantly, called the 'biopsychosocial model'. This model recognises the importance of each of the three (biological, psychological and sociological) domains; arguably, in various mental health problems, some domains are more prominent than others. Indeed, I would go further (and again this is not a unique position) and say that in a condition such as schizophrenia we are in fact dealing with a number of different syndromes. Some of these are essentially neurological diseases with very few psychological and social variables playing a part in either causation or maintenance, while at the other end of the spectrum some conditions under the umbrella term of schizophrenia are conditions in which the biological factor is no more than vulnerability, and psychological and social factors are of much more importance in causation and maintenance. Thus, there are extremely robust arguments (and indeed sources of evidence) to suggest that any reductionist model, be it biological, psychological or social, has no place in mental health care. I think it is worth pointing out that, while there has been much focus in debate on people who attempt to reduce everything to brain biology, a similar anachronistic approach may apply to various zealots in the field of psychology and sociology!

Attention deficit hyperactivity disorder

Child and adolescent mental health services (CAMHS) have long been recognised as a priority area. However, despite various government initiatives over the past two decades, most mental health professionals would agree that, although there have been some improvements, real investment in these services has been poor. As President of the UK's largest self-help organisation for anxiety disorders, *No Panic*, I know that children with a wide range of anxiety disorders, notably obsessive compulsive disorder, have little or no access to treatment. We also know that children with psychosis are often poorly managed, and the numbers of P/MH nurses specialising in this area is pitifully small.

One topic that has continued to cause significant debate is that of attention deficit hyperactivity disorder. Although there is some agreement on the central features of this condition, there are huge differences in the prevalence rates determined by the various epidemiological studies, ranging from less than 1% to more than 25% of the population. Therein lies much of the source of the debate, that is, that attention deficit hyperactivity disorder may be overdiagnosed and, thence, overtreated. There are very significant arguments (considered in an excellent debate by Timimi & Taylor 2004) that the condition is, respectively, a cultural construct or a disorder characterised by an interacting set of genetic and social factors. Both of the authors in the debate put forward very strong views to support their position on the nature of the condition, and also argue for very different treatment approaches. The P/MH nurse working in CAMHS will come across numerous children who have received the diagnosis of attention deficit hyperactivity disorder, and these children may be managed by psychiatrists and clinical teams, which operate under the influence of different models – some being at the 'cultural context' end of the spectrum, and some at the 'interaction of genetic and social factors' end. The P/MH nurse needs to appreciate the pros and cons of the various positions, as the nurse is often the primary point of contact for children and their families. The P/MH nurse, therefore, needs to have an appreciation of all of the major aetiological and treatment models. Certainly, an understanding of the biological and pharmacological factors will be essential. If the P/MH nurse, working in CAMHS, is working with children prescribed one of the medications used in this condition, it is essential that they understand the mode of action of such medication and are aware of the side-effects and adverse consequences. As in many other areas of P/MH nursing, a detailed understanding of medication is essential, as the nurse may well be called upon to provide education about the medication and its action to the child and to the family, and also have sophisticated knowledge of issues relating to dose and adherence. Furthermore, it is extremely likely that in years to come such nurses will become prescribers (see Debate 6 for the issue of nurse prescribing), and these responsibilities will then become even more central.

The immune system

Most P/MH nurses educated in modern times will know that there have been various links made between immune function and serious and enduring mental illnesses, such as depression and schizophrenia (see Weisse 1992, Chen et al 1999). However, these links are, as yet, far from clear, and currently there is no real relevance of these issues to day-to-day clinical practice. However, in other areas, knowledge of the immune system is very important for P/MH nurses. One such area is that of stress and its effects on the immune system. P/MH nurses, particularly those in primary care, should be aware of the very clear literature that exists linking excessive stress to immune system dysfunction (see, for example, Rinomhote & Marshall 2000). Once more, the P/MH nurse may have an important educative function, and the explanation of both stress and immune function requires a sound knowledge of the biology of both of these matters. It is pleasing to note that P/MH nurses have been involved in research on the immune system and its links to various stress-related conditions. Recently, a research group at the Institute of Psychiatry, London, UK, which has run a nurse-led chronic fatigue syndrome clinic for more than ten years, has produced evidence to suggest that the hypothalamic–pituitary–adrenal axis function is impaired in chronic fatigue syndrome (Roberts et al 2004). Fatigue is, of course, a very common symptom in primary care settings and is present both in specific psychological disorders and in a range of medical conditions. There are now significant numbers of nurses throughout the country, particularly those with training in cognitive behavioural therapy, who will be treating patients with chronic fatigue syndrome. Once more, it needs to be said that P/MH nurses working in this area should be aware of the biological factors that may contribute to the maintenance of chronic fatigue syndrome and its accompanying problems.

One central method of treating chronic fatigue syndrome is the use of exercise programmes. In treating such patients, it is simply not sufficient to give them vague advice about exercise. One needs to be very precise about just what is required. My experience is that clinicians need a good working knowledge of exercise physiology and, for patients with chronic fatigue syndrome, they need to use concepts, such as percentage of maximum heart rate, to set exercise regimens. An active interest in the physiological recovery of such patients is essential and a good knowledge of relevant biology is important.

In perhaps the most important disease affecting immune function, acquired immune deficiency syndrome (AIDS), it is now known that significant numbers of patients with AIDS demonstrate psychiatric syndromes. Unfortunately, because of the increased prevalence of AIDS in our society, P/MH nurses will, more and more, need to become involved in the care of thse patients. One of the most tragic consequences of AIDS is the consequent dementia. However, a wide range of psychiatric problems is associated with this condition, ranging from various psychiatric symptoms caused by specific effects on the brain, to the psychological reaction of the individual to the development of what may be an eventually fatal illness. Once more, P/MH nurses need to have an appreciation of biological aspects of this condition.

Suicide

Most P/MH nurses will have some experience of working with suicidal people during their working lives. Some 10–15% of patients with depression and schizophrenia will eventually commit suicide, and no less than 4% of all suicides in the UK occur during inpatient stays in psychiatric units (Department of Health 2001b). A recent article in the *British Journal of Psychiatry* (Heeringen & Marusic 2003) drew attention to the possible biological underpinnings of suicide. The authors, who both concentrate all their research efforts on suicides, presented a very helpful review, which demonstrated that certain brain regions may be responsible for some of the cognitive processes associated with suicide – for example, hopelessness, problem-solving and hypersensitivity to particular life events. The authors also elaborated theories based on recent research, demonstrating how the serotonin and noradrenaline neurotransmission systems may be linked to suicidal behaviour. Far from arguing that suicide is directly caused by these factors, what the authors propose is that, quite simply, some people have brains that predispose them to suicidal thinking and behaviour, and that suicide is the result of the interaction between various environmental factors, life events and brain biology. In the long term, the implications for this will be that it may be possible to identify more accurately those who possess a greater 'biological' risk, that is, those people with specific brain anomalies, who will in the future be identified by certain genetic markers. In turn, this identification may lead to the ability to intervene, perhaps using antidepressant medication, with people who may be so vulnerable.

Another area where the biological dimensions of suicide are particularly important is in the area of maternal death. For some time now, there has been a Confidential Inquiry into Maternal Deaths (Department of Health 2001a). This enquiry was set up to consider maternal deaths following a registerable live or stillbirth, at more than 24 weeks of pregnancy. Collection of these data has demonstrated that suicide is the leading cause of maternal death. Oates (2003) highlights the fact that important subgroups of women who commit suicide are those who are older and free from social adversity. These women are suffering from illnesses that are primarily biological, that is, their mood disturbance is triggered by the hormonal changes associated with pregnancy and childbirth, and the tragedy is that such conditions are, if properly detected and managed, very responsive to treatment.

Putting forth examples of how suicide may be connected to possible biological underpinnings is not to say that a great deal of suicide may be unconnected with formal psychiatric illness and that some of the major causative factors are, of course, social rather than biological. Nevertheless, it is important to appreciate all of the possible dimensions of suicide – social, psychological and biological, and in some cases (for example, altruistic suicide) the political.

Psychological treatment and its effects on brain activity

For many years now, numerous research papers have shown that cognitive behavioural therapy (CBT) often has an equivalent effect to medication in the treatment of a number of conditions. Some notable examples are depression and obsessive compulsive disorder (see, for example, the comprehensive review by Rush & Thase 1999). However, the mechanisms of action of CBT and medication have been very unclear. What one observes from clinical practice is that the thinking and behavioural changes associated with both antidepressants and CBT treatments are remarkably similar. Recently, Mayor (2004) reported on research that examined brain activity during treatment with CBT and antidepressants. The two groups of patients were scanned using positron emission tomography, before and after treatment. Both groups showed significant metabolic changes, with the group receiving CBT showing increased activity in the hippocampus and dorsal cingulate regions and decreased cortical activity. The patients treated with drugs showed metabolic changes in the opposite direction, with increased activity in the prefrontal cortex and decreased activity in the hippocampal and dorsal cingulate regions. The research team concluded that the difference in changes in brain activity reflected specific effects relating to the type of treatment. Thus, a strong suggestion is that depression may be corrected along a number of pathways, and both drugs and CBT change brain activity. One of the researchers cited in Mayor's paper, Professor Helen Mayberg, was quoted as saying, *'It's just tapping into a different component of the same depression circuit board'*. However, we do not know whether or not these changes in brain function are permanent. We do know that many patients treated with antidepressants relapse over time and, although there are strong suggestions from some authors that CBT may be a more enduring treatment than medication (see, for example, Scott 1998), there are really no good long-term studies to compare the long-term efficacy of medication and CBT. Furthermore, as many P/MH nurses know, patients with depression are often treated by both CBT and antidepressants at the same time. Although for some patients this combined approach seems to be effective, we still have no long-term follow-up studies. We do know, as noted above, that in some patients with depression psychological treatments do have a chemical effect. This, of course, begs the questions: how are psychological problems caused, and how do the environment and developmental experiences interact with genetic factors? P/MH nurses need to appreciate all of these dimensions.

One burgeoning area of the clinical application of CBT is for people with schizophrenia. The recent UK National Institute for Clinical Effectiveness (NICE) guidelines on schizophrenia have provided support for the view that CBT should be part of mainstream approaches and aimed at ameliorating the terrible distress that this disease causes (NICE 2002). Although there is widespread acceptance that the umbrella term 'schizophrenia' covers a number of disorders, some of which have an underlying biological base, the efficacy of CBT in this condition, taken together with the findings on the biological impact of CBT for depression, suggest quite strongly that at least some of the biological abnormalities created by the 'schizophrenic condition' may be modified by a purely psychological treatment. Once more, the research evidence that is available to us is based on studies with a short follow-up period, and the design and methodological problems of researching schizophrenia are well known. It may, therefore, be many years before we are able even to begin answering the question about the exact biological impact of CBT alone, and of CBT in combination with medication, for schizophrenia.

Drug-induced psychiatric problems

Another dimension of the biological underpinning of mental illness is to be found in drug use. The legalisation, or otherwise, of illicit drugs is the topic of huge public debate. In the narrower field of psychiatry, this debate has concentrated on different interpretations of the evidence. In an excellent review, Arseneault et al (2004) examined five well designed studies based on population-based registers or cohorts, which used prospective measures of cannabis use and adult psychosis. These five studies used four samples: three cohort studies and one longitudinal population-based survey. These samples were drawn from populations of Swedish conscripts, a Dutch population-based sample, and two birth cohorts from Christchurch and Dunedin (both in New Zealand). This review demonstrated that cannabis use appeared to be neither a sufficient nor a necessary cause for psychosis, but that it was an important part of the constellation of factors leading to psychosis. The authors went on to argue that, if cannabis use could be eliminated, the incidence of schizophrenia would fall by 8%. Once more, as with other areas reviewed in this chapter, the research indicated that the biological factor (i.e. cannabis) was important in the causation of serious mental illness.

One other drug worthy of consideration is Ecstasy. There is widespread acknowledgement that the use of Ecstasy is endemic (Winstock et al 2001). Ecstasy is now being used increasingly in liquid form (Rodgers et al 2004) and this seems to have quite complex and profound effects on brain chemistry, notably on the fatty acids in the hypothalamus and basal ganglia. Liquid Ecstasy seems to produce tolerance and physical dependence, and there is a growing acknowledgement that this drug, and drugs like it, will have a major impact on psychiatric services because of the problems associated with adverse psychological effects and withdrawal syndromes.

People presenting with a combination of problems related to drug/alcohol use and mental illness are a population that preoccupies every P/MH nurse working in community mental health teams and in patient wards. (Editors: A combination termed 'dual diagnosis' or 'co-morbidity' depending upon which side of the Atlantic one comes from.) I will not reiterate the facts of dual diagnosis, other than to say that, in the opinion of most commentators, the phenomenon probably represents the greatest single challenge to contemporary mental health services. In the past few years, my department at the Institute of Psychiatry has been at the forefront of developing training programmes for P/MH nurses and other mental health professionals working with this population, and has also been involved in epidemiological and treatment research studies. In the course of this extensive work, which has involved literally thousands of nurses, it has become clear to me that P/MH nurses working in this area must have knowledge of how drugs and alcohol affect brain function and contribute to mental illness. In turn, it is essential that P/MH nurses, in their roles as educators, are able to relay this information to patients, families and other carers.

Serious and enduring mental illness

Space confines me merely to sketching out the importance of biology in the area of serious and enduring mental illness, and at the same time the reader needs reminding of my comments made earlier in this chapter regarding the interaction of biological, psychological and social factors. In particular, it is worth restating the principle that I set out above, that any attempt to reduce issues of causation to single factors should be viewed as anachronistic. It also bears repeating that this applies as much to those who reduce everything to the social or psychological (or indeed to a mixture of the two) and discount the biological. I am somewhat saddened to see continuing publication of texts that call for new taxonomies, based on the social and/or psychological, without attempting to grasp the nettle of dealing with all three essential factors, including the biological. Indeed, I would go further. Having had significant experience in the former Soviet Union, I would say that the debate regarding causation and diagnosis needs to also take account of the political.

This chapter is certainly not the place to attempt to review the hugely significant research on the biology of schizophrenia and major affective disorders. However, I think it is worth noting that, while it is true that the early promise of finding a single gene responsible for these conditions will most likely never materialise, biological research, year on year, produces vast amounts of evidence to demonstrate biological underpinnings. However, as time goes on, the interaction of the biological factors between themselves, let alone the interaction of other social and psychological factors with the interacting biological factors, is revealed to be extremely complex. In order to take part in any debate about biological contributions to causation, today's graduate of P/MH nursing needs to be equipped with a sophisticated account of brain biology, so that they can keep up to date with the burgeoning state of knowledge. It seems to me that, for the foreseeable future, there will be considerable debate about the respective contributions of various causes. I think that this is exemplified in matters connected with drug use and the role of culture, race and ethnicity. Without knowledge of the biological, P/MH nurses will not be in a position to make significant contributions. My own view is that many undergraduate programmes in the UK today compare very poorly with similar undergraduate programmes in the USA in terms of content concerning biology.

Although one explanation is that there is insufficient curricular time available, I fear that blatant prejudice is another explanation. Perhaps simple ignorance of brain biology on the part of teachers may also be explanatory. I know from my own experience that P/MH nurses do not have access to comprehensive sources of biological knowledge, and as a discipline I think that we need to be honest about the shortcomings of our educational system.

Conclusion

In this chapter I have attempted to demonstrate, via my observation and comment on six particular topics, the importance of appreciating biological factors in the practice of P/MH nursing. I realise that, on a day-to-day basis, none of us in clinical practice is conscious of theoretical issues for much more than a few nanoseconds. This perhaps contrasts with those who have spent many of their working years in academic life, with no real contact with patients. For my own part, I have been pleased that, in my relatively brief academic career since 1992, I have continued to see patients and experienced the real environments of the NHS for a significant proportion of my time at work. The reality is that, in most of my patient encounters, I am doing my best to apply my experience, knowledge and skills to a range of distress – anything from panic attacks to abnormal sensory experiences. During these encounters, I do not for a moment dwell on particular theories relating to the causation, maintenance or treatment of mental health problems. I think I share the experience of the vast majority of practitioners insofar as we are all involved in care and treatment regimens with multiple perspectives. The biological is one of these perspectives, and although, as this chapter emphasises, it has major importance, it cannot be divorced from others.

References

Arseneault L, Cannon M, Whitton J, Murray R 2004 Causal association between cannabis and psychosis: examination of the evidence. British Journal of Psychiatry 184:110–117.

Chen C, Chiu Y, Wei F 1999 High seroprevalence of Borna virus infection in schizophrenic patients, family members and mental health workers in Taiwan. Molecular Psychiatry 4:33–38.

Department of Health 2001a Why mothers die. Confidential Enquiries into Maternal Deaths in the United Kingdom, 1997–1999. RCOG Press, London.

Department of Health 2001b Safety first: five-year report of the National Confidential Inquiry into Suicide and Homicide by People with Mental Illness. Department of Health, London.

Heeringen C, Marusic A 2003 Understanding the suicidal brain. British Journal of Psychiatry 183:282–284.

Mayor S 2004 Cognitive behaviour therapy affects brain activity differently to anti-depressants. British Medical Journal 328:69.

National Institute for Clinical Excellence 2002 Guidelines for the treatment of schizophrenia. NICE, London.

Oates M 2003 Suicide: the leading cause of maternal death. British Journal of Psychiatry 183:279–281.

Rinomhote A S, Marshall P 2000 Biological aspects of mental health nursing. Churchill Livingstone, London.

Roberts A, Wessley S, Chalder T, Papadopoulos A, Cleare A 2004 Salivary cortisol response to awakening in chronic fatigue syndrome. British Journal of Psychiatry 184:136–141.

Rodgers J, Ashton C, Gilvary E, Young A 2004 Liquid Ecstasy: a new kid on the dancefloor. British Journal of Psychiatry 184:104–106.

Rush A, Thase M 1999 Psychotherapies for depressive disorders: a review. In: Maj M, Sartorius N, eds. Depressive disorders. Wiley, New York: p 161–206.

Scott J 1998 Where there's a will . . . Cognitive therapy for people with chronic depressive disorders. In: Tarrier N, Wells A, Haddock G, eds. Treating complex cases. Wiley, Chichester, p 81–104.

Timimi S, Taylor E 2004 ADHD is best understood as a cultural construct. British Journal of Psychiatry 184:8–9.

Weisse C 1992 Depression and immunocompetence: a review of the literature. Psychological Bulletin 111:475–489.

Winstock A, Griffiths P, Stewart D 2001 Drugs and the dance music scene: a survey of current drug use patterns among a sample of dance music enthusiasts in the UK. Drug and Alcohol Dependence 64:9–17.

Michael Clinton

Biological psychiatry versus humanism: why taking meaning seriously in mental health practice is not inferior

Irrespective of whether we are concerned with psychiatry, psychology or psychiatric/mental health (P/MH) nursing, mental health practice raises significant philosophical questions. We ask questions not only about how scientific, sociocultural, evaluative, therapeutic, practical and other presuppositions impact on our understanding of mental disorders (Sadler et al 1994), we also worry about whether or not these and other forms of intelligibility are unavoidable preconditions for mental health practice. While both kinds of question are ultimately concerned with the relationship between one's mind and the world, I shall focus only on those of the second kind. This is because the argument I shall develop is concerned mainly with problems of intelligibility. At issue is whether some ways of understanding (and the associated responses to) mental disorder are more primitive than others. To believe that they are is to privilege some ways of thinking about psychopathology. For example, it has become commonplace to suppose that scientific reasoning is the highest form of human rationality and that any modes of reasoning that do not live up to its canons are necessarily inferior. Accordingly, humanistic perspectives in mental health practice are thought of as a poor relation to scientific psychiatry. The purpose of this chapter is to reject this view by arguing that motivated humanistic reasoning is sufficiently objective and essentially causal. Although I shall be concerned with only one humanistic perspective – life-story methodology – my argument applies quite generally to other humanistic views. A truism about clinical practice provides a convenient place to start.

Falling back into more natural ways of thinking

Mental health practitioners work with people who are *'grief stricken, demoralized, and angry'* (McHugh & Slavney 1998, p 256) and who are otherwise subject to the full range of human emotions and suffering. The problem for scientific psychiatry is that few of these people have a mental disorder that can be explained by physical causes. McHugh & Slavney (1998) claim that, when faced with this anomaly, mental health practitioners depart from science to fall back on a more natural way of thinking – one that exemplifies forms of intelligibility characteristic of historical reasoning. (In 1998 when the second edition of their book was published Paul McHugh was Henry Phipps Professor and director of the Department of Mental Health Practice and Behavioural Sciences and Phillip Slavney was Eugene Meyer III Professor of Mental Health Practice and Medicine at the Johns Hopkins University School of Medicine. The purpose of the second edition, like that of the first, was to introduce approaches to psychiatric reasoning by focusing on the application of explanatory methods. The first edition rapidly became popular with academic mental health practitioners in the USA and was heralded as a brilliant book by the New England Journal of Medicine. The eminence and influence of McHugh and Slavney justifies this examination of one of their key assumptions.)

The structure of this argument is clear. The science of mental health practice is concerned with the study and treatment of mental disorders. However, people experiencing a range of human emotions seek psychiatric help. Unless they have a mental disorder that is amenable to interventions that can be explained in terms of underlying physical causes and effects, mental health practitioners have to depart from science in order to understand and help them. This form of understanding is not only different from that used in the science of mental health practice, it is inferior to it, in the sense of being less objective, less universal, and less explicable in terms of laws of cause and effect, which I shall from now on refer to as the realm of law.

Examining McHugh & Slavney's (1998) notion of 'falling back' requires clarification of the distinction between explanations of mental disorder that rely on assumptions about the effects of natural laws and those that take seriously the meanings people give to the distress and other emotional experiences that accompany misfortune. Clarification of this important distinction permits analysis of two prominent perspectives in contemporary psychiatric thinking: the disease concept and life-story methodology. The crux of this distinction is the difference between regarding a person as an object for scientific study and as a subject with beliefs, desires and intentions (Sellars 1956). I associate or liken the first approach to scientific psychiatry, the second to humanistic perspectives in mental health practice. If the two perspectives cannot be reconciled, mental health practitioners could have grounds for privileging scientific objectivity over understanding what it means to be a person, or, more accurately, over what it means to be a person with a mind. With these matters clarified, it will be possible to show why taking meaning seriously does not involve 'falling back' on a more primitive way of reasoning.

Taking up these matters requires pointing out that McHugh & Slavney's notion of 'falling back' implies a broadly naturalistic view of mental health practice that allows explanations of mental disorder, assimilated to the physical realm, to be privileged over those that are likely to drop out of significance as science and technology advance. At issue is whether McHugh & Slavney (1998) are justified in what appears to be their position on naturalism. The answer depends on answers to two underlying questions:

1 Can everything that mental health practitioners need to understand about mental disorder be explained within (or by) the realm of (physical/biological) law?
2 And, if not, does going beyond what can be explained within (or by) the realm of law involve a more primitive form of reasoning?

McHugh & Slavney (1998) answer 'no' to the first question and 'yes' to the second. I agree with their answer to the first question, but reject their second answer because, as I shall show, it is based on a limited (and restrictive) view of naturalism. Therefore, much of what follows is concerned with rejecting what I take to be McHugh & Slavney's overly external position on naturalism. My disagreement with them follows McDowell's (1994) argument in rejecting what he calls 'bald naturalism' in favour of what he regards as 'naturalised platonism'. With these preliminaries out of the way, it will be possible to follow McDowell's (1994) reasoning in distinguishing between the realm of law and the space of reasons – or those forms of intelligibility that presuppose a world regulated by causal relations, including strict nomological or causal laws, and the world of meaningful relations.

The disease concept

Assumptions about the relevance of the realm of law to the scientific status of mental health practice underpin what McHugh & Slavney (1998) call the disease concept of mental disorder. McHugh & Slavney appear to accept all four of the following propositions:

1 Symptoms of mental disorder are effects of disturbed neurophysiological functioning.

2 Psychiatric symptoms correspond to genuine laws of cause and effect that reflect natural events of the kind found in brain states.

3 These regularities reflect laws that are strongly deterministic, but other regularities are possible in which lower levels of probability are involved.

4 The weakest laws involved in psychopathology are grounded in only accidental generalisations that must not be mistaken for genuine laws.

In this view, at least some mental disorders are afflictions in which abnormalities of the brain, or disturbances of neurophysiological function, result in characteristic psychopathology. Such disease reasoning involves a categorical way of differentiating between mental disorders by attributing them to underlying abnormalities, which themselves are regarded as having specific causes. However, McHugh & Slavney (1998) recognise that this way of thinking about mental health practice is particularly problematic because such notions of mental disorder presume the identification of neurophysiological mechanisms that not only permit the identification and description of clinical syndromes, but also support claims to a rational basis for treatment and prognosis. The problem is that the neurophysiological mechanisms implicated in mental disorders are seldom identifiable, and, irrespective of whether they are, or even can be, treatments that are effective for some patients demonstrably fail with others. Moreover, judgements about prognosis often turn out to be wrong.

Irrespective of its success in promoting accurate diagnosis and effective treatment, the disease concept has two fundamental flaws. It cannot be made to take into account the specific vulnerabilities of individuals, and it encourages the erroneous expectation of a neurophysiological explanation for every aspect of mental suffering (McHugh & Slavney 1998). Nevertheless the disease concept facilitates an ordering of mental disorders from those that can be explained causally, such as delirium and dementia, to those such as major depression and schizophrenia that have this potential. The credibility of such ordering depends on the ability to make accurate diagnoses. Consequently, it is necessary to consider what is involved in diagnosing a mental disorder.

Diagnosing

Psychiatric diagnosis proceeds by correlating a particular form of psychopathology to a specific syndrome. The next and crucial step is the presumption of a causative agency predicated on discoveries in the neurosciences. Relevant aetiological agency is reflected in phenomena such as *'neurotoxicology, genetic mutation and its influence on neuronal development and degeneration, neuropharmacology, and so on'* (McHugh & Slavney 1998, p 51). Therefore, diagnosis involves the application of a three-step model of psychopathology. First, clinical syndromes are identified and described. Second, they are then explained with reference to increasingly sophisticated descriptions of neurophysiological or other pathological processes. Finally, causal factors are sought to account for these abnormalities. Such reasoning offers not only an explanation for the clinical features of categories of mental disorder, it also provides a rationale for prevention and, depending on advances in the neurosciences, ultimately cure (McHugh & Slavney 1998).

This approach to *making sense* of mental disorders is exemplified by psychiatric conditions with known neuropathology. Examples include delirium, dementia, Huntington's disease, Korsakoff's syndrome and aphasia, and syndromes considered secondary to poisoning, genetic predisposition, vascular damage, alcoholism, infection, neoplasia and trauma. More problematic are those mental disorders to which the concept of disease is applied with less certain knowledge of neurophysiological dysfunction. Examples are the mentally challenging conditions of bipolar disorder(s) and schizophrenia(s). Although bipolar disorder can be understood from the standpoint of the disease concept, there is as yet an insufficient psychopathology of affect. Advances in neuroscience are required to help explain the onset and natural history of the syndrome, including how it is to be distinguished from affective reactions such as grief, and its response to treatment (McHugh & Slavney 1998).

Problems are even more obvious when trying to understand schizophrenia from within the perspective of the disease concept. As a category schizophrenia is so disjunctive (the term disjunctive is used here in a way that follows McHugh & Slavney's (1998, p 34) usage by referring to categories of clinical syndromes made up of heterogeneous and, therefore, non-additive criteria) as to make it difficult to grasp its conceptual essence beyond reference to the fact of insanity. Although there is evidence of a failure of executive function linked to dysfunction of the frontal lobe, and damage to particular neurological regions is implicated in hallucinatory experiences, there is as yet insufficient evidence to explain the relationship between symptoms of schizo-phrenia, underlying neurophysiological processes and developmental factors (McHugh & Slavney 1998). Although the disease concept might be a useful way of thinking about schizophrenia and its causation, there is still a long way to go before any underlying causal laws can be identified. Furthermore, it is difficult to conceive of causal laws that would be relevant to understanding the 'aboutness' of intentionality that is as much a feature of the consciousnesses of people with schizophrenia as it is of the consciousness of anyone else.

The use of the concept of intentionality implies the importance of the beliefs, desires, hopes and fears of people with a mental disorder, their aspirations and disappointments. The concept is significant when considering explanations of mental disorder and the forms of intelligibility they rely on in that, following Brentano, philosophers generally claim that intentionality is central to any efforts to define or refute the distinction between mental and physical phenomena (Chisolm 1960). Whereas Brentano argued that only mental phenomena could have the quality of intentionality, eliminative materialists and others claim that the mind is nothing more than the brain. Brentano's irreducible thesis is relevant here because at issue in McHugh & Slavney's (1998) assumption is the nature of the intelligibility that mental health practitioners rely on when *making sense* of the subjective experiences of people with a mental disorder.

Life-story methodology

McHugh & Slavney (1998) identify life-story methodology as the perspective in which mental health practitioners are best able to understand the discouragement, hopelessness, loneliness, de-moralisation and human despair their patients experience. Therefore, the life-story approach has a place in contemporary mental health practice precisely because it helps to *make sense* of human experience in ways that offer practical solutions to current and future life events. However, the process involves more than a chronological description of events. Like all stories, narratives of distress have a setting, sequence and outcome, but this structure is a construction. For that reason, experiences embedded in the facts of a human life can be understood in many ways. Consequently the interpretations placed on them are primarily constructed to *make sense* to those involved. Therefore, there is a sense in which life stories are a fiction (McHugh & Slavney 1998), although no less important for that. The act of structuring human experience forces facts and experiences into neat structures that are contrived for the purposes at hand – to relieve human suffering by offering the person a wider range of choices for the future.

Another difficulty is that life stories differ in the extent to which they write themselves. According to McHugh & Slavney (1998), it is easy to piece together an account of demoralisation that arises from a recent loss or traumatic experience. But human lives are complex, and narratives often require layers of assumptions and nuance necessarily transcending descriptions of personal experience, however rich the account of misfortune. Moreover, only what can be put into words is available for a life-story account, and people in general, including mental health practitioners, can and do neglect important factors in their explanations. People are also likely to misjudge the impact of those factors of which they are aware (McHugh & Slavney 1998). Furthermore, the meanings given to such narratives do not stand totally outside the disease concept and other psychiatric perspectives. Narratives can complement understandings of psychopathology predicated on the disease concept, and matters of intelligence, temperament and drive can be, and often are, invoked in the subtext of life-story accounts.

Although McHugh & Slavney (1998) claim that life-story methodology gives the clearest understanding of the human predicament of people with a mental disorder and other people who consult mental health practitioners, they recognise that the approach has problems as well as power. The principal limitation is that any method involving intelligibility, of the kind invoked by what Sellars (1956) and McDowell (1994) call the space of reasons (sets of meanings), is not one from which a steady advance in human knowledge and irrefutable discoveries can be expected. Furthermore, any attempt to grasp meanings in the space of reasons can provoke disagreements about where the 'best' explanation lies for a particular set of circumstances. Unlike the disease concept of mental disorder, there is no linear process of causation between the elements in the life-story method. However, as will be shown later, McHugh & Slavney (1998) are not strictly correct to claim that the chain of causes of pathology to symptomatology, in the realm of law, has no counterpart in the narrative structure of setting to sequence to outcome. Consequently, symptomatology understood as an outcome of misfortune cannot be causally attributed to a particular setting or sequence of events. Neither can a sequence of events be attributed to only the characteristics of a particular setting. Still less can knowledge of a setting or a sequence predict the outcome of psychiatric treatment in any strong sense (McHugh & Slavney 1998).

Therefore, McHugh & Slavney (1998) claim that mental health practitioners 'fall back' on a more natural way of thinking when they depart from the disease concept to adopt a life-story approach to understanding the suffering of their patients. It follows that McHugh & Slavney appear to think that there is a hierarchy of reasoning in which scientific reasoning is superior because it is different. What seems to set scientific thinking apart on this view is a form of what McDowell (1994) calls the disenchantment of science. Two false assumptions made by McHugh & Slavney (1998) in this regard are that intentionality and, therefore, subjectivity is irrelevant to naturalism, and that only scientific reasoning is nomological. McDowell's (1994) naturalised platonism refutes both assumptions.

Naturalised platonism

The dilemma that needs to be resolved in McHugh & Slavney's (1998) views on thinking about mental health practice is how to recognise the differences between mental disorder seen from the disease concept perspective and in the life-story approach, without assuming that reasoning in the space of reasons (about meanings) is inferior to reasoning about the realm of law (science). The problem can be posed in the terminology of McDowell (1994) by asking how mental health practitioners can reconcile the desire for justifying their empirical understandings of mental disorder in possible ultimate contacts between mental life and the world, while maintaining that the way they understand the empirical world is not separable from their conceptualisations of it?

Putting the question this way helps to clarify the philosophical problems implicit in the position that McHugh & Slavney (1998) take on in privileging understandings of the realm of law over those within the space of reasons. In other words, a way is needed of countering McHugh & Slavney's assumption that those understandings of mental disorder that fall within the realm of law, connect with the experiences of mental health practitioners and with the world, unproblematically. Whereas those that fall within the space of reasons do not because they depend on interpretations of meaning. An example can help to bring out this contrast, and is provided in Box 21.1.

The logical space in which such reasoning takes place (the active process through which CD and EF reflect on AB's request, and without which that request would be meaningless) is not something that can be understood from a scientific point of view. Nevertheless, according to McDowell (1994), CD and EF's ability to understand AB's request is part of their animal nature as humans and, in this sense at least, their

---

BOX 21.1 Contrasting understandings of mental disorder

AB is a person with a long history of mental illness, punctuated with varying periods of hospitalisation and treatment over many years with various antipsychotic compounds. Such interventions have been supported with psycho-education and the long-term support of a community psychiatric nurse, CD. Last week AB asked CD to speak to the doctor, EF, about a reduction in medication. CD's reasoning about AB's request went like this:

'AB is making progress. The psycho-educational sessions have clearly helped. AB understands the significance of the onset of acute symptoms, and is clearly willing to take on more responsibility. AB seems well at the moment, so I will speak to EF and follow up with AB more often to see how things are going.'

Subsequently, CD raised the question of AB's medication with EF. EF reasoned:

'AB has a long history of paranoid ideation. I know from the notes that previous requests for reductions in medication have been associated with loss of insight and an increase in positive symptoms. I will need to be careful here. Although CD thinks AB is well, I'd better do an evaluation to see whether the current level of medication needs to be increased.'

reasoning is a natural process. Therefore, McDowell's (1994) conceptualisation of the natural (what exists in nature), unlike that of McHugh & Slavney, is not limited to what can be understood by scientific reasoning. McDowell's idea is that spontaneity can be conceived of as a *sui generis* (specific and unique) mental power that actualises human nature. Consequently, McDowell (1994) defends a Kantian (1998) notion of spontaneity, which provides mental health practitioners with grounds for rejecting McHugh & Slavney's (1998) assumption that the only kind of naturalism we should be concerned with is confined to the realm of law (that which can be subjected to scientific investigation).

McDowell's (1994) key move is to bring responsiveness to meaning (CD and EF's understanding of AB's request) into the notion of naturalism, thereby putting meaning at the centre of what they make of it. But, as we have seen, their spontaneity in doing this cannot be captured scientifically, unless the notion of what is natural is extended beyond that which McHugh & Slavney (1998) associate with the realm of law. However, McDowell's (1994, p 78) position does not require that the contrast between the realm of law and the space of reasons be blurred. It only requires that we follow him in recognising that:

'To see exercises of spontaneity as natural, we do not need to integrate spontaneity-related concepts into the structure of the realm of law; we need [only] *to stress their role in capturing patterns of living.'*

In other words, EF has a pattern of living, including a way of practising, in which the notion of recovery colours interpretation of AB's request, whereas CD's understanding is predicated on a form of practice in which psychopathology is presupposed in the absence of clinical assessment. Therefore, McHugh & Slavney (1994) and EF's false privileging of the realm of law over the space of reasons can be dismissed by accepting McDowell's (1994) argument as a tenable view of the relationship between mind and world, that is, the relationship between CD and EF's interpretations and AB's request. McDowell's position makes it possible to clarify the representational content of experience in mental disorder and the conceptions through which it is understood in life-story methodology. At stake is the defensibility of a conception of empirical thinking in which there is sufficient scope for constraints from outside the conceptual sphere (a sufficient degree of objectivity), while at the same time denying that the only ultimately tenable view of mental disorder is that which presupposes its place within the realm of law. In other words, the view recommended by McDowell (1994) allows rejection of McHugh & Slavney's (1998) views on the primitiveness of reasoning within life-story methodology on the basis that all empirical reasoning is grounded in a reality external to thought, even if that reality is *primarily* located in the space of reasons. That is, CD's reasoning is no less empirical that that of EF.

Further challenge to McHugh & Slavney

McDowell's (1994) position requires that McHugh & Slavney (1998) give up their assumption about the relative primitiveness of reasoning about meaning because it presupposes an oversimplification of the Kantian notion of cooperation between receptivity (hearing AB's request) and spontaneity (making sense of it). Thus, it is important to note that receptivity is understood as an experience that is not and cannot be separated from the reasoning that makes it intelligible. This is because experiential intake, what Kant (1998) calls 'intuition', is not and never can be a bare getting of an extra-conceptual given, in the sense implied by what McDowell (1994) refers to as the Myth of the Given, and which McHugh & Slavney (1998) appear to take for granted in what they refer to as the disease concept of mental illness. Understanding of what is given to experience is always already conceptualised, in the sense that intelligibility is predicated on the assumption that *'things are thus and so'* (McHugh & Slavney 1998, p 9).

In other words, any invocation of a disease concept in psychopathology involves what McDowell (1994) regards as the 'Myth of the Given' (by which McDowell (1994) means the mistaken belief that anything in the world can be regarded as having existence independent of the way in which sense is made of it). As a result, it is a mistake to suppose with EF that AB's request is a feature of a mental disorder that has a reality independent of EF's conception of it. This is not to say that mental disorders do not exist, but to stress that their existence is not something independent of the way they are understood.

The Kantian spontaneity with which receptivity cooperates is the capacity that empowers CD no less than EF to take charge of the way AB's possible reduction in medication is to be thought about – a capacity that goes all the way to the limits of perceptual experience itself. This capacity is fundamental to all reasoning. Yet the perspectives on mental health practice described by McHugh & Slavney (1998) imply that understandings of mental disorders rely on reasoning that is separable into forms of intelligibility associated with the natural sciences and those that fall within the 'logical space of reasons'. This suggests an unnecessary and untenable tension in thinking about psychopathology that divides attempts to make mental disorder intelligible from the standpoint of natural laws from those that recognise and bring into play what McDowell (1994, p 71) calls *'the kind of intelligibility that is proper to meaning'*.

However, the space of justification or warrant extends more widely than the conceptual sphere within which an object of sensible intuition is understood (McDowell 1994). Yet the space of justification cannot be allowed to exceed that which cannot be justified without recourse to the objects of sensible intuition. That is, all forms of empiricism are grounded in an assumption about what McDowell (1994) refers to as the 'given', the object of intentionality (the object or state of affairs that is construed to have existence outside the person); the neurophysiology associated with mental disorders in general, but not the conceptualisation of the observer; the 'patterns of life' through which CD and EF make sense of AB's request. The dualism of scheme (the framework within which an object is intuited, CD's predication of recovery, EF's predication of psychopathology) and content (AB's request) is intended as a guarantee that empirical understanding extends beyond itself to encompass something substantial (something that is not just a figment of the imagination of the observer), that is possible grounds for an empirical justification (McDowell 1994). Therefore, in order to be justified in a belief about mental disorder, a mental health practitioner needs to abstract out the right weight to be given to the empirical evidence, something best done in partnership with the person.

There is another good reason for rejecting the notion that adopting life-story methodology or any other humanistic perspective in mental health practice involves a more primitive form of reasoning than that found in conceptualisations of psychopathology that invoke the disease concept. The life-story method depends on a narrative structure that follows a sequence of events in which what happens at each stage is, in part at least, somewhat dependent on what happened previously to a limit at which a happening, event or set of circumstances is regarded as materially significant. According to Hempel (1965), such genetic reasoning involves descriptions of some initial stage that leads on to an account of second and subsequent stages that are regarded in part as causally related. To the extent that parts of the materially relevant circumstances at each stage are looked upon as dependent on at least some of the characteristics of the previous stage, the stages are regarded as nomologically linked. Hence the nomological or causal reasoning implicit in the disease concept, or in any other perspective on psychiatric thinking that relies on assumptions about the realm of law, is found also in what McHugh & Slavney (1994) regard as the more primitive reasoning associated with life-story methodology.

Nevertheless, McHugh & Slavney (1994) are correct to think that there is something questionable about psychiatric explanations that presuppose the space of reasons. One way of bringing out the relevant worry is to consider the relevant aspect of life-story methodology. When CD or EF and AB help each other to *make sense* of AB's request, it becomes necessary to explain pertinent events by motivating reasons. In other words, part of the conversation is likely to involve not only explanations of why AB should or should not have less medication, but also consideration of why this request was made. Explanations of the second kind are likely to rely on how AB understands the relevant circumstances, why he understood them in that way, and what he intended or hoped to achieve. If explanations are sought for these motivating reasons, they are likely to be found in explanations of both the relevant circumstances and in attributions of character: a request for a reduction in medication was made because AB perceived the situation in a particular way and acted on that basis.

Consequently explanations of motivating reasons are in part likely to be found in attributions of character. Therefore, McHugh & Slavney (1998) are correct in thinking that historical explanations of the kind uncovered in the life-story method are different from those that typify the disease concept of mental disorder. However, they are different only in that they are normative. They are not different in that they depend on other than objective and nomological or causal reasoning. Such explanations remain objective for the reasons I have given, and nomological because all explanations that involve sequences of materially relevant events and attributions to character cannot be other than causal (Hempel 1965).

This problem, which Hempel (1965) includes in what he describes as the difficulty of explanation by motivating reasons, supports the realism found in McDowell's (1994) naturalised platonism, which entails that any reference to the rationale for AB's request conforms to a probabilistic form of nomological reasoning based on character. In other words, McHugh & Slavney's (1998) 'falling back' claim misses the point that explanations uncovered by the life-story method are necessarily nomological because any normative principles of action are at some stage likely to be replaced by statements of a dispositional kind. These arguments gain support from McDowell's (1994) notion of second nature, because all arguments from character as well as those from what Hempel (1965) calls genetic reasoning are essentially nomological. In other words, the processes of shaping our lives that we use to build our characters in the direction of our preferences for the kind of people we want to become are necessarily nomological, as is the reasoning that enables the pursuit of professional, therapeutic or personal goals. Consequently, CD's interpretation of AB's request is no less nomological than that of EF. Therefore, CD's reasoning cannot be inferior on nomological grounds.

Conclusion

Only in a partial view of reality can explanations of mental disorder be regarded as separate from conceptualisations of them. As reality has no intrinsic character that can be understood only by the natural sciences, there can be no brute facts about mental disorders, nor any purely objective accounts of mental disorder. Therefore, mental health practice that relies on life-story methodology and other humanistic perspectives is on a par with scientific psychiatry because it is not based on an inferior kind of reasoning.

The important implication for practice is that the person with a mental disorder can be legitimately thought of as sharing in a common humanity in which the capacity for meaning is no less part of nature than neurophysiology. As a result, all approaches to practice that emphasise the central importance of meaning are licensed by the certainty that reframing is as important in caring as therapeutic compounds are in treatment. Furthermore, those practitioners who rely primarily on meaning as a resource for helping others need not be embarrassed by the mistaken assumption that they rely on some inferior kind of reasoning.

References

Chisolm R 1960 Realism and the background of phenomenology. Free Press, Glencoe, Chicago, Illinois.

Hempel C G 1965 Aspects of scientific explanation and other essays in the philosophy of Science. Free Press, New York.

Kant I 1998 Critique of pure reason (Guyer P, Ward A W, translators and editors) Cambridge University Press, Cambridge.

McHugh P R, Slavney P R 1998 The perspectives of mental health practice, 2nd edn. Johns Hopkins University Press, Baltimore.

McDowell J 1994 Mind and world. Harvard University Press, Boston.

Sadler J Z, Wiggins O P, Schwartz M A 1994 Philosophical perspectives on psychiatric diagnostic classification. Johns Hopkins University Press, Baltimore.

Sellars W 1956 Essays in philosophy and its history. In: Freigl H, Scriven M, eds. Minnesota studies in the philosophy of science. University of Minnesota, Minneapolis, p 253–329.

Commentary

Bryn Davis

Introduction

On looking at the recent psychiatry/mental health (P/MH) nursing literature, it does seem that this topic is still very much alive. I found sixty papers debating the topic from the last few years of the *Journal of Psychiatric and Mental Health Nursing* alone. However, is there anything more to say? It seems to me that there are several meanings hidden within or behind the title of this debate that were also reflected in the recent literature referred to above. First, we have the question of a scientific knowledge base (biopsychosocial) versus another kind of knowledge base. Then there is the issue of different kinds of research generating that knowledge base. Linked with this is the question of dealing with knowledge referring to people in general, and knowledge about a particular person. This then leads on to those professionals apparently working from a more scientific knowledge base and those working from a different kind of knowledge base – doctors and nurses, curing and caring. This is tied up with differing levels of autonomy in practice and subsequent issues of power and control. Accordingly, it appears as though there remains much to explore and, similarly, more worth saying.

Commentary on the papers

The first chapter, 'Psychiatric/mental health nursing: biological perspectives' (Ch. 20), although written by someone who generally operates from a biopsychosocial perspective, does identify a range of mental health issues that are clearly identified with pathophysiological changes and warrant an understanding of these by P/MH nurses. This is particularly the case when dealing with the administration of various drugs, and in the future perhaps with the prescription of medications. The question of possible genetic influence on behaviour, emotions and thought processes is also raised. Another aspect of this that is considered is the possible interaction between pharmacological and psychological interventions with either genetic or environmental factors. In addition, there is much current interest/research into monitoring brain function through PET scans and similar processes.

An important point raised is that of poisoning through substance misuse and abuse; in this substantive area, a clear link between the cause of the mental health problems and pathophysiology is posited. The major conclusion of this paper is that the P/MH nurse, if he or she is to be able to make a useful and substantial contribution to the care of those with mental health problems, in association with other health care professionals, must have the ability to comprehend and comment on such problems and possible interventions from a biological as well as a psychological and sociological perspective. This is supported by the fact that all P/MH nurses are prepared according to a syllabus that uses a biopsychosocial model as its basis. P/MH nurses do not work in isolation from other mental health professionals, and in many instances act in a coordinating role for the P/MH team. They are expected to care for those with problems in a holistic way and to practise their skills from this model. At different times, of course, one or other of these three areas (biology, psychology and sociology) may predominate, but it should never be to the total exclusion of the others. Perhaps a weakness of this paper is that there are few suggestions as to how this biological insight might be incorporated into everyday practical situations. However, acknowledging the limitations of the space allocated to the paper, one can expect that serious readers will be able to make that jump for themselves.

The second chapter, 'Biological psychiatry versus humanism: why taking meaning seriously in mental health practice is not inferior' (Ch. 21), addresses the topic from a very different angle, and attempts to demonstrate that there is no big difference between the scientific way of thinking and dealing with client-centred narratives. The main argument is that people, when dealing with descriptions and explanations of particular situations, use the same processes as the scientist attempting to describe and explain. In other words, perhaps, the individual is as scientific in their description and explanation of their *particular* situation as the scientist is in formulating *general* descriptions and explanations that might apply to all.

These two words, the general and the particular, are perhaps at the nub of the whole issue. On what evidence do we draw to arrive at our understanding of an individual's mental health problem? The general, scientific explanations or those presented by the particular individual? In other words, it is argued, the individual's experiences of their mental health problem and their attempts to describe and explain it are as valid and as rigorous as the professional's attempts to describe and explain them from a scientific point of view. However, I feel that, in the example given, both professionals used the same scientific reasoning to come to opposite conclusions. It seems to me that the client's judgement that he or she is better is not accepted at face value as a valid judgement in itself, but as one that conforms or not with scientific expectations. The nurse sees the client's statement as a symptom/outcome of the science-based psycho-educational intervention, whereas the doctor sees it as a symptom/outcome of (the scientific understanding of) the mental health problem.

Nevertheless, the author here has clearly identified a major issue: the relative value and validity of evidence drawn from a general scientific base and that provided by an individual about his or her particular experiences and explanations. It is increasingly the case that we should be including the client in decision-making about diagnosis, treatment and care. It does seem, therefore, of paramount importance that this situation should be clarified. I shall return to this aspect below.

Commentary on the literature

As indicated above, I have been aware of tensions within the psychiatric/ mental health nursing discipline as revealed in commentary papers published in the *Journal of Psychiatric and Mental Health Nursing* over the last six or seven years. Let me also add that I was the editor of the journal during that period in association with my assistant editors for that section. Humanism seems to have started life as a movement in the Renaissance period whereby there was an attempt to break away from the view of the world ordained by the church based on the Bible and supernatural explanations for events or the subjective experiences and preachings of 'wise men' or gurus. This applied to illnesses and, in particular, mental health problems. The sufferers were possessed by the devil or affected by bad spirits conjured up by witches. The humanists sought other explanations for things based on human reasoning. This led, over the centuries, to the development of the sciences as we know them. However, there are still attempts to invoke spiritual or mystical factors in explanations of events, and the idea that illness or particular problems are punishments still holds in some quarters. Indeed, some of those who experience mental health problems do explain it to themselves and others by invoking God or the devil, or ideas of punishment.

Ironically, those calling themselves the humanists in this debate are those rejecting scientific explanations. Humanism now seems, for some, to involve concentration only on the emotions and relationships as described by the individual. However, this scientific knowledge base is expected of P/MH nurses, who are educated to the requirements of the Nursing and Midwifery Council which registers them to practise. Along with these sciences is a study of relevant legal and ethical issues. This allows a more holistic approach. Another aspect of the education and training involves interpersonal skills so that the individual needs of the client can be identified in the light of this knowledge base and a suitable individual service plan or care pathway developed in conjunction with other mental health colleagues.

Some of the ire of the humanists (anti-biologists) has been focused against suggestions that nurses should be aware of new medications (Gray et al 1997), and that nurses should be aware of the extrapyramidal side-effects of some medications and participate in monitoring them and discussing the implications with medical colleagues (Gray &

Gournay 2000). The responses indicated that some nurses felt that such medication and its management was not necessary and that, even if it was, nurses should not be involved with it (see, for example, Clarke 2000, Long 2001). Some nurses seem to advocate an 'interpersonal relationships' model as being sufficient to inform P/MH nursing practice. This is seen as being more holistic, helping the clients to explore the 'lived experience' of their mental health problems (Graham 2001, Long 2001, Wilkins 2001). Nurses are encouraged to reject the medical model and to *enter the pathless woods of madness'* (Wilkins 2001, p 119). Mental illness is seen as a product of the medical desire for control, and the special scientific languages used are part of their technique of control. Different knowledge bases for nurses are preferred, such as tacit knowledge – the nurse's own personal knowledge of experience as a person, or ethics and human rights (Welsh & Lyons 2001). This rejection of the biopsychosocial knowledge base of evidence about the experience of mental health problems and evaluations of interventions, in order to concentrate solely on 'the lived experience' of the sufferer, seems to me to be very 'reductionist', and not at all 'holistic'.

This question of medical diagnosis is interesting. Over a long period of time the 'lived experiences' reported by clients have been recorded by professionals, together with observations by others including relatives and friends. From these qualitative data, clusters of symptoms, experiences and behaviours have been identified and a classification system of mental health problems has been created. This has been modified over the years as further analysis of these 'lived experiences' has been undertaken. These patterns of symptoms and so on guide the practitioner in their approach to a particular client. I believe that this process has a methodological similarity with Grounded Theory, developed inductively (Glaser & Strauss 1967). Further questions have arisen about this descriptive classification of mental health problems. These include the questions of 'What causes these problems?' and 'How can the client be helped?'.

The subsequent deductive phase follows, where hypotheses are generated about causation or therapeutic interventions, and research is undertaken to test them. This is where the biopsychosocial model comes from. A range of evidence has been generated offering insights into the causation of some mental health problems, and of the relative effectiveness of various interventions, from this model. The evidence has been gained from the qualitative experiences of the sufferers and from experimental and quasi-experimental studies drawing on quantitative and qualitative data. Unfortunately there have been arguments about the way in which such research should be undertaken following the paper by Gournay & Ritter (1997) advocating a controlled experimental approach. It pains me to read eminent academic nurses discussing qualitative versus quantitative research, as if there is only one valid type of datum. If the question is inductive, and attempts to build a descriptive picture of the situation, either qualitative or quantitative data can be used. If the question is deductive, and attempts to test hypotheses or to evaluate developments, then it is somewhat easier to answer the question with quantitative data, although in theory it should be possible to use qualitative data.

Words are very important in generating theories about people's experiences, but most qualitative research seems to be inductive and to reduce the information from several individuals to a list of general categories, or types of experience. It is difficult, though not impossible to find any qualitative research that attempts to evaluate possible causative factors or interventions, without the introduction of quantitative concepts such as 'more' or 'less' or 'frequency'. The postmodernist approach, frequently with reference to the work of Foucault (1977), is used to justify a rejection of the 'scientific' approach. This is based on the belief that rational forms of knowledge are mechanisms of control; there is no one perspective, and that 'reality' as proposed by science (a 'commonality' of perspectives between members of a group or society) does not exist. Thus, it is argued, the perspective of the client is more valid, more real than a scientific knowledge base, and therefore is all that is needed for the mental health nurse. The nurse brings her or his own perspective (tacit knowledge) to interact meaningfully with the client, who leads the process. This would seem unnecessarily to deprive the client of valuable sources of help. One of the factors driving this approach seems to be a desire for more autonomy for nurses, with a claim that doctors are concerned only with 'curing' whereas nurses are the only ones who 'care for' the client.

The original humanist approach was based on human reasoning, that is an inductive–hypotheticodeductive model. This is well described, in modern terms by George Kelly (1955) in his Personal Construct Theory, and as expanded by such as Fransella & Bannister (1977). This follows to some extent the Piagetian approach of assimilation and accommodation. Kelly proposed that all human beings perceive the world in their own way, generating a series of constructs about the world and their place in it. These constructs are, in effect, an inductive theory. This is then tested as the individual acts on or with the world and finds the original perceptions confirmed or not. If not, then adjustments are made to the construct system. Importantly, in order to be able to interact meaningfully with others it is necessary that individuals have a certain degree of commonality with others in the way they make sense of the world. They can then share their construct systems and work together to build up a shared working model, confirming their dealings with it, through an inductive–hypotheticodeductive process. The knowledge base can be codified and archived and then shared with others, newcomers to the world.

The biopsychosocial knowledge base informing nursing practice is part of the common shared knowledge base generated by and on behalf of our society. This knowledge base comprises information from both quantitative and qualitative data. In any particular situation where a new problem is tackled – geological change, astronomical event, behavioural or emotional change/distress – the information about the new situation (for example a personal construct system, the individual's experiences) is then dealt with in the light of the current body of knowledge (common construct system, for example the biopsychosocial knowledge). Similarities and differences can be identified and an explanation relevant to that new situation offered. This explanation then leads to any necessary interventions or further investigations, based on the common knowledge base. The choice of intervention or further investigation may depend on particular aspects of the new situation (the client's personal construct system) as well. Information provided by the client is most important in helping to evaluate the effects of any intervention and in providing clues as to other possible interventions.

Thus I feel that P/MH nurses hold a unique and most important position in the mental health team in that they work to this holistic approach, that is, one based on a common biopsychosocial knowledge base (guided by ethical and human rights principles which are also shared construct systems) together with their insights into the client's own personal experiences of the problem and interventions or further investigations through the practice of their interpersonal skills. To practise as a P/MH nurse with an emphasis only on biological psychiatry or on the client's own perceptions of their situation is poor practice. Gallop & Reynolds (2004) have argued this eloquently, and offer a biopsychosociocultural model in illustration, similar to that proposed by Davis (2000) regarding the 'lived experience' of pain. To deny the client the benefits of insights from the scientific knowledge base, or for the professional to deny themselves insights from the client's own experiences, seems to me to be most unprofessional, unethical and not consistent with human rights.

References

Clarke L 2000 Nursing and extrapyramidal symptoms: a critical commentary. Journal of Psychiatric and Mental Health Nursing 7:467–474.

Clarke L 2002 Doubts and uncertainties in the nursing profession. Journal of Psychiatric and Mental Health Nursing 9:225–229.

Davis B D 2000 Caring for people in pain. Routledge, London.

Foucault M 1977 Madness and civilisation: a history of insanity in the age of reason. Random House, London.

Fransella F, Bannister D 1977 A manual of repertory grid technique. Academic Press, London.

Gallop R, Reynolds W 2004 Putting it all together: dealing with complexity in the understanding of the human condition. Journal of Psychiatric and Mental Health Nursing 11:357–364.

Glaser B G, Strauss A 1967 The discovery of grounded theory. Aldine
    Publishing, New York.
Gournay K, Ritter S 1997 What future for research in mental health nursing?
    Journal of Psychiatric and Mental Health Nursing 8:227–230.
Graham I W 2001 Seeking a clarification of meaning: a phenomenological
    interpretation of the craft of mental health nursing. Journal of Psychiatric
    and Mental Health Nursing 8:335–345.
Gray R, Gournay G 2000 What can we do about acute extra-pyramidal
    symptoms? Journal of Psychiatric and Mental Health Nursing 7:205–212.
Gray R, Gournay K, Taylor D 1997 New drug treatments for schizophrenia:
    implications for mental health nursing. Mental Health Practice 1:20–30.
Kelly G A 1955 The psychology of personal constructs, Vols I & II. Norton,
    New York.
Long A 2001 Have we embraced the right to deny people their right to
    embrace their emotional pain? Journal of Psychiatric and Mental Health
    Nursing 8:85–92.
Welsh I, Lyons C M 2001 Evidence-based care and the case for intuition and
    tacit knowledge in clinical assessment and decision making in mental
    health nursing practice: an empirical contribution to the debate. Journal
    of Psychiatric and Mental Health Nursing 8:299–306.
Wilkins P E 2001 From medicalisation to hybridisation: a post-colonial
    discourse for psychiatric nurses. Journal of Psychiatric and Mental Health
    Nursing 8:115–120.

Subject Index

A

Abuse (of patients), 236
Advocacy role, 7, 11, 13
  nurse prescribing and, 76–77, 212
  standardisation of care and, 281
Affective disorder, 346, 353
  see also Depression
Aggressive/violent patients,
    management
  control and restraint *see* Control and
    restraint (C&R)
  crisis aggression and limitation and
    management (CALM), 183
  de-escalation *see* De-escalation/
    defusing
  risk assessment, 64–65, 173, 174,
    268–269
  staff attitudes, 166
  verbal, 185, 186
  'whole systems' approach, 197–198
AIDS, 349
Alcohol abuse, 229, 352–353, 360
Allmark, Peter, 71
Altschul, Professor Annie, 35
Alzheimer's disease, 345
  see also Dementia
Anticonvulsants, 228
Antidepressants, 228, 295, 350–351
  adverse effects, 30
  patient non-compliance, 31, 229,
    236
  suicidal clients, 243
Antipsychiatry movement, 27, 57, 78–
    80, 342, 344
  see also Psychiatry/psychiatric
    medicine
Antipsychotics, 17–18, 228, 295, 330,
    363
  adverse effects, 27
'Antisocial behaviour,' 67
Anxiolytics, 228
Aphasia, 360
'Apprenticeship model' *see* Education/
    training
Argument, development through
    debate, 8
Asphyxia, positional, 189
'Assertive outreach,' 64

Assistant mental health practitioner
    programme, UK, 87
Asylumdom, 57–58, 62
Attention deficit hyperactivity
    disorder, biological *vs.*
    humanistic perspectives, 346,
    347–348
Australia
  generic nurse preparation, 92, 102
  suicidal clients, care of, 265–266
Autism, 190
Autonomy
  patient, 28, 29
  professional, 59, 369
Aversion therapy, 13, 14

B

Bennett, David, 195
Benzodiazepines, 295
Bernard, Claude, 346–347
Biological perspective, 344–355, 358–
    361
  diagnosis and, 359–361, 370, 372
  humanistic *vs. see* Biological *vs.*
    humanistic perspectives
Biological *vs.* humanistic perspectives,
    341–375
  attention deficit hyperactivity
    disorder, 346, 347–348
  diagnosis and, 359–361, 370, 372
  drug-induced mental illness, 352–
    353, 369
  immune function, 348–349
  life-story methodology, 356, 357,
    361–362, 366–367
  naturalised platonism, 362–364,
    367
  psychological treatments, 350–352
  schizophrenia, 346, 347, 348, 353–
    354
  suicidal clients, 349–350
  see also Psychiatry/psychiatric
    medicine
Bipolar disorder, 229, 360
Bloom's 'taxonomy of educational
    objectives,' 155–156
Brain imaging, 17–18

Breakaway skills training, 184, 186–187, 191, 192
    see also Control and restraint (C&R)
Bright Futures, 41

C

Call systems, 'voice verification,' 64
CALM (crisis aggression and limitation and management), 183
CAMHS (child and adolescent mental health services), 347, 348
Canada
    education/training, 93, 107–109, 144–145
        Ponoka Psychiatric Nursing Training Program, 117
        preceptorship, 153–154
        practice standards, 307–308
        suicidal clients, 245
        terminology, 48–50
Canadian Federation of Mental Health Nurses (CFMHN), 93, 307, 308
Cannabis, 332, 352
'Care and responsibility,' 170
    learning disability field, 183
    see also Control and restraint (C&R)
'Care in the community' *see* Community care
'Care maps,' 308–309
Care pathways, 86
    standardisation *see* Standardisation (of care)
Care programme approach (CPA), 302–303
Caring practice, 71–72, 84, 134, 315
Cartesian mind-body dichotomy, 24, 347
CBT (cognitive behavioural therapy), 81–82, 147, 349, 350–352
CFMHN (Canadian Federation of Mental Health Nurses), 93, 307, 308
Child and adolescent mental health services (CAMHS), 347, 348
Children, 41
    hospitalisation, 13, 14
    mental health services, 347, 348
Chronic fatigue syndrome, 348–349
Citizenship skills, 10
Clarke, Liam, 147
Clay, Trevor, 126
Client satisfaction, service user evidence, 95–96, 100–101, 104
Clinical decision-making, 283

Clinical nurse specialist (CNS) role, USA, 25, 26
Clinical practice standards, 283–284, 307–308
    see also Standardisation (of care)
Clinical Resource and Audit Group, Scottish Executive, 332
Clinical standards, 283
    see also Standardisation (of care)
Clinical supervision, 162
'Close observations,' suicidal clients *see* Suicidal clients, approaches/perspectives
Clunis, Christopher, 302
CNS (clinical nurse specialist) role, USA, 25, 26
Cognitive behavioural therapy (CBT), 81–82, 147, 349, 350–352
Collaboration, 100–101
Communication (nurse–patient), 112
Communication skills, development through debate, 8
Community care, 59, 222, 298
    care programme approach, 302–303
Co-morbidity, 352–353
Competence, professional, 87, 152, 154
Compliance, pain-controlled, 171, 179, 190–191, 196
    see also Control and restraint (C&R)
Compulsory detention, 64, 98, 135
Confidential Inquiry into Maternal Deaths, UK, 350
Control and restraint (C&R), 165–202
    aim, 178
    breakaway skills, 184, 186–187, 191, 192
    definitions, 170–171, 182, 192
    education/training, 181–194, 200–201
        benefits, 183–184
        outcome research, 183–184, 192
    elements, 171, 189–191
    ethical issues, 177–178
    evidence-base, 173–177
    guidelines, 179
    history, 169–170
    learning disabled clients, 183, 184, 190
    locking procedures, 191, 192
    managers, challenges for action, 198–200
    pain-controlled compliance, 171, 179, 190–191, 196
    progressive, 182
    prone postures, 189–190, 192
    rationale, 171–173
    research, 183–184, 192

risks associated, 188, 189–190, 192, 197

self-defence and, 187–188

social validity, 191

staff confidence and, 172–173, 184, 196

traditional, 182

see also specific methods

Core competencies, 87

see also Competence, professional

Counselling, 172

CPA (care programme approach), 302–303

C&R (control and restraint) *see* Control and restraint (C&R)

Criminal justice system, UK, 64–65

Crisis aggression and limitation and management (CALM), 183

Critical thinking, education/training, 135, 137–138, 153

The Crown I Report (1989), 221

The Crown II Report (1999), 221

Culture, role in perceptions of mental illness, 40

D

Death, maternal, 350

Debate/debating, 1–19

definitions, 1, 2–3, 15

forms/types, contemporary, 2–6

Karl Popper, 3, 6, 8

Lincoln–Douglas, 3–4, 5, 6

parliamentary, 3, 5–6

policy, 3, 4–5, 6

heckling, 6

historical origins, 1–2, 6

misconceptions associated, 14–16

scientific certainty and, 16–18

value/function, 11–14

communication skills development, 8

educational, 7–10

see also specific topics

Decision-making, clinical, 283

De-escalation/defusing, 172–173, 175, 176

skills training, 184–186, 196, 197

see also Control and restraint (C&R)

Defensive practice, 268–269

Delirium, 359, 360

Dementia, 229, 345

in AIDS, 349

disease concept, 359, 360

Demosthenes, 2

Depression

'care maps,' 308

cognitive behavioural therapy, 350–351

disease concept, 359

immune function and, 348

postnatal, 318

prevalence, 229

inter-country variation, 160

treatment, adverse effects, 30

Detention, compulsory, 64, 98, 135

Diagnosis

biological *vs.* humanistic perspectives, 359–361, 370, 372

DSM criteria, 318

'dual,' 352–353

Diagnostic and Statistical Manual (DSM) IV, 318

Diazepam, 13

Discourse, definition, 318–319

Disease concept, of mental illness, 358–359, 360, 362

Drug abuse, 229, 352–353, 369

Drug treatments *see* Psychopharmacological treatments

'Dual diagnosis,' 352–353

E

Ecstasy, 352

ECT *see* Electroconvulsive therapy (ECT)

Eczema, 316–317

Education/training, 37, 89–128

'apprenticeship model,' 146, 148, 156

theory and *see theory–practice interface (below)*

assessment, 115–116

in Canada *see* Canada

career perspective, 161–162

'close observations' training, 262, 264

communication issues

nurse–patient, 112

written/verbal assessment, 115–116

control and restraint *see* Control and restraint (C&R)

critical thinking/analytical skills, 135, 137–138, 153

curriculum, 37–40

biological content, 353–354

relevance, 114

sociological content, 74

theory–practice interface *see theory-practice interface (below)*

evidence-based programmes, 139

in Finland, 158, 160, 161

focus, 26–28, 42, 289

theory *vs.* practice *see theory–practice interface (below)*
gender issues, 134
generic, 90, 92–127
  advantages, 112–113
  specialist *vs. see below*
generic *vs.* specialist, 89–128
  assumptions, 112
  collaborative component, 100–101
  historical perspective, 107–110
  'human focused' skills, 99–100
  integrative model, 102, 107–118
  role ambiguity and, 120, 121, 126–127
  service user evidence, 95–96, 100–101, 104
history, 36–37, 47–49, 132–133
integrative model, 102, 107–118
interprofessional, 137
nurse prescribing and, 214, 224–226, 231, 237
policy issues, 41–42, 159–161
  theory *vs.* practice *see theory–practice interface (below)*
preceptorship, 111, 153–154, 262
professional identity and, 70–71, 94–95, 141
Project 2000 *see* Project 2000
research dissemination, 115
specialist, 90, 92–127
  challenges, 113–115
  generic *vs. see generic vs. specialist (above)*
  limitations, 112–113
standardisation of care and, 289
student feedback, 116
technology, use of, 115
terminology issues, 34, 37–42, 44, 141
theory–practice interface, 129–163
  clinical experience and, 144–148, 152–156
  higher education and, 132–143, 148–152, 154–156
  historical context, 147–150
  synthesis, need for, 156, 158–162
UKCC review, 92
in USA, 107, 108, 226
Electroconvulsive therapy (ECT), 54
  adverse effects, 27
  suicidal clients, 243, 296
Electronic panopticon, 64
Empathy, 72, 82, 98, 99, 100, 213
  suicidal clients, 248, 266
Empowerment (of clients), 101
'Engagement and hope inspiration' approach, suicidal clients *see*

Suicidal clients, approaches/perspectives
Engaging people, observation of people with acute mental health problems, 332
English National Board for Nursing, 170
Epistemology, 57, 72–74, 134–135, 373
  research and, 315–321, 336
  see also Knowledge
Ethical issues
  control and restraint, 177–178
  research, 319
  standardisation of care, 289, 309
Ethics committees, 319
Evidence-based practice, 312, 314
  control and restraint, 173–177
  education/training and, 139
  guidelines, 86
  standardisation of care and, 288–289, 290
  see also Research

F

Finland
  education/training, 158, 160, 161
  health care costs, 160
Fitness for Practice report (1999), 38
'Floor restraint' methods, 189
Foucault, Michel, 57, 342

G

Gender issues, 147
  education/training and, 134
  role dissonance, 56
Gene isolation, 17–18
Generic education/training *see* Education/training
Gournay, Professor Kevin, 253
Grounded Theory, 372
GTP-binding proteins, 29

H

Health and Social Care Act (2001), 222
Health care
  as commodity, 300
  economic issues, 101, 160
Health policy
  education/training and, 159–160
  nurse prescribing and, 207–208, 215–216
  standardisation, 294–296

Health promotion, 32, 41, 78
Higher Education Funding Council, 325
Holding, therapeutic, 183, 190
Holistic practice, 374
    attributes, 71–74, 112–113
    general nurses/nursing, 71–74, 80, 81
    nurse prescribing and, 208
    standardisation of care and, 287
Homeostasis, 346
Humanistic perspective, 356–368, 370–374
    biological perspectives *vs. see*
        Biological *vs.* humanistic
        perspectives
    life-story methodology, 356, 357,
        361–362, 366–367
Huntington's disease, 360

I

Iatrogenic harm, 13–14, 27, 30, 235,
    236
Immune system, biological *vs.*
        humanistic perspectives, 348–349
Inpatient care
    research, 332–333
    see also Patient(s)
Integrative model, education/training,
    102, 107–118
Intentionality concept, 360–361, 366
Internal markets (in health care), 101
'Interpersonal relationships' model,
    372
Interpersonal Relations in Nursing, 150
Interpersonal theory, 26, 139, 150, 287,
    372

J

Jay Committee, 81
Jingoism, 12
Journalism, 12
*Journal of Psychiatric and Mental Health
    Nursing*, 34

K

Karl Popper debates, 3, 6, 8
Kelly, George, 373
Knowledge
    forms/generation in nursing, 134–
        135, 138–139

postmodernism and, 39, 320–321, 373
scientific hegemony, 13–14, 16–18
theory/epistemology, 57, 72–74, 134–
    135, 138–139, 373
    research and, 315–321, 336
Korsakoff's syndrome, 360

L

Laing, R, 27, 344
Learning disabled clients, 80–81, 97
    control and restraint training
        systems, 183, 184, 190
Lecturer-practitioners, 140
Life-story methodology, 356, 357, 361–
    362, 366–367
Lincoln–Douglas debates, 3–4, 5, 6
Lithium, 243
Locking procedures, 191, 192
    see also Control and restraint (C&R)
Lunacy Act (1845), 57

M

Managers, challenges associated with
        control and restraint, 198–200
Maternal death, 350
'McDonaldisation,' 296–300
McHugh, Paul, 357
Media, 12
Medicalisation, 37
    nurse prescribing and, 223
    professional identity and, 60
    social control and, 62–63
Medication *see* Psychopharmacological
        treatments
'Medication management programme,'
    231
Medico-Psychological Association
        (MPA), 47, 48
Mental health
    definitions, 40
    nurses/nursing contribution, 95–96,
        100–101
    see also Nurses/nursing (psychiatric/
        mental health)
Mental Health Act Commission, 264
Mental Health Act, Scotland (2003),
    121
Mental Health Act, UK (1983), 296
Mental Health Foundation (England),
    41
    'Strategies for living' report (2000),
        212

Mental Health Foundation report (2000), 96
Mental health nurses *see* Nurses/ nursing (psychiatric/mental health)
Mental hospitals, history, 57–59
Mental illness
    aetiology, 54–55
    biological perspective *see* Biological perspective
    criminalisation, 289
    culture, role in perceptions of, 40
    definitions, 40
    disease concept, 358–359, 360, 362
    drug-induced, 352–353, 369
    humanistic perspective *see* Humanistic perspective
    medicalisation *see* Medicalisation
    prevalence, 229
    stigma associated, 43
    see also specific conditions
Mind–body dichotomy, 24, 347
'Money therapy,' 215
Monoamine oxidase inhibitors, 30
Mood stabilisers, 228
Moral Treatment Movement, 36
MPA (Medico-Psychological Association), 47, 48
Myth of the Given, 365

N

NAPPI (non-aversive psychological and physical interventions), 183
Narratives *see* Life-story methodology
The National Health Service Plan, 222
National Institute for Clinical Excellence (NICE)
    control and restraint guidelines, 179
    medication prescribing standards, 297
    schizophrenia management guidelines, 351
National Institute for Mental Health England (NIMHE), 86–87
National Institute of Mental Health (NIMH), USA, 26
National Prescribing Centre (NPC), 221
National Psychiatric Morbidity Survey, 295
National Service Framework for Mental Health, 41, 176, 224, 295
Naturalised platonism, 362–364, 367
Natural therapeutic holding, 183, 190
Nerve membrane potentials, 26

Netherlands
    education/training, 107, 111, 116
    patient aggression, staff attitudes, 166
Neuroimaging, 17–18
Neuroleptics *see* Antipsychotics
Neuropsychiatric research
    history, 29–32
    see also Research
New World Order, psychiatry and, 57, 65–67
NHS Direct, 295, 299–300
NICE (National Institute for Clinical Excellence) *see* National Institute for Clinical Excellence (NICE)
Nightingale, Florence, 146, 148–149
NIMH (National Institute of Mental Health), USA, 26
NIMHE (National Institute for Mental Health England), 86–87
NMC (Nursing and Midwifery Council), 170
Non-aversive psychological and physical interventions (NAPPI), 183
No Panic, 347
NPC (National Prescribing Centre), 221
Nurse behaviour therapists, 86
Nurse practitioners (NPs), 227–228
    prescriptive practice *see* Nurse prescribing
Nurse prescribing, 76–77, 81, 115, 135, 203–238
    advocacy role and, 76–77, 212
    definition, 221
    education/training issues, 214, 224–226, 231, 237
    efficacy, 227–228
    future of, 230–231
    history, 221–222
    holistic practice and, 208
    iatrogenic harm and, 235, 236
    medicalisation and, 223
    nurses' perceptions, 222–223, 230
    patient advocacy and, 76–77, 212
    policy issues, 207–208, 215–216
    professional identity and, 208–211
    scientific hegemony and, 213–214
    service users
        acceptance, 226–227
        expectations and needs, 212–213
    USA practice, 217–218, 220–221, 230
    see also Psychopharmacological treatments

Nurses/nursing (general)
  caring role, 71–72, 84, 134, 315
  clinical judgement, 75–76
  definitions, 70–77, 81, 100
    Royal College of Nursing, 75
  history, 145–146
  holistic practice, 71–74, 80, 81
  professional identity, 76, 141
  status, 61
Nurses/nursing (psychiatric/mental
    health)
  alliance with psychiatry/psychiatric
      medicine see Professional
      identity
  autonomy, 59, 369
  biological perspective see Biological
      perspective
  definitions, 81, 84–86, 124, 286–287,
      325, 337
  education/training see Education/
      training
  history, 11, 22, 68, 281
  humanistic perspective see
      Humanistic perspective
  knowledge generation see Knowledge
  'McDonaldisation,' 296–300
  mental health, contribution to,
      service user evidence, 95–96,
      100–101
  practice standards, 283–284, 307–
      308
    see also Standardisation (of care)
  professional identity see Professional
      identity
  research see Research
  role
    advocacy see Advocacy role
    ambiguity, 120, 121, 126–127
    collaborative, 100–101
    deviancy, 57
    human component, 99–100
    'invisibility' of, 98
    key elements, 96–99
    prescribing see Nurse prescribing
    social control, 27, 62–65, 67–68,
        97–98
  standardisation see Standardisation
      (of care)
  terminology, 21–51, 35–37, 46–50
    Canada, 48–50
    confusion associated, 25–26, 34
    education/training issues, 34, 37–
        42, 44, 141
    euphemisms, 35
    historical aspects, 26–32, 35–37
    postmodernism and, 34, 42–43, 44

professional status and, 43–44
research and, 29–32
suicidal clients, 259
USA, 25–32, 46–47, 48–50
world shortage, 263
Nursing and Midwifery Council
    (NMC), 170
Nursing models
  history, 37, 80
  'interpersonal relationships,' 371
  professional identity and, 70–77, 80–
      82, 325
  research and, 325, 330–332

O

'Observation'
  suicidal clients see Suicidal clients,
      approaches/perspectives
  'supportive,' research, 332–333
Obsessive–compulsive disorder, 229,
    347
  cognitive behavioural therapy, 350
Office of Technology Assessment
    (OTA), USA, 227
Oral communication skills,
    development through debate, 8
OTA (Office of Technology
    Assessment), USA, 227
Outreach, 'assertive,' 64

P

Pain-controlled compliance, 171, 179,
    190–191, 196
  see also Control and restraint (C&R)
Panopticon, electronic, 64
Paranoid ideation, 363
Parliamentary debates, 3, 5–6
Patient(s)
  abuse of, 236
  aggressive/violent see Aggressive/
      violent patients, management
  autonomy, 28, 29
  narratives see Life-story methodology
  non–compliance in medication
      regimes, 31, 229, 236
  nurse–patient communication, 112
  satisfaction with services, 95–96,
      100–101, 104
  suicidal see Suicidal clients,
      approaches/perspectives
Peplau, Hildegard, 26, 35, 149–150,
    287

Personal Construct Theory, 373
Personality disorder, 64
Pharmacological agents *see*
    Psychopharmacological
    treatments
Phenothiazine, 13
Physical restraint, 189
Platonism, naturalised, 362–364, 367
PNAC (Project for a New American
    Century), 66
PNPs (psychiatric nurse practitioners)
    see Psychiatric nurse
    practitioners (PNPs)
Policy debates, 3, 4–5, 6
Ponoka Psychiatric Nursing Training
    Program, Canada, 117
Poor Law Amendment Act (1834), 57
Popperian debates, 3, 6, 8
Positional asphyxia, 189
Postmodernism, 74, 317–318
    knowledge and, 39, 320–321, 373
    research and, 337–338
    terminology and, 34, 42–43, 44
Postnatal depression, 318
Post-traumatic stress disorder (PTSD),
    330
Practice standards, 283–284, 307–308
    see also Standardisation (of care)
Practitioner-researchers, 140
Preceptorship, 111, 153–154, 262
PRICE (protection of rights in care
    environments), 183
Professional autonomy, 59, 369
Professional competence, 87, 152, 154
Professional identity, 53–88
    antipsychiatry movement and, 78–80
    'close observations' approach to
        suicidal patients and, 267
    dominance of psychiatry, 59–61
    education/training and, 70–71, 94–
        95, 141
    gender-role dissonance and, 56
    general nurses/nursing, 76, 141
    historical aspects, 57–59
    medicalisation and, 60
    New World Order and, 57, 65–67
    nurse prescribing and, 208–211
    nurses/nursing (general), 76, 141
    nursing models and, 70–77, 80–82,
        325
    role deviancy and, 57
    social control and, 62–65, 68
    standardisation of care and, 280,
        284–285, 287–288
    uncertainty, 114
    uniqueness, 101–105, 119–123

Project 2000, 133, 136, 146, 151
    changes associated, 41
    common foundation programme, 38,
        101, 103
    effects, 153
The Project for a New American
    Century (PNAC), 66
Prone postures, in control and
    restraint, 189–190, 192
Protection of rights in care
    environments (PRICE), 183
Psychiatric nurse practitioners (PNPs),
    221, 230
    see also Nurse prescribing; Nurses/
        nursing (psychiatric/mental
        health)
Psychiatric nurses *see* Nurses/nursing
    (psychiatric/mental health)
Psychiatry/psychiatric medicine
    antipsychiatry movement, 27, 57,
        78–80, 342, 344
    biological perspective, 344–355,
        358–361
        diagnosis and, 359–361, 370, 372
        humanistic *vs. see* Biological *vs.*
            humanistic perspectives
    history, 11, 22, 57–59, 68
    New World Order and, 57, 65–67
    professional dominance issues, 13–
        14, 59–61
    psychiatric nursings' alliance with *see*
        Professional identity
    role review, 87
    social control and, 27, 62–65, 67–68
Psychological treatments
    brain activity effects, 350–352
    research, 336–337
    see also specific therapies
Psychopharmacological treatments
    administration, 76–77
    concordance promotion, 330
    efficacy, 27, 211
    expansion of use, 59, 229–230
    gene expression effects, 54
    iatrogenic harm, 13–14, 27, 30, 235,
        236
    'medication management
        programme,' 231
    nurse prescribing *see* Nurse
        prescribing
    patient non-compliance, 31, 229,
        236
    polypharmacy, 236
    prescribing standards, 297
    research trials, 326
    see also specific drugs/drug types

Psychosis, 301, 347, 352
　see also Schizophrenia
Psychosurgery, 27
Psychotherapy, 328
　interpersonal interaction, 26
　stigma associated, 31
PTSD (post-traumatic stress disorder), 330
Publication Manual of the American Psychological Association, 116

Q

Qualitative research *see* Research
Quality (of care), 285–286, 294–296
　suicidal clients, 303–304
　　see also Suicidal clients, approaches/perspectives
　　see also Standardisation (of care)
Quantitative research *see* Research

R

Randomised controlled trials, 314–315, 326, 327–328, 329
Readings, Bill, 293, 294, 303
Research
　assessment, 324–326
　control and restraint, 183–184, 192
　definitions, 9
　dissemination, 115
　ethics committees, 319
　history, 29–32
　inpatient care, 332–333
　knowledge generation and, 134–135, 138–139
　methodology determination, 323–324, 329–330, 334, 338–339
　nursing models and, 325, 330–332
　postmodernism and, 337–338
　psychological treatments, 336–337
　psychopharmacological treatments, 326
　qualitative, 314–322, 323–324, 336–338
　　bias and, 324
　　paradigms underpinning, 319–320, 372–374
　　quantitative *vs. see below*
　qualitative *vs.* quantitative, 311–339, 372–374
　　epistemological hegemony and, 315–321, 336
　　language, ambiguity in, 317–318

　　methodology determination, 323–324, 329–330, 334, 338–339, 344
　　validity issues, 320, 370–371
　quantitative, 323–335, 338–339
　　as decision-making aid, 333
　　paradigms underpinning, 319–320, 372–374
　　qualitative *vs. see above*
　　randomised controlled trials, 314–315, 326, 327–328, 329
　resource allocation, 325–326, 327
　skills development through debate, 8–9
　standardisation of care and, 286–287
　suicidal clients, approaches to, 247, 260, 264, 266
　'supportive observations,' 332–333
　terminology, 29–32
　validity issues, 320, 370–371
　vested interests, 331
　see also Evidence-based practice
Research ethics committees, 319
Restraint *see* Control and restraint (C&R)
Review of prescribing, supply and administration of medicines, 222
Richards, Linda, 26
Risk assessment, 64–65, 173, 174, 268–269
Ritchie inquiry, 176
Ritzer, George, 294, 297, 303
Rogers, Carl, 27
Royal College of Nursing, 151
　nursing definition, 75

S

Sainsbury Centre for Mental Health, 264
Schizophrenia, 229, 288, 302
　biological *vs.* humanistic perspectives, 346, 347, 348, 353–354
　cannabis use and, 352
　diagnostic uncertainty, 95
　disease concept, 358–359, 360
　immune function and, 348
　management, 135, 139
　　cognitive behavioural therapy, 351–352
　　guidelines, 351
　　nurse–patient relationship, 288
　see also Antipsychotics

prevalence, inter-country variation, 160
Scientific hegemony, 13–14, 16–18
    nurse prescribing and, 213–214
    see also Knowledge
SCIP (Strategies for Crisis Intervention and Prevention), 183
ScotCRAG, 332
Selective serotonin reuptake inhibitors (SSRIs), 17–18, 30
Self-defence training, 187–188
    see also Control and restraint (C&R)
Sex offenders, registration, 64
Slavney, Phillip, 357
Smail, David, 211
Social control, 27
    medicalisation and, 62–63
    professional identity and, 62–65, 68
    psychiatric/mental health nurses/ nursing as agent, 27, 62–65, 67–68, 97–98
    psychiatry as agent, 27, 62–65, 67–68
'Social prescribing,' 211
    see also Nurse prescribing
Standardisation (of care), 277–310
    advocacy role and, 281
    definitions, 282–283, 292–294
    education/training and, 289
    elements, 283–284
    ethical issues, 289, 309
    evidence-based practice and, 288–289, 290
    health service administration and, 294–296
    holistic practice and, 287
    professional identity and, 280, 284–285, 287–288
    quality and, 285–286, 294–296
    research and, 286–287
    resistance to, 280–281
    technology role, 299–300
    therapeutic relationship and, 307
Standing Nursing and Midwifery Advisory Committee, 252
Status issues, 61
    preparation and see Education/ training
Stigma, 31, 43
Strategies for Crisis Intervention and Prevention (SCIP), 183
'Strategies for living' report (2000), Mental Health Foundation (England), 212
Stress, immune function and, 348–349
Studio III, 183

Study on the Therapeutic Management of Violence (2001), 179
Substance abuse, 229, 352–353, 369
Suicidal clients, approaches/ perspectives, 229, 239–276
    antidepressant medication, 243
    biological vs. humanistic, 349–350
    'close observations,' 240–246, 251–253, 257–275
        criticisms, 272–274
        education/training and, 262, 264
        nursing leadership and, 261–264, 268
        practical application, 261
        professional identity and, 267
        research, 260, 264, 266
        risk culture and, 268–269
        terminology issues, 259
        therapeutic intentions, 258
    electroconvulsive therapy, 243, 296
    'engagement and hope inspiration,' 242–243, 246–254
        criticisms, 251–254
        emphasis, 240, 274–276
        research, 247
        therapeutic value, 246–249
    quality of care, 303–304
    standards, 295–296
Supervision, clinical, 162
Supervision registers, 64
Supplementary prescribing, 222, 230–231
    see also Nurse prescribing
'Supportive observations,' 332–333
Szasz, Thomas, 27, 344

T

'Tagging,' 64
'Taxonomy of educational objectives' (Bloom's), 155–156
Teamwork, development through debate, 8
Technology
    education/training role, 115
    standardisation of care and, 299–300
Terminology, nurses/nursing (psychiatric/mental health see Nurses/nursing (psychiatric/ mental health)
Therapeutic holding, 183, 190
Therapeutic relationship
    aggressive/violent patients, management see Patients
    social control and, 63

standardisation of care and, 307
　　see also Standardisation (of care)
Thorn initiative, 139
Timian training, 183
Training *see* Education/training
Tranquillisers, 13–14, 28
　　see also specific drugs
Treatment approaches
　　biological *vs.* humanistic *see*
　　　　Biological *vs.* humanistic
　　　　perspective
　　psychological *see* Psychological
　　　　treatments
　　psychopharmacological *see*
　　　　Psychopharmacological
　　　　treatments
Tricyclic antidepressants, adverse
　　effects, 30

U

United Kingdom Central Council
　　(UKCC)
　　education/training review, 92
　　Study on the Therapeutic
　　　　Management of Violence (2001),
　　　　179
Universities UK, 136
USA
　　clinical nurse specialist (CNS) role,
　　　　25, 26
　　education/training, 107, 108, 226
　　gender issues, 147
　　New World Order and, 65–66

nurse prescribing, 217–218, 220–221,
　　230
Office of Technology Assessment
　　(OTA), 227
terminology, 25–32, 46–47, 48–50

V

Value-driven (Lincoln–Douglas)
　　debates, 3–4, 5, 6
Verbal aggression, 185, 186
Victims, 64
Violent patients *see* Aggressive/violent
　　patients, management
'Voice verification' call systems, 64

W

Welsh centre method, 183
Welsh Debate Federation, 9–10
Wikipedia.org website, 4, 5, 6
Workforce Action Team 2001, 213

Y

York Retreat, 47

Z

'Zero tolerance,' 168
　　see also Control and restraint (C&R)